*I*ntegrating

Conventional

& Alternative

Therapies

Holistic Care for Chronic Conditions

Charlotte Eliopoulos, RNC, ND, PhD
Specialist in Holistic Chronic Care
President, Health Education Network
Glen Arm, Maryland

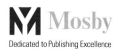
Mosby
Dedicated to Publishing Excellence

Editor: Barry Bowlus
Developmental Editor: Barbara Watts
Project Manager: Gayle Morris
Manuscript Editor: Linda Wendling
Layout Artist: Ken Wendling
Manufacturing Manager: Betty Mueller
Cover and Page Design: Laura Kangrga
Cover Photo: Beatriz DaCosta

Copyright © 1999 by Mosby, Inc.

Printed in the United States of America
Composition by Wordbench
Printing/binding by Mulligan

Mosby, Inc.
11830 Westline Industrial Drive
St. Louis, Missouri 63146

International Standard Book Number 0-8151-2793-6

98 99 00 01 02 / 9 8 7 6 5 4 3 2 1

Reviewer
Johanne A. Quinn, PhD, RN
Executive Director
American Holistic Nurses Association
Raleigh, North Carolina

This book is dedicated to
George Considine,
business coach and husband *extraordinaire*

Preface

Some of us open our minds to new knowledge and practices because we want to keep current and be on the cutting edge, while others face change and innovation kicking and screaming; I was of the latter group. After a couple of decades of nursing, I felt secure in my clinical knowledge. I read current professional literature, attended continuing education programs, networked, stayed abreast of new developments in my specialty.

But often, we don't know what we don't know. Although I could implement the nursing practice and recite conventional treatments for major chronic conditions, there was an entire field of interventions of which I was significantly ignorant: alternative and complementary therapies. Certainly I had heard about acupuncture, herbal therapies, imagery, and the like; I had even taken a course and practiced (although discreetly!) therapeutic touch. But I had an attitude that practitioners of these therapies were on the fringe, remnants of the flower children of the sixties. No respectable, mainstream practitioner who used these therapies could be taken seriously. Without learning about the realities of alternative and complementary therapies, I maintained my tunnel vision as I continued down my path of conventional nursing practice.

Then crisis struck my life—or several crises, I should say. Within an eighteen-month period my fifty-four-year-old husband and twenty-five-year-old sister-in-law developed different, but equally aggressive and ultimately fatal cancers; my mother forfeited her driver's license due to cataracts; and my community-based grandmother became totally dependent. All of these individuals were receiving state-of-the-art medical care; that was the easy part. However, the most challenging and time-consuming demands arose from the needs that weren't being met through conventional health care practices. None of the fine conventional practitioners could lift my husband's depression and hopelessness as he faced trials of chemotherapy for a cancer that was known to be unresponsive to treatment. The physicians and nurses responded with discomfort to my sister-in-law's emotional anguish as she faced the reality of leaving her toddler motherless. The isolation accompanying my mother's subtly shrinking social world was never identified by the eye clinic staff who saw her regularly. Not a soul addressed my grandfather's insecurity, inexperience, and frustration as he had to assume caregiving, housekeeping, and cooking responsibilities for the first time in his eighty plus years. These loved ones had needs that exceeded the usual prescriptions for medications, surgery, and radiation, and I was impressed at how little the conventional health care system could offer them. In desperation to help, I searched anything and everything I could; thus began my journey into the realms of alternative and conventional therapies and my understanding of holistic nursing.

The further along the path I traveled the more embarrassed I felt about the attitude I had held and my limited understanding of alternative and complementary therapies. I became aware that many of these therapies have been practiced successfully for centuries and are used by most of the world, including a significant number of Americans. I began to understand the difference between treating a disease and healing a person. I learned of the political and economic reasons for the limited research supporting alternative and complementary therapies. Most important, my eyes were open to the reality that these therapies offered hope and help when conventional care couldn't, particularly for chronic and terminal conditions.

If we as clinicians are committed to holistic care of our patients/clients, we must utilize all approaches and modalities that can benefit the body, mind, and spirit. Learning about and utilizing alternative and complementary therapies are essential to this effort. This is not to imply that conventional treatments shouldn't be respected and used, but rather, that conventional treatments be used appropriately and selectively, and in collaboration with alternative and complementary therapies when possible. If noninvasive, nonpharmacologic interventions can effectively and safely improve a condition, it makes sense to try these interventions first or as an enhancement to conventional treatments. For example, if progressive relaxation and yoga can aid in reducing hypertension, these interventions should be tested before a client begins using an antihypertensive drug that carries the risk of adverse reactions. Likewise, if guided imagery can encourage a state that enhances a medication's circulation throughout the body, this intervention should accompany the drug's administration to maximize its benefits. We will serve our patients/clients best when we help them use the best of both conventional and alternative/complementary therapies.

This book is a supplement to the existing knowledge base of clinicians from various disciplines who work with clients who have chronic conditions. It certainly is not all inclusive, but may shed new light on approaches that can enhance practice. In an era when health care is highly influenced by high-tech interventions and reimbursement, perhaps the approaches described in this book can encourage clinicians to revisit the basic, and very important, essence of their healing role in serving clients.

Peace and Blessings,

Charlotte

Contents

Holism and Healing

Consumers are influencing changes in the conventional health care system in the United States. The recognition of their rights, spiraling health care costs, and a dissatisfaction with the paternalistic attitude of some providers have caused many consumers to take a more active role in their health care. Disillusioned with an emphasis on high-tech treatment, many clients want more personalized services. The emergence of a world community has made more Americans familiar with acupuncture, medicinal herbs, and other time-tested alternative therapies that have been used successfully in other countries. Often without their traditional health care providers' knowledge or consent, consumers have sought the services of acupuncturists, homeopathic practitioners, osteopaths, hypnotherapists, and other alternative practitioners. And this practice continues, despite criticisms from traditional health care providers; in fact, more than one-third of all Americans have used alternative healing measures (Eisenberg et al., 1993). In 1992, acknowledging this growing trend, Congress established the Office of Alternative Medicine within the National Institutes of Health as a vehicle for evaluating alternative therapies.

The paradigm is shifting from an impersonal, expensive, high-tech health care delivery system that is physician-directed to one that recognizes the need for clients to be empowered to direct their own care activities as well-informed decision-makers. Under this new model, clients take responsibility for mobilizing inner and external resources to achieve high levels of wellness and to heal from illness (Box 1-1). In this new arena, clinicians from a wide range of disciplines have opportunities to reframe their relationships with clients as they integrate scientific medical advancements with ancient healing traditions.

History of Healing

Healers have existed since ancient times. Primitive tribes considered illness the work of evil spirits and, consequently, believed these spirits needed to be driven away by incantations, spells, and other rituals. As average tribespeople found the growing body of healing lore becoming too complex and extensive for them to remember and use, they selected individuals to serve as masters of these healing traditions. These individuals came to be known as "medicine men and women" and "shamans."

Early shamans demonstrated many talents such as singing, dancing, storytelling, drawing, and jesting. They used these talents to communicate with the spirit world. In addition, shamans achieved altered states of consciousness to assist in their healing rituals. Their communications with the spiritual world helped them to gain a position of respect and power within their tribes. Shamans did not separate the body, mind, and soul, but saw these components as part of an integrated whole. Cave drawings as early as 20,000 B.C. show the activities of shamans, demonstrating the early origins of this healer role (Achterberg, 1985). Although the spread of modern medicine throughout the world has provided new treatment

---

BOX 1-1   **Features of the New Paradigm of Health and Medical Care**

The client:
- is viewed as an autonomous individual who has an active role in health promotion and illness-related care
- assumes responsibility for self-care, health promotion, and illness management
- utilizes inner and external resources to promote wellness, manage illness, and heal
- is seen as a dynamic member of other systems (e.g., family, community) that influence are influenced by the client's health status

The health care professional:
- promotes a relationship with the client in which they are partners in the achievement of health-related goals
- appreciates the client's mind, body, and spirit as interrelated variables affecting health and illness and considers these variables in assessing, planning, delivering, and evaluating services to clients
- values subjective data as a highly important adjunct to objective data in assessment and evaluation
- utilizes natural, noninvasive techniques before employing aggressive, high-tech, or high-risk interventions
- respects the client's self-healing capabilities and strengthens and assists the client in healing
- recognizes that the health care professional's self and energy play a part in the therapeutic relationship and uses these factors to facilitate the client's healing

---

options for people, many cultures continue to rely primarily on shamans for healing.

Ancient Greece was the site of early temples dedicated to the art of healing. These healing institutions were known as Asclepions, named after Aesculapius, the god of healing (see Box 1-2), and used music, dream interpretation, drama, massage, humor, baths, herbs, and rest to complement the scientific treatments of the day (Sanford, 1977). The Asclepion centers created a healing environment that addressed the physical, mental, and spiritual aspects of individuals.

While the Asclepions offered healing to the Greeks, Chinese medicine was developing in the Far East. Chinese healers recognized the movement of life energy, or ch'i, along a system of meridians (see Figure 5-2 in Chapter 5). This system, still in use today, asserts that illness occurs when energy flow is blocked. Various methods to unblock energy, including acupuncture and herbal therapies, were developed, most of which are used today and are gaining increasing credibility among Western allopathic practitioners.

The Indian healing system of ayurveda also developed during this early period. It promoted the unity of the mind, body and spirit and developed methods of treating illness according to theories of the five elements (ether, air, fire, water, and earth), and the body tissues, humors, and excretions. Ayurveda taught that whenever Energy

Coronis, a beautiful young maiden of Thessaly, was loved by the god Apollo, but the girl took a fancy to a mortal man. Upon learning that Coronis was pregnant by the man, Apollo became livid and arranged for Coronis' death, but he did save the baby, who was ready to be born. Apollo named the male child Aesculapius and turned him over to the old Centaur Chiron to be raised.

Chiron was well skilled in the use of herbal remedies and incantations and schooled Aesculapius in the healing arts. Soon Aesculapius developed healing abilities that surpassed his master. People came from throughout the land to be healed as Aesculapius' reputation as an outstanding physician grew. But when the great healer raised a man from the dead for a fee, he drew the wrath of Zeus, who did not look kindly upon a mortal demonstrating such power and brought about Aesculapius' death by a thunderbolt. Angered by his son's death, Apollo forged the thunderbolts and killed the Cyclops who made them. For his revengeful deed, Apollo was condemned to become a slave for King Admetus.

Aesculapius' influence did not end with his death, however. Temples honoring him were built that attracted the ill and disabled who came to be healed. After offering a sacrifice and praying, the ill would sleep and in their dreams receive instructions from Aesculapius on how to be cured of their maladies. People left the temples believing they were healed. Thus the temples survived for hundreds of years after Aesculapius' death as centers for health and healing.

---

fields, or *chakras*, were blocked, they caused illness. Yoga and other measures could stimulate the energy centers and promote healing.

The birth of Christianity also promoted the integration of body, mind, and spirit in the physical healing process. The Bible offers evidence of the spiritual dimension to restoring physical health in descriptions of Jesus Christ healing through touch and through spiritual healing. Examples include the following:

- a paralytic man healed by forgiveness of sins (Matthew 9:2)
- a woman with a twelve-year-long bleeding disorder healed by touching His cloak (Luke 51:43-44)
- the sick and tormented healed by extraction of evil spirits (Acts 5:16)

Many people brought the sick to Jesus and begged Him to allow them to touch the edge of His cloak in order to be healed. It was not medicine, but belief in God's work and spiritual healing that helped the ill.

With the advent of the scientific revolution, any event considered illogical or unexplainable by objective evidence was viewed with skepticism. By the 19th century, physicians and nurses separated themselves from the early healing practices and moved toward a scientific basis for practice. The healing arts and the role of the mind and spirit in health status were considered more folklore than fact, and hardly within the sphere of scientific medical practice. Illness was seen as a pathophysiologic occurrence that could be treated with chemicals, surgery, or radiation. The mentality shifted from helping ill people use their own resources to heal themselves and regain wholeness and balance, to doing things "to" the patient to fight the illness. Although the concept of caring for the total person was articulated by many health professions, actual practice often reflected treatment of the pathogen and physical symptoms.

To her credit, Florence Nightingale promoted a holistic approach to caring for the ill in her *Notes on Nursing* (1859) despite the shift to scientific medical care. She stated that nursing's concerns should be to attend to the response of the patient, touching the patient, fostering a healthy environment, and care more than curing. (Box 1-3) The female-dominated profession promoted "feminine" qualities such as caring, compassion, nurturance, and intuition until the twentieth century, when the movement toward increased emphasis on the scientific approach made these characteristics seem unprofessional, inexact, and even embarrassing.

An interest in psychology and spirituality throughout the sixties and seventies influenced the health care system to develop a new sensitivity to the relationship of mind, body, and spirit. At the same time, an awareness of health as more than the absence of disease propelled an interest in wellness and prevention. During this period, nursing and other health professions began to articulate theoretical frameworks that described their clinical activities. These theories varied in their degree of

---

BOX 1-3   Words of Wisdom from Florence Nightingale

- All disease is more or less a reparative process, an effort of nature to remedy a process of poisoning or decay.
- Symptoms and sufferings considered inevitable and incident to the disease are very often not symptoms of the disease at all, but the result of want of fresh air, or light, or warmth, or quiet, or cleanliness, or punctuality and care in the administration of the diet, or all of these things.
- The effect in sickness of beautiful objects, of variety of objects, and brilliancy of color is hardly appreciated at all.
- You can have no idea of the relief which manual labor is to you or of the degree to which the deprivation of manual employment increases the peculiar irritability from which many sick suffer.
- A sick person enjoys hearing good news.
- The power of forming any correct opinion about the patient must entirely depend upon inquiry into all the conditions in which the patient lives, not just the physical signs.
- Pathology teaches the harm that disease has done, but it teaches nothing more. Nothing but observation and experience will teach us the ways to maintain or to bring back the state of health.
- Medicine and surgery can remove obstructions; however, nature alone cures.
- Nursing has been limited to signify little more than the administration of medicines and application of poultices; it ought to signify the proper use of fresh air, light, warmth, cleanliness, quiet, and proper selection and administration of diet.

From: Nightingale, F: *Notes on nursing*, London, 1859, Harrison and Sons.

abstraction and scientific testing, but most communicated concepts that addressed the relationship of the discipline, the client, health, and the environment. A sampling of some theories is offered in Box 1-4. The choice of a theory to guide professional practice is an individualized process based on the unique characteristics and preferences of the clinician.

BOX 1-4   Theories Useful in Holistic Chronic Care

Orem's Self-Care Theory (Orem, 1978)
- Promotes responsibility and independence of client in meeting self-care needs
- Works from assumptions that individuals value independence

Rogers' Theory of Life Processes (Rogers, 1991)
- Sees human beings as highly complex fields of various forms of life energy
- Discusses highly complex energy exchange, interrelationships, and resonance that occur between the clinician and client in the healing process

Newman's Theory of Health as Expanding Consciousness (Newman, 1994)
- Builds on Rogers' theory
- Considers nursing a caring profession moving to an integrative role
- Sees client as a dynamic field of energy that is continuous with a larger energy field
- Asserts that health is a state of expanding consciousness that includes the client's total pattern

Roy's Adaptation Model (Roy, 1970)
- Based on belief in adaptation to stressors and achieving state of health as a state of homeostasis or balance
- Identifies four modes of adaptation:
  physiologic needs
  self-concept
  role mastery
  interdependence
- Views client as adaptive system; clinician's role is to help client develop positive response to stimuli (i.e., adapt)

Modeling and Role-Modeling Theory (Erickson, Tomlin, and Swain, 1983)
- Focuses on client as holistic being with interacting subsystems (biological, psychological, social, cognitive), inherent genetic bases, and spiritual drives; health is a dynamic equilibrium between these subsystems
- Asserts that clinician individualizes health care by creating a model of the client's subjective world

---

Watson's Humanistic Theory (Watson, 1988)
- Reinforces the humanistic characteristics of nursing that combine with scientific knowledge to create highly interpersonal human-to-human care
- Sees health as a subjective state in which there is harmony; illness exists as disharmony

Leininger's Cultural Care (Leininger, 1991)
- Views nursing as a culturally congruent activity that assists clients in regaining state of well-being or coping with handicapping condition or approaching death

Antonovsky's Salutogenic Model (Antonovsky, 1972)
- Sees inability of client or family to cope with stressors over prolonged period leading to breakdown and development of chronicity; accumulated effects of stressful demands threatens individual's balance and increases risk of health problems
- Asserts that breakdown can be alleviated by promoting sense of self, fostering socialization and social support, supporting effective coping behavior, and affirming client-clinician relationship

---

Finally, in recent years, nonconventional (nonallopathic) modalities to promote health and treat illness have begun being rediscovered and developed as important complements to traditional Western medicine. This movement is supported by scientific evidence demonstrating the positive effects of prayer, therapeutic touch, herbal remedies, acupuncture, biofeedback, and other healing practices, coupled with consumers' desires for more natural, personal care that recognizes the important relationship of mind, body, and spirit. Professional associations representing clinicians committed to holistic practice have been established, such as the American Holistic Nurses' Association, American Holistic Medical Association, and American Holistic Health Association. These have provided standards and principles of practice (Boxes 1-5 and 1-6) to facilitate high-quality services.

Healing vs. Curing

The incurable nature of chronic illness requires that the focus of care and the evaluation of the success of interventions consider factors other than the *elimination* of the disease. These factors include adjustment to living with the disease and wholeness of the individual (i.e., quality of life, sense of well-being, comfort, integration of the body-mind-spirit). Appropriately, healing becomes the objective of care. Healing, as used in this framework, means *to use the body, mind, and spirit to control disease, promote a sense of well-being, and enhance the quality of life.* Figure 1-1, page 12, illustrates the Bio-Psycho-Social-Spiritual Model, frequently applied to chronic care.

| BOX 1-5 | American Holistic Nurses' Association (AHNA) Standards of Holistic Nursing Practice Core Values |

PART I: DISCIPLINE OF HOLISTIC NURSING PRACTICE

Core Value I. Holistic Philosophy, Foundation, and Education

Holistic Philosophy and Foundation

1. Holistic nurses are committed to the continuing development of the philosophy and foundation and the art and science of holistic nursing practice.

Holistic Education

1. Holistic nurses acquire and maintain current knowledge and competency in holistic nursing practice.

Core Value II. Care For the Caregiver

1. Holistic nurses are committed to holism as related to personal development.
2. Holistic nurses seek to understand and develop the process and state of the "nurse as an instrument of healing."

Core Value III. Holistic Ethics, Theories, and Research

Holistic Ethics

1. Holistic nurses adhere to a professional ethic of caring and healing that seeks to preserve the dignity and support the wholeness of the person who is receiving care.

Holistic Nursing Theories

1. Holistic nurses recognize that holistic nursing theory provides the framework for all aspects of professional holistic nursing practice.
2. Holistic nurses recognize that holistic nursing care is grounded in one of the many theories of nursing practice.
3. Holistic nurses seek to identify a nursing theory or theories consistent with holistic thinking upon which to ground their nursing practice.

Holistic Nursing and Related Research

1. Holistic nurses provide care and guidance to clients and aggregates through nursing interventions and holistic therapies based on research findings.
2. Holistic nurses discuss holistic application to clinical situations where rigorous research has not been done.

PART II: CARING AND HEALING OF CLIENTS AND AGGREGATES

Core Value IV. Holistic Nursing Process

1. Assessment: Clients are assessed holistically and repeatedly.
2. Problems;/patterns/needs identified: Client actual and high-risk problems/patterns/needs and opportunities to enhance health and well-being shall be identified and prioritized based upon collected data.
3. Client Outcomes: Client's actual or high-risk problems/patterns/needs or opportunities to enhance health and well-being have appropriate outcomes specified and revised as appropriate.
4. Therapeutic Care Plan: Clients have an appropriate plan of holistic nursing care formulated focusing on health promotion or health maintenance activities.
5. Implementation of Care: Client's plan of holistic nursing care is prioritized and holistic nursing interventions will be implemented accordingly.

6. Evaluation: Client's response to holistic nursing care is regularly and systematically evaluated.

Core Value V. Therapeutic Communication, Therapeutic Environment, and Cultural Diversity

Therapeutic Communication

1. Clients and aggregates experience the presence of the nurse as a shared humanness that includes a sense of connectedness and attention to them as unique persons.
2. Clients and aggregates experience the presence of holistic nurses as authentic and sincere practitioners who provide and value them as individuals.

Therapeutic Environment

1. Clients and aggregates receive care in an environment that is safe.
2. Clients and aggregates shall receive care in an environment that is respectful and healing.
3. Clients and aggregates are cared for in as healthy an environment as possible (e.g., clean air and water, nutritious food, with environmentally "friendly" life-sustaining practices).

Cultural Diversity

1. Clients and aggregates receive care consistent with their cultural backgrounds, health beliefs, sexual orientation, and values.
2. Clients' and aggregates' cultural diversity and its importance to the global community are respected, protected, and supported.
3. Clients and aggregates receive care that is consistent with their values and beliefs.
4. Clients are cared for as whole, spiritual beings.
5. Clients and aggregates receive support for their spiritual growth.

Core Value VI. Client Self Care

1. Clients and aggregates are supported in managing self-care to maximize quality of life (e.g., treatments and side effects, activities of daily living, changes in relationships and life style).
2. Clients and aggregates are offered the information and resources needed for ongoing holistic health care.
3. Clients receive care aimed at empowering them to accept responsibility for their own health and well-being.
4. Clients and aggregates receive the knowledge they want and need in order to be involved in decisions about health care, work, home life, and recreation.
5. Clients and aggregates receive health care based on priorities of care that contribute to desired outcomes.
6. Clients and aggregates are included as active partners in health care planning and decision making based on individual desires.
7. Clients and aggregates recognize patterns that place them at risk for health problems (e.g., personal habits, personal and family health history, age-related risk factors).
8. Clients and aggregates practice preventive measures (e.g., immunizations, breast self-exam, fitness/exercise programs, appropriate nutrition, belief practices [prayer]).

From the American Holistic Nurses' Association, P.O. Box 2130, Flagstaff, AZ 86003, Revised 1998.

BOX 1-6	American Holistic Medical Association: Principles of Holistic Medical Practice

1. Holistic physicians embrace a variety of safe, effective options in diagnosis and treatment, including:
   a) education for lifestyle changes and self-care;
   b) complementary approaches
   c) conventional drugs and surgery
2. Searching for the underlying cause of disease is preferable to treating symptoms alone.
3. Holistic physicians expend as much effort in establishing what kind of patient has a disease as they do in establishing what kind of disease a patient has.
4. It is preferable to diagnose and treat patients as unique individuals rather than as members of a disease category.
5. When possible, lifestyle modifications are preferable to drugs and surgery as initial therapeutic options.
6. Prevention is preferable to treatment and is usually more cost-effective. The most cost-effective approach evokes the patient's own innate healing capabilities.
7. Illness is viewed as a manifestation of a dysfunction of the whole person, not as an isolated event.
8. In most situations, encouragement of patient autonomy is preferable to decisions imposed by physicians.
9. The ideal physician-patient relationship considers the needs, desires, awareness and insight of the patient, as well as those of the physician.
10. The quality of the relationship established between physician and patient is a major determinant of healing outcomes.
11. Physicians significantly influence patients by their example.
12. Illness, pain and the dying process can be learning opportunities for patients and physicians.
13. Holistic physicians encourage patients to evoke the healing power of love, hope, humor and enthusiasm and to release the toxic consequences of hostility, shame, greed, depression and prolonged fear, anger, and grief.
14. Unconditional love is life's most powerful medicine. Physicians strive to adopt an attitude of unconditional love for patients, themselves, and other practitioners.
15. Optimal health is much more than the absence of sickness. It is the conscious pursuit of the highest qualities of the spiritual, mental, emotional, physical, environmental and social aspects of the human experience.

From the American Holistic Medical Association, 6728 Old McLean Village Drive, McLean, VA 22101, 1998.

The Healer Role

Historically, nurses, physicians, and other clinicians have assumed a role of healer—one who restores health or makes a person whole again. Compassion, empathy, touch, and caring have long been the hallmarks of the helping professions. These are particularly significant attributes of the clinician who works with the chronically ill. With the orientation of healer, the clinician uses a variety of modalities to promote a client's self-care in normal activities of daily living and the additional demands imposed by illness, recognizing that the client's level of independent function and subsequent need for assistance can fluctuate (Figure 1-2).

Scientific knowledge and skill in performing caregiving activities are important foundations to a healing relationship, but they must be supplemented by other healing approaches. For instance, healing actions of the health care professional may include any combination of the following: nurturing and caring; facilitating growth and development; modeling and supporting positive health and self-care practices; assisting with transitions; promoting and restoring balance of the mind, body, and soul; guiding self-discovery, self-awareness, and spiritual development; encouraging optimal function and quality of life; coordinating with community resources; performing clinical procedures that exceed the client's self-care capabilities. In addition, the holistic health care provider should develop personal attributes that enable him or her to do all of the following: respect clients' self-determination and decisions; empower clients; listen attentively; provide time; use and trust intuition; share insights; engage in an exchange of healing energies; and demonstrate sensitivity, honesty, love and compassion.

Implicit in all these approaches is the clinician's ability to:

- recognize his or her own strengths and limitations
- model positive health practices
- understand the role of body, mind, and spirit in the healing process

As a healer, the clinician must recognize that *the quality of self that he or she offers may be more significant to the healing process than the procedures that are performed.* The presence of the clinician—not merely the physical presence but the inner qualities—can have a therapeutic effect. The interconnectedness of the energy fields of the clinician and client influence healing. This is not to imply that conventional treatment procedures are irrelevant, but rather, that the love, caring, concern, and compassion displayed by the clinician can enhance the effects of treatments and affect the quality of the client's life. The healer must be willing to give of self. In accord with this thinking, the healer must be willing to take care of self to be in a position to be most therapeutic to the client. Some of the ways the clinician cares for self to optimize a healing relationship are listed in Box 1-7.

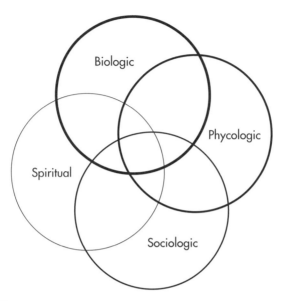

FIGURE 1-1

The Bio-Psycho-Social-Spiritual Model.

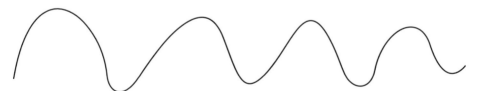

Optimal wellness – Maximum independence – Minimal intervention

Maximum symptoms – Total dependence – Extensive intervention

FIGURE 1-2

Fluctuating nature of care needs of chronically ill individuals.

BOX 1-7   The Clinician's Self-Care Practices to Optimize the Healing Relationship

- Eat a well-balanced diet
- Exercise several times each week
- Engage in relaxing activities daily
- Obtain sufficient sleep and rest
- Self-assess health regularly
- Obtain check-ups at recommended intervals
- Limit alcohol intake
- Avoid tobacco and recreational drugs
- Work in moderation
- Schedule time for rest and relaxation
- Meditate, schedule personal private time
- Express views and needs openly and honestly
- Enjoy hobbies, leisure pursuits
- Learn new skills, develop new interests, continue to grow
- Develop and nurture meaningful relationships
- Socialize
- Be open to new or different views
- Respect rights of self and others
- Accept faults of self and others
- Be optimistic
- Enjoy and use humor
- Clarify values
- Set goals
- Engage in positive self-talk, affirmations
- Form linkage with God or other higher power

References

Achterberg J: *Imagery in healing*, Boston, 1985, New Science Library.

Antonovsky A: Breakdown: a needed fourth step in the armamentarium of modern medicine, *Social Science and Medicine* 6:537-544, 1972.

Eisenberg DM et al: Unconventional medicine in the United States: prevalence, costs, patterns of use, *New Engl Med* 328(4):246-52, 1993.

Erickson H, Tomlin E, and Swain MA: *Modeling and role-modeling: a theory paradigm for nursing*, Lexington, SC, 1983, Pine Press.

Leininger M: *Cultural care diversity and universality: a theory of nursing*, New York, 1991, National League for Nursing.

Newman M: *Health as expanding consciousness*, ed 2, New York, 1994, National League for Nursing.

Nightingale F: *Notes on nursing*, London, 1859, Harrison.

Nightingale F: *Notes on nursing: What it is and what it is not*, New York, 1969, Dover Publishing.

Orem D: *Nursing: concepts of practice*, ed 2, New York, 1980, McGraw-Hill.

Rogers M: *An introduction to the theoretical basis of nursing*, Philadelphia, 1991, F.A. Davis.

Roy SC: The Roy adaptation model. In JP Riehl, SC Roy (editors): *Conceptual models for nursing practice*, (ed 2), New York, 1970, Appleton-Century-Crofts.

Sanford JA: *Healing and wholeness*, New York, 1977, Paulist Press.

Watson J: *Nursing: human science and human care*, New York, 1988, National League for Nursing.

Recommended Readings

Dossey BM: *Core curriculum for holistic nursing*, Gaithersburg, MD, 1997, Aspen Publishers.

Dossey B et al: *Holistic nursing: handbook for practice*, ed 2, Gaithersburg, MD, 1995, Aspen Publishers.

Dreher H: Proven mind/body medicine: scientific approaches provide hope for those suffering from chronic conditions, *Natural Health* 23(3):86-96, 1993.

Dunkle RM: Parish nurses help patient: body and soul, *RN* 59(5):55-58, 1996.

Gordon S and Fagin CM: Commentary: preserving the moral high ground, *Amer J Nurs* 96(3):31-32, 1996.

Joel LA: Alternative solutions to health problems, *Amer J Nurs*, 95(7):7, 1995.

Kane RL: Health perceptions: real and imagined, *American Behavioral Scientist* 39(6):707-717, 1996.

Keegan L: *The nurse as healer*, Albany, NY, 1994, Delmar Publishers.

Keegan L and Cerrato PL: Nurses are embracing holistic healing, *RN* 59(4):59-61, 1996.

Krieger D: *Accepting your power to heal*, Santa Fe, 1993, Bear and Company Publishing.

Lubkin IM: *Chronic illness: impact and interventions*, ed 3, Boston, 1995, Jones and Bartlett Publishers.

McConnell EA: The daughter is a nurse, *Amer J Nurs* 96(1):46-47, 1996.

Miller JF: *Coping with chronic illness: overcoming powerlessness*, ed 2, Philadelphia, 1992, F.A. Davis Co.

Moore JD: Nurses' patient-care outlook grim, *Modern Healthcare* 26(25):44, 1996.

Plawecki JA: Holistic nursing: moving beyond a professional commitment, *Journal of Holistic Nursing* 14(3):171-173, 1996.

Plawecki HM: The advancement of holistic nursing practice, *Journal of Holistic Nursing* 14(2):83-84, 1996.

Rew L: *Awareness in healing*, Albany, NY, 1995, Delmar Publishers.

20 Overview of Chronic Care

*W*hether it's the senior citizen who has limited mobility due to arthritis, the expectant mother who requires close monitoring because she is diabetic, the child who is challenged by Down syndrome, the trauma victim, or the individual struggling with a heart condition and schizophrenia, persons with chronic illnesses penetrate every clinical service. Naturally, even more individuals are affected by persons with chronic illnesses either in their family, school, work, or social settings. This is not surprising when one looks at the statistics concerning the extent to which chronic illnesses affect Americans. The U.S. Census Bureau reports that 30% of all Americans have a chronic illness and that:

- 4.1 million are under age 25
- 33.3 million have arthritis
- 27.8 million have hypertension
- 23.7 million are hearing impaired
- 21.5 million have heart conditions
- 13.4 million suffer from chronic lung disease
- 12.3 million have asthma
- 10.6 million suffer from migraines
- 9.2 million have developmental disabilities
- 7.4 million are living with diabetes

As Table 2-1 shows, the rate of chronic illness rises with age and results in a majority of older adults possessing at least one chronic condition. Although better health status caused the rate of chronic illness among seniors to decline in the past decade, the growing number of people achieving advanced years will increase the presence of chronically ill individuals in that age group.

Although this growth of the older population offers some explanation for the high prevalence of chronic illness, other factors that affect the burgeoning of the chronically ill population include our increased understanding of disease processes, improved control of infectious diseases, as well as a variety of technological, pharmacological, and surgical advancements. Prenatal detection and early correction of congenital anomalies that used to consistently end in miscarried pregnancies and premature deaths for previous generations of children are now common; diseases once considered hopeless can now be prevented and eliminated; and complications that would have been fatal in the past have become correctable or avoidable. All of these changes mean that persons with chronic conditions will be a significant component of the population for a long time to come and demand specialized services to meet their unique needs.

Defining Chronic Illness

Most clinicians probably would be able to describe chronic illnesses as long-term conditions; however, the characteristics of these diseases complicate the clearest definition. For instance, nearly a half century ago, a definition of chronic diseases was provided by the Commission on Chronic Diseases (Roberts, 1955) as:

> *All impairments or deviations from normal that have one or more of the following characteristics: permanency, residual disability caused by nonreversible pathological alteration, require rehabilitation or require a long period of supervision, observation, or care.*

This definition was expanded by the National Conference on Care of the Long-Term Patient to include a time frame (Roberts, 1955):

> *A chronic disease or impairment requiring a continuous or prolonged period of care of at least 30 days acute hospitalization or 3 months of medical supervision and/or rehabilitation in another caretaking setting.*

These definitions addressed the nature and time period associated with chronic illnesses but did little to consider the psychosocial dynamics of these conditions. It was not until the 1970s that definitions emerged that discussed the need for general adaptation (Abram, 1972) and included the psychosocial impact by defining chronic illnesses as (Feldman, 1974):

> *ongoing medical conditions with potential social, behavioral, and economic complications that require personal and professional attention.*

Finally, the disruption to daily life arising from chronic illness was discussed by Reif (1975), who identified the general features of chronic illness as:

> *disease symptoms that interfere with many normal activities and routines, limited effectiveness of the medical regimen, and treatment that contributes to a disruption of the usual patterns of living.*

As time progressed, the role and responsibilities of the client began to be seen in the definitions, as in Mazzuca's (1982) description of a chronic illness, as a condition requiring a high level of self-responsibility for day-to-day management.

With this history and a current awareness of the scope of chronic illness, we can develop an understanding of a chronic disease as a condition that:

- is neither curable nor reversible.
- is of a long-term duration.
- requires ongoing contact, supervision and care over a long period of time.
- imposes new self-care requirements (e.g., monitoring of condition, taking medications, performing treatments).
- potentially can affect the physical, emotional, socioeconomic, and spiritual well-being of the client and the client's family.

TABLE 2-1

Rates of Chronic Illness in Adults by Age (per 1,000 Population)

CHRONIC CONDITION	CONDITIONS (1,000)	RATE[1]							
		Male				Female			
		-45	45-64	65-74	75+	-45	45-64	65-74	75+
Arthritis	33,317	26.1	199.2	364.8	417.2	42.2	315.9	508.7	611.2
Dermatitis, including eczema	10,146	32.6	32.1	33.5	37.9	48.6	50.1	49.0	24.8
Trouble with—									
Dry (itching) skin	5,383	14.5	19.8	25.4	35.3	20.7	31.5	34.3	49.1
Ingrown nails	6,273	21.6	26.1	28.3	29.0[2]	17.0	35.9	47.2	75.7
Corns and calluses	4,433	6.5	24.3	13.9[2]	44.4	11.2	41.4	51.2	58.9
Visual impairments	8,976	31.1	66.0	96.6	131.9	14.5	33.1	49.6	99.4
Cataracts	6,721	2.5	18.7	112.5	193.2	1.7[2]	32.3	137.1	245.2
Hearing impairments	23,777	44.3	216.2	322.3	452.7	30.4	96.9	204.3	392.9
Tinnitus	7,779	11.4	75.2	95.5	113.7	13.5	45.1	77.1	84.6
Deformities or orthopedic impairments	31,605	102.1	181.8	154.9	185.8	100.5	167.4	167.1	243.0
Ulcer	4,408	11.1	23.2	38.4	31.8[2]	13.4	29.5	34.0	26.9
Hernia of abdominal cavity	5,228	11.5	39.0	61.5	64.8	6.5	34.1	57.4	67.5
Frequent indigestion	6,374	19.0	37.9	56.0	34.4	16.9	42.0	43.4	35.7
Frequent constipation	4,296	4.8	12.6	24.9	40.9	16.0	28.2	40.9	88.8
Diabetes	7,417	6.1	52.5	119.6	96.8	9.0	59.2	109.2	110.2
Migraine	10,627	26.0	18.4	15.3[2]	8.4[2]	60.8	80.6	35.4	21.7
Heart conditions	21,584	25.7	150.8	334.7	408.5	32.9	120.3	220.6	401.2

High blood pressure (Hypertension)	27,816	37.5	231.0	341.4	314.7	30.2	222.1	377.7	374.3
Varicose veins of lower extremities	7,281	5.3	26.7	34.3	56.3	24.2	76.9	84.4	101.0
Hemorrhoids	9,562	19.0	77.3	63.9	56.7	30.5	65.6	51.6	68.9
Chronic bronchitis	13,494	41.0	43.6	76.6	40.1	58.0	71.9	80.0	65.9
Asthma	12,375	50.7	32.4	28.9	35.7	53.5	56.6	55.9	32.8
Hay fever, allergic rhinitis without asthma	25,698	102.4	98.2	61.5	63.7	109.2	104.8	103.0	90.5
Chronic sinusitis	36,659	108.5	152.7	123.9	120.2	155.0	219.3	185.4	183.6

1 Conditions per 1,000 persons.
2 Figure does not meet standards of reliability or precision.

From US Department of Commerce. Statistical abstract of the US. 113th ed. Washington, DC: Bureau of the Census, 1993:140.

Impact of Chronic Illness

A chronic illness potentially can affect every aspect of a client's life (Figure 2-1). These diseases can alter mobility, breathing, digestion, and elimination, as well as mood and cognition. These alterations affect self-care ability, body image, activity level, and general well-being.

Roles and responsibilities may need to be changed or forfeited to accommodate the effects and demands of the disease. The chronically ill adult may be unable to maintain a job, care for a child, or participate in social activities. The chronically ill child may have poor academic achievement due to the effects of the disease or time absent from school, be limited in participation in recreational activities, and be rejected or ridiculed by peers. Even in the absence of real symptoms that limit function, an individual's roles and responsibilities may nevertheless be limited by others who make assumptions about the client's limitations based on stereotypes or misinformation.

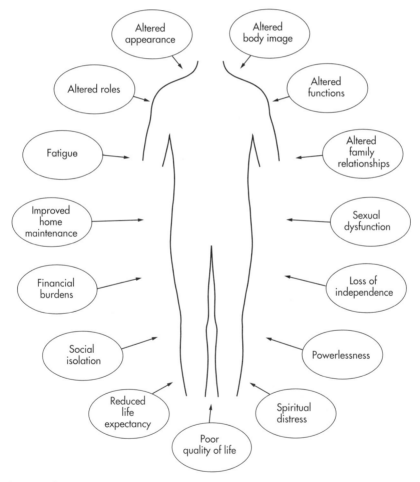

FIGURE 2-1

Potential impact of chronic illness on the client.

The emotional costs of living with a chronic disease can be significant. The chronically ill person can fear becoming dependent, suffering, or dying. There may be anxiety and concern about losing the love of or being abandoned by significant others. The ability to give and receive affection may be lessened. Grief may be experienced over the loss of function, appearance, roles, relationships, and responsibilities. Guilt and embarrassment can result if one perceives that he or she was responsible for causing the illness or if the disease carries a social stigma. Anger can be manifested as the individual asks, "Why me?" Optimism may be replaced by pessimism. If one charts the emotional responses to a diagnosis of a chronic illness, it could show a rocky path as the individual adjusts to living with this new challenge (Figure 2-2).

From this point, it is not hard to imagine how a chronic illness can challenge one's faith. Confusion, anger, and resentment can surface as the chronically ill individual and his or her family ask, "Why has God done this?" Guilt can arise as an illness is interpreted as punishment for a wrongdoing. For example, a person who has become blind may believe this was repayment for years of reading pornographic literature; a parent may attribute a child's disability to some action such as

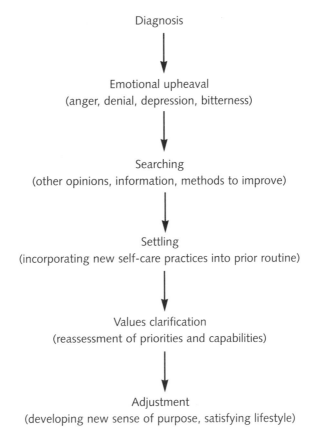

Diagnosis

Emotional upheaval
(anger, denial, depression, bitterness)

Searching
(other opinions, information, methods to improve)

Settling
(incorporating new self-care practices into prior routine)

Values clarification
(reassessment of priorities and capabilities)

Adjustment
(developing new sense of purpose, satisfying lifestyle)

FIGURE 2-2

Emotional responses to chronic disease diagnosis.

unfaithfulness to a spouse. As prayers for cure or improvement of a chronic disease are unanswered, one's belief system can be shattered.

Looking at more external effects, we become aware of how economic hardships can arise from a chronic illness. The management of a chronic disease can necessitate frequent visits to a health care provider, the purchase of medications and supplies, and special diets—all of which cost money. Symptoms and care requirements can cause time to be lost from a job. In some circumstances, the client may feel unable to meet the demands of the job; likewise, the employer may have concern as to the safety hazards, risks and costs associated with a chronically ill employee.

In the larger, social sphere, the client's chronic illness can change the way in which others view him or her. A spouse may begin to view a chronically ill partner as a burden and develop resentment, or treat the spouse as incapable and promote unnecessary dependency. There may be reduced sexual interest from the partner. Concern about the client's premature death can cause significant others to disengage from the chronically ill individual. Others may fear that they may risk contracting the disease if in contact with the chronically ill individual.

In fact, every member of the family is affected by the chronic illness. Additional responsibilities may fall on the spouse as the chronically ill individual is unable to be employed, maintain a household, or care for children. Sexual, leisure, and social activities may be curtailed or discontinued. The chronically ill parent may be unable to engage in activities with children and can be limited in the amount of care and nurturing afforded to children. Children may miss the opportunity for normal sibling relationships if their brother or sister is chronically ill. The presence of a symptomatic relative can serve as a deterrent to having guests in the home. Family members may need to become caregivers to the chronically ill person (see Chapter 3).

Finally, chronic illness also has an impact on society. The United States spends hundreds of millions of dollars on chronic disease control activities. Chronically ill people may place demands on the government for health, housing, educational, social, and economic assistance. Furthermore, limitations imposed by chronic diseases reduce the ability of this population to be productive members of society.

A variety of interventions, such as those listed below, must be utilized with the client, family and caregivers to minimize the impact of chronic illness:

- management of the disease to achieve as much improvement as possible and to stabilize or delay unavoidable decline
- control of symptoms
- coordination and support
- knowledge and skills training
- motivation for compliance and maximum self-care
- protection from complications and hazards to health and well-being
- identification and referral to resources
- promotion of hope, normalcy, control, and self-determination
- ongoing evaluation and planning for needs

Specific interventions will be discussed later in this book.

Chronic Care Goals

Most health care professionals were educated and socialized in a system that emphasized the acute care model, in which the goals were to diagnose, treat, and cure. Most care measures were directed toward ridding the patient of the problem: for example, resetting a broken bone, eliminating an infection, or restoring the body's electrolyte balance. The aim was sometimes to solve the problem with the assumption that the patient should live happily ever after.

Chronic conditions are a different story. They are long-term, present for life. Diagnosis and treatment are essential and important aspects of care, but these measures are just the beginning. Care measures must empower and enable the person to live with the condition, emphasizing more appropriate goals, like these:

- effectively manage the disease
- develop and stimulate the body's own healing abilities
- prevent complications
- achieve the highest possible quantity and quality of life, and
- die with peace, comfort, and dignity

Managing the Disease

To effectively manage the disease, individuals must understand their conditions. This implies becoming informed about the diagnosis, the pros and cons of various treatments, lifestyle adjustments (e.g., diet, exercise, rest patterns), and intended and adverse effects of medications and other treatments. Chronically ill persons must develop skill in fulfilling the demands imposed by illness, such as changing a dressing or giving an injection, or they must arrange for someone to assist them in meeting these care requirements.

Knowledge and skill mean little if one isn't motivated to comply with or engage in necessary care activities. For example, a client may know that a high-calorie, high-fat diet is not advantageous to her hypertension management. However, she may make a conscious decision to risk complications so that she can consume all the foods she enjoys. Likewise, a client may be depressed and see little reason to administer medications that sustain his life. These factors are important for clinicians to consider when assessing persons with chronic conditions.

Boosting the Body's Healing Abilities

An often overlooked aspect of chronic care is to develop and stimulate the body's own healing abilities. The body has tremendous abilities to fight disease, control symptoms, and prevent complications, and there are numerous ways that people can stimulate these activities naturally. In many situations, healing can be promoted by using alternative approaches such as biofeedback, herbal therapies, progressive relaxation exercises, and acupuncture. These alternative approaches can be used to supplement conventional treatments or, in some instances, to substitute for conventional treatments (as is done when relaxation exercises are used instead of tranquilizers). In most situations, the client's possession of a positive mindset and sense of control over self and the disease can positively influence healing.

Preventing Complications

Three basic levels of prevention are considered in health care: primary, secondary, and tertiary prevention. Primary prevention includes efforts to reduce the risks that could lead to the development of a disease; such efforts include anti-smoking campaigns, exercise promotion, nutrition education, and early prenatal care. Next, efforts to detect and manage disease in an early stage comprise secondary prevention; mammograms and cholesterol screening are examples of this type of prevention. Finally, tertiary prevention efforts address the needs of persons who possess diseases; these efforts aim toward maximizing function and preventing avoidable complications. Although tertiary prevention is significant to persons with chronic illnesses, all levels of prevention play a role in the promotion of health and maximum independence.

Chronic diseases and many of the conventional treatments used to manage them can increase the risk for infections, injuries, and other complications. For example, the person with chronic lung disease removes secretions from the lungs ineffectively and is easily susceptible to pneumonia; the medications used to control hypertension can produce dizziness and cause the individual to fall; and the inability to read small print can lead the visually impaired person to administer a medication incorrectly. Prevention of complications must be an active goal in chronic care.

In some situations, decline and disability cannot be prevented despite excellent attention to care. For instance, a progressive condition such as Alzheimer's disease will result in continued decline for the client. The challenge in caring for this client is to delay or slow the decline and disability that is experienced through preventive measures.

Maximizing the Quality and Quantity of Life

The achievement of a regular heartbeat or electrolyte balance means little if one must sacrifice a decent quality of life to obtain these outcomes. The control of a chronic illness can require significant lifestyle changes: habits, such as drinking or smoking may need to be discontinued; plain diets may need to be substituted for the exotic foods long enjoyed; a carefree existence may be burdened by the need to administer medications and perform treatments at specific times. The acceptance of uncertainty of the disease is necessary (e.g., not knowing how one will feel tomorrow, the effect of the illness on life expectancy, future ability to support or care for self).

Life is seldom the same once one possesses a chronic illness. Although a chronic illness can require lifestyle adjustments, care must be taken to ensure that the illness is controlled in harmony with the client's lifestyle, rather than controlling the client's life. The person possessing a chronic illness must not only effectively manage the disease, but also strive to achieve the greatest possible length and the highest quality of life despite the presence of the condition. This could result in less than ideal care choices in some cases; these choices are not always simple. For instance, a person with cancer may make an informed decision to discontinue chemotherapy and enjoy whatever lifetime remains without chemotherapy-related adverse effects, rather than accept uncomfortable side effects to gain several additional months of life. On the other hand, every possible care option that could lengthen life or improve function should be made available to the chronically ill individual. An important aspect of chronic care is to help the client find meaning and joy in the present, rather than grieve for the past that will never again be or the future that holds many uncertainties beyond control.

Dying with Peace, Comfort, and Dignity

Some chronic conditions result in a premature death regardless of the treatment options employed. Further, because the prevalence of chronic illness increases with age, most people who live a full life will possess at least one chronic illness by the time they die. A realistic and necessary goal of chronic care, therefore, is to die with peace, comfort, and dignity. This includes providing support to persons as they are dying, using effective pain control techniques, clarifying and respecting wishes regarding life-sustaining measures, and ensuring that the body, mind and spirit are adequately cared for as death approaches.

Clinicians are reminded that client's goals and the priority of various goals can change when there are changes in the status of the disease, the support system, and the client's level of coping and adaptation.

Factors Affecting the Care of Chronic Conditions

The medical treatments prescribed for chronic illnesses constitute only a part—and perhaps a small part—of the care outcomes. A variety of factors influence the success of the treatment plan and the quality of life chronically ill clients experience. Some of these include:

Type of Chronic Condition

Some chronic diseases are better understood than others and, subsequently, can influence the reactions of clients and others. For example, arthritis and Huntington's chorea are both chronic illnesses. While most people have enough familiarity with arthritis to engage in a conversation about the disease and not be concerned about exposure to the arthritic individual, many people do not understand Huntington's chorea. As a result, they could be uncomfortable engaging in a conversation with a person affected by the disease or even be concerned as to their own risks if they have contact with the client. Likewise, a disease like diabetes mellitus can elicit a different reaction than a disease such as AIDS.

Nature of Symptoms

Some chronic conditions may cause no noticeable symptoms, while others can result in deformities, incontinence, abnormal speech patterns, skin eruptions, altered cognition, and impaired mobility. Symptoms can influence the reactions of the client and others.

Experience with The Chronic Condition

Suppose a newly diagnosed diabetic individual is aware of a coworker who possesses the disease while living an active, productive life. This knowledge is likely to give him a more positive view of diabetes than if his only contact with another diabetic was a friend who suffered an amputation and was unsuccessful in keeping her diabetes under control.

Age, Lifestyle, Responsibilities

Lifestyle modifications to accommodate treatments, special diets, symptoms, and other factors associated with the disease can have a moderate to high impact on a client, depending on age and lifestyle. Imagine the difference in impact these factors are likely to have on a young professional who has significant career and family demands as opposed to a retiree who has flexible and ample time. Likewise, the retiree may accept the diagnosis itself differently than a person who is just beginning his or her life's journey.

Resources

A chronic disease can create a host of needs, and the physical, emotional, socioeconomic, and spiritual resources of the client can affect care outcomes (Figure 2-3). For instance, knowledge of the disease and its management, money to pay for care and medications, time to engage in special activities related to the disease, and the support and perhaps assistance of significant others are needs that often arise.

Because of the significance of the many variables affecting client outcomes, clinicians need to assess these factors along with items customarily included in the assessment. Factors to consider in assessing persons with chronic illnesses are discussed in Chapter 4.

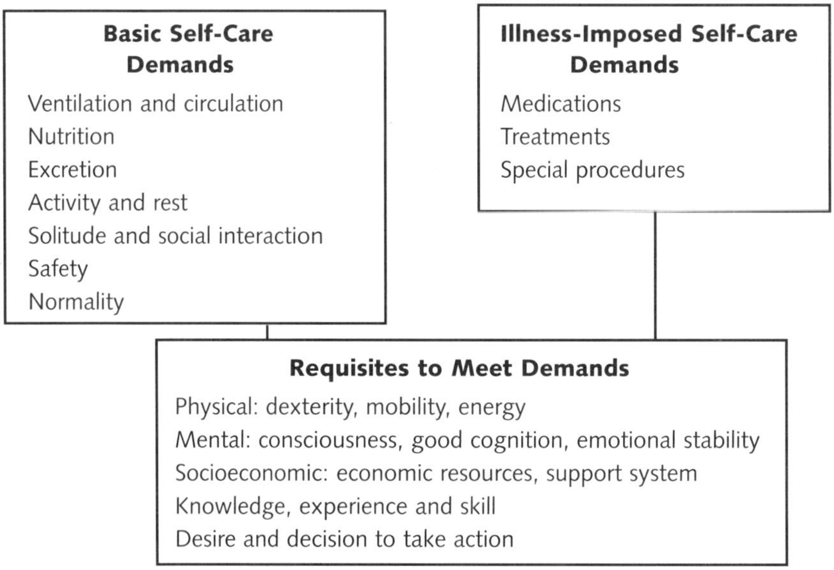

Basic Self-Care Demands

Ventilation and circulation
Nutrition
Excretion
Activity and rest
Solitude and social interaction
Safety
Normality

Illness-Imposed Self-Care Demands

Medications
Treatments
Special procedures

Requisites to Meet Demands

Physical: dexterity, mobility, energy
Mental: consciousness, good cognition, emotional stability
Socioeconomic: economic resources, support system
Knowledge, experience and skill
Desire and decision to take action

All human beings must meet basic needs in order to maintain life and achieve a sense of well-being; these needs are expressed as basic self-care demands. When people possess an illness, additional needs may have to be met; these illness-imposed self-care demands could become essential for the maintenance of life and achievement of a sense of well-being. A variety of factors, the requisites to meet needs, influence the degree to which these demands are fulfilled. When a self-care deficit has been identified, further assessment is necessary to determine the factors contributing to the deficit in order to plan care appropriately.

FIGURE 2-3

Requisites to meet self-care demands.

Chronic Illness Trajectory

A trajectory implies progressive movement in a predictable path, as a planet in its orbit. In the 1960s Glaser and Strauss (1968) introduced the concept of illness trajectory as it related to dying individuals. They found that dying takes time, and there were many strategies used by professionals, families, and dying individuals to manage and shape the dying course. They identified some predictable phases and patterns along the path of dying that affected the dying individual and others immediately involved (Corbin and Strauss, 1993). From this work, a specific framework of phases (Box 2-1) was proposed to represent expected changes in status of a chronic condition over its course.

Although there can be a potential course predicted for each illness, the illness course varies among individuals and illnesses, and often is uncertain. Individuals will possess their own trajectory projection and views on how it should be shaped. The trajectory framework offers a structure to direct care of the chronically ill.

Challenges for Clinicians

The problems and needs of chronically ill individuals are dynamic and complex, representing physical, emotional, spiritual, and socioeconomic dimensions. The expertise and collaboration of a wide range of professional disciplines ensure that these multifaceted needs are met. Crucial to this is an openness to a new profile of the health care team, one in which conventional disciplines are complemented by practitioners of alternative therapies. The development of new colleageal relationships and practice models are needed as a result.

As we consider new trends in chronic care, some may view the incorporation of alternative therapies into practice as a detour from the main road of medical treatments. As with any deviation from the main highway, the unfamiliar new territory of alternative therapies may be resisted and criticized as inappropriate, inefficient, ineffective, and incorrect by those who have known only the popular route. However, some of the most exciting and fruitful destinations are those not found on the beaten path.

BOX 2-1	**Trajectory Phases**
Pretrajectory:	Preventive phase before illness course begins
Trajectory onset:	Presence of signs and symptoms
Crisis:	Life-threatening situation
Acute:	Immediate medical attention and hospitalization is required to prevent deterioration or death
Stable:	Illness/symptoms are either controlled by regimen, in remission, or changing so slowly that few signs are present
Unstable:	Illness/symptoms are not controlled by regimen
Downward:	Progressive deterioration with increasing disability or symptoms
Dying:	Immediate period preceding death

Modified from Corbin J and Strauss A: A nursing model for chronic illness management based upon the trajectory framework. In Woog P (ed): *The chronic illness trajectory framework*, New York, 1992, Springer.

References

Abram H: The psychology of chronic illness (editorial), *Journal of Chronic Diseases* 25:659-664, 1972.

Feldman D: Chronic disabling illness: A holistic view, *Journal of Chronic Diseases* 27:287-291, 1974.

Glaser B and Strauss A: *Time for dying*, Chicago, 1968, Aldine.

Mazzuca S: Does patient education in chronic disease have therapeutic value? *Journal of Chronic Diseases* 35:521-529, 1982.

Reif L: Beyond medical intervention strategies for managing life in face of chronic illness. In Davis M, Kramer BJ, and Strauss A (editors): *Nurses in practice: A perspective on work environments*, St Louis, 1975, CV Mosby.

Roberts D: The overall picture of long-term illness, *Journal of Chronic Diseases* 8(2):149-159, 1955.

Straus AL and Glaser BG: *Chronic illness and the quality of life*, St Louis, 1975, Mosby-Year Book.

Recommended Readings

Allert G, Sponholz G, and Baitsch H: Chronic disease and the meaning of old age, *The Hastings Center Report* 24(5):11, 1994.

Benet A: A portrait of chronic illness: inspecting the canvas, reframing the issues, *American Behavioral Scientist* 39(6):767-777, 1996.

Blackwood F: Holistic health care enters mainstream; but business is wary of going with the flow, *San Francisco Business Times* 7(32):4A-7A, 1993.

Budd MA: New possibilities for the practice of medicine, *Advances, The Journal of Mind-Body Health* 8(1):7-16, 1992.

Callahan P: Alternative health: an office for studying unorthodox medical practices, *Omni* 16(1):20, 1993.

Consumers Union: Working out chronic illness, *Consumer Reports on Health* 7(10):113, 1995.

Davidson D: Partners in change are ready to roll, *Hospitals and Health Networks* 69(8):58, 1995.

Dossey B, Keegan L et al: *Holistic nursing: handbook for practice*, ed 2, Gaithersburg, MD, 1995, Aspen Publishers.

Dreher H: Proven mind/body medicine: scientific approaches provide hope for those suffering from chronic conditions, *Natural Health* 23(3):86-96, 1993.

England M and Artinian B: Salutogenic psychosocial nursing practice, *Journal of Holistic Nursing* 14(3):174-195, 1996.

Erdal KJ and Zautra AJ: Psychological impact of illness downturns: a comparison of new and chronic conditions, *Psychology and Aging* 10(4):570, 1995.

Fraley AM: *Nursing and the disabled across the lifespan*, Boston, 1992, Jones and Bartlett Publishers.

Green L: Build it and they might come: if a seamless system of care is ever created, it will be the best thing that's ever happened to the chronically ill, *Hospitals and Health Networks* 70(11):50-54, 1996.

Hawkins AH: Reforming the biomedical model: finding a successor model or going beyond paradigms? *Advances, The Journal of Mind-Body Health* 10(1):55-56, 1994.

Hornbrook MC and Goodman MJ: Chronic disease, functional health status, and demographics: a multi-dimensional approach to risk adjustment, *Health Services Research* 31(3):283-308, 1996.

Joel LA: Alternative solutions to health problems, *Amer J Nurs* 95(7):7, 1995.

Kane RL: Health perceptions: real and imagined, *American Behavioral Scientist* 39(6):707-717, 1996.

Keegan L: *The Nurse as Healer*, Albany, NY, 1994, Delmar Publishers.

Keegan L and Cerrato PL: Nurses are embracing holistic healing, *RN* 59(4):59-61, 1996.

Lorig K, Holman H, Sobel D et al: *Living a healthy life with chronic conditions*, Palo Alto, CA, 1994, Bull Publishing Co.

Lubkin IM: *Chronic illness: impact and interventions*, ed 3, Boston, 1995, Jones and Bartlett Publishers.

Mandelker J: Managing chronic disease, *Business and Health* 12(11):45-48, 1994.

Marwick C: Advisory group insists on 'alternative' voice, *Journal of the American Medical Association* 272(16):1239-41, 1994.

Marwick C: Another health care idea: disease management, *Journal of the American Medical Association* 274(18):1416-18, 1995.

Miller JF: *Coping with chronic illness: overcoming powerlessness*, ed 2, Philadelphia, 1992, F.A. Davis Co.

Moore JD: Nurses' patient-care outlook grim, *Modern Healthcare* 26(25):44, 1996.

Perrin EC, Newacheck P, Pless BI et al: Issues involved in the definition and classification of chronic health conditions, *Pediatrics* 91(4):787, 1993.

Plawecki HM: The advancement of holistic nursing practice, *Journal of Holistic Nursing* 14(2):83-84, 1996.

Rew L: *Awareness in healing*, Albany, NY, 1995, Delmar Publishers.

Shoor R: Looking to manage care more closely, *Business and Health* 11(10):46-52, 1993.

Suber R: Chronic care in ambulatory settings: components of an integrated care system, *American Behavioral Scientist* 39(6):665-676, 1996.

Turner DC: The role of culture in chronic illness, *American Behavioral Scientist* 39(6):717-729, 1996.

Wichramaekera IE: Diagnosis by inclusion: the perspective of a behavioral medicine practitioner, *Advances, The Journal of Mind-Body Health* 8(1):17-30, 1992.

Woog P (ed): *The Chronic Illness Trajectory Framework: The Corbin and Strauss Nursing Model*, New York, 1992, Springer Publishing Co.

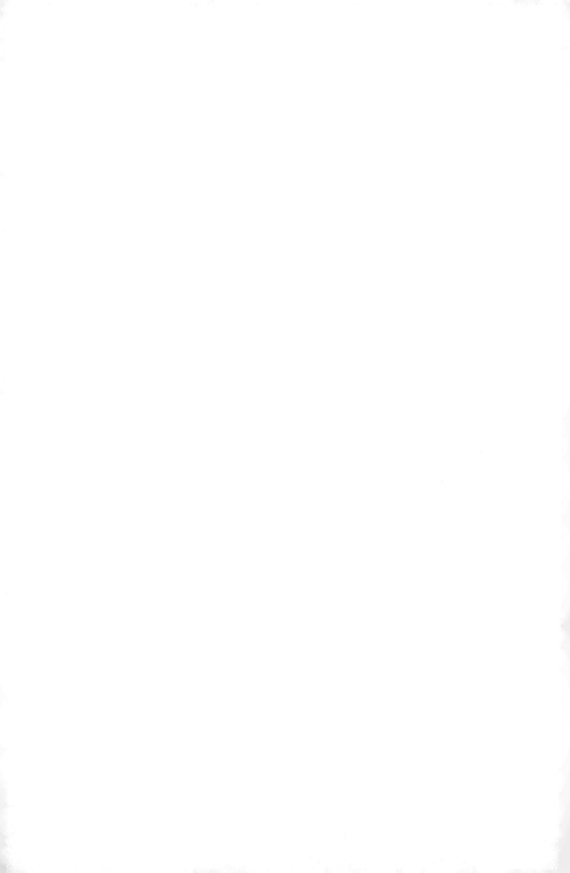

Chronicity and the Family

*C*hronic illness is a family affair. The parents of a profoundly disabled infant face a different future from what they expected when they first learned of the pregnancy and fantasized about the adventures they would have with their beautiful, active, and *normal* child. The middle-aged daughter who looked forward to opportunities to self-actualize now that she is free of child-rearing responsibilities may have to postpone her plans so that she can care for a parent who has suffered a stroke. A healthy child's needs may take back burner to the needs of a sibling who has diabetes. The young husband may feel torn between his desire to engage in physically challenging recreational activities and the lifestyle modifications imposed by his wife who has lupus. The retiree may feel resentment in having to forfeit long-awaited leisure pursuits to care for a spouse with Alzheimer's disease. An adult child of an abusive parent may experience guilt at refusing to accept caregiving responsibilities for the parent. The reactions, care demands, lifestyle modifications, financial burdens, and role changes of the chronically ill individual can have an impact on the entire family unit.

Who Is the Family?

Families come in many forms (Box 3-1). They can range in complexity from individuals, childless couples, and couples with children to grandparents and grandchildren, siblings, groups of unrelated individuals, or a single parent and child. A family structure can be formed through blood relationship, marriage, or emotional bonds. In chronic care, the functions fulfilled by individuals can be more relevant to identifying family than formal relationships. It is important to be broad in defining the family to ensure that all significant others who serve as family to the chronically ill client are included appropriately in care activities. To assist in identifying individuals who perform family functions, clients can be asked who:

- sees or speaks with the client daily?
- can be depended upon to help?
- is consistently trusted to share feelings and problems?
- helps with these problems?
- accompanies the client to health and social agencies?
- provides care during illness?
- assists in decision-making?
- should be contacted in the event of an emergency?

BOX 3-1	Family Structures

Single individual living alone
Several single unrelated individuals living together
Several single related individuals living together
Married couple without children
Married couple with children
Single parent with children
Step-parent, parent and children
Unmarried couple without children
Unmarried couple with children
Extended family
Compound (individual with several spouses)
Several couples living together with or without children
Group marriage (group of individuals sharing all spouses and children)
Homosexual couple without children
Homosexual couple with children

Family Dynamics

Each family is unique in its dynamics, and one way in which this is manifested is through the roles various family members fill. Some possible roles could include the following (Eliopoulos, 1990):

- *Decision-maker:* The person who is granted or assumes responsibility for making important decisions for the family. This individual may not be geographically close or in daily contact with family members; however, he or she is consulted before major decisions are made.
- *Problem-solver:* The crisis manager who, like the decision-maker, may not be geographically close or in regular contact with the family.
- *Caretaker/caregiver:* Usually a daughter, daughter-in-law, or wife who performs daily tasks such as cooking, cleaning, shopping, and personal care activities to dependent members. Although in a responsible role, this individual may not necessarily be given responsibility for decision-making.
- *Dependent:* An individual who, due to age, health status, preference, or family expectations, relies on other family members for physical, emotional, or socioeconomic well-being.
- *Victim:* A person who, by choice, situation, or force, forfeits his or her legitimate rights; this individual may be physically, emotionally, socially, or economically abused by family members.
- *Deviant:* The "problem child" who strays from family norms and may cause embarrassment, problems, or burdens for the family; may serve as family scapegoat, provide sense of purpose, or be used as excuse for actions or inaction of family members.

It is crucial for the clinician to understand family roles in order to plan and provide realistic care. For example, if a social worker has been coordinating arrangements for nursing home placement with the client's "caregiver" daughter but has not involved the "decision-maker" son, the son can stop the plans at the eleventh hour due to his objection to institutional care. This can result in unnecessary stress for the client, and guilt and frustration for the daughter. Likewise, if a nurse views the client's dependent, irresponsible adult child as a burden from which the client should distance herself, but the client enjoys the adventures and feelings of being needed arising from this relationship, the client may reject the nurse's advice (and could even reject the nurse!).

A family has norms or rules that guide its behavior as to right or wrong, acceptable or unacceptable. These are influenced by experiential, cultural, racial, religious, and socioeconomic factors. For instance, families can differ as to whether they:

- hide or share problems with persons outside the family unit.
- ask for help or limit problem-solving and assistance to the family unit.
- are proactive or crisis-oriented.
- confront each other with problems and concerns or avoid confrontation.
- respect or discourage each other's individuality and privacy.
- allow or discourage independence.
- accept responsibility or place blame.

Family norms can influence the manner of communication, acceptance of professional interventions, expectations, and other dynamics.

Chronic Illness and the Family

As mentioned earlier, chronic illness is a family affair. Seldom are relatives untouched by the illness of a loved one. Roles and relationships may change, caregiving may be required, social and recreational activities may need to be curtailed, household maintenance may suffer, finances may dwindle.

The family requires a realistic view of the course of the illness to effectively make preparations and cope. For example, the family will need to take different actions if they are informed that the client could remain stable for many years than if they are told the client can be expected to be totally dependent within one year. This is not to imply that individual variation and hope do not influence the trajectory, but rather, that there is some predictability to the course of illness.

Clinicians need to assess the impact of chronic illness on the family unit (Box 3-2) and identify diagnoses (Box 3-3) in need of intervention. Although specific interventions are applicable to each diagnosis, there are some general measures that can be of value.

BOX 3-2   **Factors to Consider in Assessing the Impact of Chronicity on the Family**

Reaction to diagnosis
Knowledge and experience with condition
History of illness within family
Usual coping mechanisms
History of and potential for abuse
Health of members
Socioeconomic resources
Roles and responsibilities
Expectations and motivations of members
Dependencies and interdependencies
Living arrangements
Sacrifices resulting from illness
Faith, spiritual beliefs

BOX 3-3   **Potential Diagnoses of the Family**

Activity intolerance
Anxiety
Altered family processes
Ineffective family coping
Fatigue
Grieving
Altered health maintenance
Impaired home maintenance management
Hopelessness
Risk for injury
Impaired verbal communication

Knowledge deficit
Noncompliance
Parental role conflict
Altered parenting (risk for or actual)
Powerlessness
Altered sexual dysfunction
Sleep pattern disturbance
Impaired social interaction
Social isolation
Spiritual distress
Risk for violence

Education

Facts about the disease, its management, course, and expected prognosis should be presented. The family should be provided with literature to supplement verbal explanations. Introducing the family to other individuals who are coping with a similar condition can prove helpful, as can referral to support groups. Just as the client can benefit from learning assertiveness skills (see Chapter 4), the family can be aided in learning how to communicate and behave assertively (e.g., expressing needs, setting limits, responding to inquiries about the client, voicing dissatisfaction to health care professionals). Laws that affect the chronically ill person and his or her family should be reviewed also (Box 3-4).

Counseling

Family members need to be prepared for the feelings they and the client could experience. If they hear that anger, guilt, resentment, jealousy, and depression often occur in the course of living with a chronic illness, they may be less distressed by these feelings when they do occur and perhaps understand measures that can be taken to cope effectively. They may require periodic reminders that the client's responses and behaviors directed to them are most likely attributable to reactions to the illness rather than feelings toward them.

BOX 3-4   Laws of Interest to the Disabled and Their Families

Americans with Disabilities Act (PL 101-336)

Enacted in 1990; protects disabled people from discrimination in employment, public transportation, stores, and theaters.

Fair Housing Amendments Act (PL 100-430)

Enacted in 1988; forbids discrimination due to disability by realtors and landlords; requires all new buildings of four units or more constructed after March 13, 1991, to be accessible and adaptable for people with disabilities.

Individuals with Disabilities Education Act (PL 101-476)

Enacted in 1975, amended in 1990; enforces free and appropriate public education to every child with a disability until the child graduates from high school or reaches age 22.

Rehabilitation Act (PL 93-112)

Enacted in 1973, amended in 1974, 1978, 1983 and 1986; forbids discrimination on basis of disability by federal agencies and any recipient of federal grants or federal contracts.

Technology-Related Assistance for Individuals with Disabilities Act (PL 100-407)

Enacted in 1988; provides federal funds to states for technology services and devices for the disabled.

The clinician can initiate and guide discussions between a couple as to the impact of a partner's chronic disease on the other partner. The clinician's input can be essential in helping the couple reorganize and adjust to the effects of the illness on the client's ability to maintain the current lifestyle, fulfill parental responsibilities, retain a job, engage in social activities, and enjoy a mutually satisfying sexual relationship.

The parents of a chronically ill child must consider the distribution of labor between them, particularly if the child has a condition that requires continuous attention or causes significant disability. A variety of issues can be addressed, such as the manner in which:

- the child's care needs can be balanced with the demands of a parent's job.
- two employed parents will share responsibilities for taking the child for medical appointments and staying at home when the child is ill.
- the parents will allocate time for themselves and each other.

If other children are in the home, the impact of the chronically ill child on them and measures to ensure that their needs aren't shortchanged should also be considered.

Finally, the family needs to understand the important role they have in promoting the client's positive self-esteem and self-worth. It will be difficult for the chronically ill individual to feel that he or she is whole and of value if family members convey the message that the client is incapable, an embarrassment, or unneeded. The client with poor self-esteem may be less able to cope with the stresses of the illness, display more dependency than is necessary, deal with problems ineffectively, suffer poor relationships with loved ones, and be nonassertive, self-depreciating, and unrealistic in expectations. Families can be guided in ways to facilitate a positive self-concept in the client by using measures such as:

- helping the client control symptoms and manage the illness.
- focusing on realistic goals.
- encouraging the client's independence and assertiveness.
- setting limits on maladaptive behaviors.
- identifying and reflecting self-depreciating and negative behaviors.
- recognizing and praising the client's accomplishments.
- suggesting and supporting professional intervention as needed.

Reactions of Children

Children of chronically ill parents are not immune to the effects of the illness. The children's age, developmental stage, and health status of their parents are major factors in determining the way in which children cope with chronicity.

Toddlers and preschoolers, normally concerned with their own needs above all others', may fear losing the people on whom they depend, become angry that the needs of ill relatives occasionally interfere with their own needs being met, and feel guilty that perhaps they are responsible for their loved ones' poor health status. These children may regress, experience sleep problems, or withdraw. They may be fearful of being apart from their families. Promoting a sense of security and trust can be helpful, and this can be facilitated by developing routines and offering truthful, basic explanations.

School-age children may experience similar feelings, but in addition, they may have reactions associated with having family members or a lifestyle different from their peers. They may be embarrassed about a relative's condition, resentful of the economic and social restrictions illness imposes on the family, or angry that their family relationships and activities are not similar to those of their friends. They may become depressed, do poorly in school, and withdraw. Some of these children may assume responsibility for housekeeping, caregiving, and babysitting of siblings, and be robbed of their own normal childhood. Parents might be wise to consider getting household assistance to avoid placing excess responsibilities on children, and honest talks about the illness and feelings toward it are helpful. These children should be informed that their feelings are normal and can be freely expressed.

Children's worries over peers' reactions to the illness are intensified in the teen years. Adolescents may be embarrassed at the different appearance or function of chronically ill relatives and at the same time, may feel guilty about having these feelings. They need to be encouraged to discuss their feelings. Developing relationships with individuals outside the family unit may help compensate for deficits resulting from the relative's illness. Also, honest discussions about the disease may be necessary to alleviate anxieties about their own risks of developing similar illnesses (Figure 3-1).

Parents must ensure that their children are not excessively depended upon for caregiving assistance. There is nothing wrong with a child learning responsibilities and assisting with tasks, but not to the extent that he or she is forfeiting normal educational, social and recreational needs for an ill relative. Parents also must ensure that the illness isn't used as a means to influence children's behavior (e.g., "You need to make something of your life to make up for what your sister can't do") or instill guilt ("You've upset me so much I'm having chest pain"). Professional counseling could prove beneficial.

Reactions of Older Adults

Retirement, the death of loved ones, relocation, and forfeiture of social roles are some of the losses that paint the landscape of old age. Living with a chronic illness introduces additional losses to the lives of older individuals. Energy, mobility, continence, and anatomical normality are among the physical losses that can arise from a chronic disease. The freedom of eating whatever one likes, achieving a full night's sleep, and taking an unhampered stroll can be lost. Symptoms associated with the illness can rob one of the ability to enjoy significant people and activities; social isolation may be experienced. Mood and cognition can be altered. There may be a need to become dependent on one's children and grandchildren. Institutionalization can be a real risk.

It is not uncommon for fear, anxiety, anger, and depression to be outgrowths of the effects of chronic illness on older adults. They may question why they had to be struck with an illness at the point in their lives when they have the opportunity to enjoy leisure pursuits. They may be resentful that after sacrificing and provid-

Knowledge of one's family medical problems is useful to anyone and can be particularly beneficial to family members who have had a history of serious or chronic illness. A valuable resource that can be given to young family members is a family tree that includes relatives' health history. Interviews with older relatives can aid in learning about medical conditions that plagued recent ancestors, as can causes of death listed on death certificates (copies of death certificates can be obtained through the vital records departments of state health departments; records prior to 1920 may be available from the National Archives, which kept census records by family name until that time). Further research can be done by searching records of the churches family members attended and obituaries (the Social Security Death Index, available in some libraries, lists zip codes of people who have died since 1963, which can assist in identifying areas in which their obituaries may have been published). Data searches also can be done using the Internet. The information obtained can be organized in a manner similar to a family tree for ease in retrieval and review; an example is shown below.

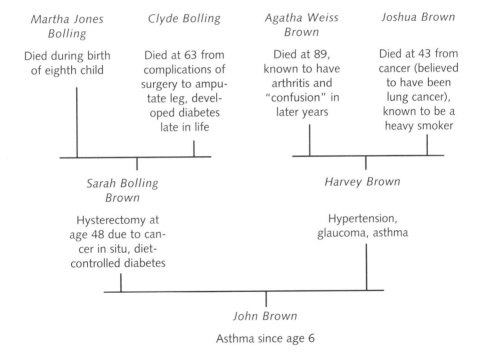

FIGURE 3-1

Family Health History.

ing for their children, their children are not caring for them, but rather, placing their care in the hands of professional caregivers. They may feel insecure that the people on whom they depend will withdraw support and assistance. They may be uncertain of what lies ahead.

Explanations of the disease and its probable consequences can be useful in helping older adults make plans and view their conditions realistically. It is important for older adults to take an active role in their care and decision-making. Advising them of the range of resources available to assist can alleviate some of the anxiety they feel. Encouraging and guiding family discussions of current and anticipated care needs can prove beneficial also. The clinician should serve as an advocate in ensuring that not only the quantity but, more important, the quality of the remaining years of the elderly are considered in the management of chronic illnesses.

Caregiving

There are times when the family will be called upon to do more than offer the client support; they may need to provide "hands-on" caregiving assistance. Thirty-one percent of the total population provide long-term care to a family member or friend; one in sixty full-time workers is a caregiver, and one in twelve is a potential caregiver (Shellenbarger, 1996). In addition, many homemakers and retirees provide caregiving assistance. Caring for a relative is a more natural than unique event for most families.

Many families ease into caregiving responsibilities gradually, and often subtly. For example, consider the following scenario:

> Marjorie lived in another town from her widowed mother, Francis Blake, who had been diagnosed with a chronic illness. At first, Marjorie would telephone several times weekly to check on her mother's status. Mrs. Blake was able to visit the physician independently and would report the physician's recommendations to Marjorie. As the months progressed, Marjorie could detect that her mother was anxious about visiting the physician alone and would forget to discuss important issues, so Marjorie began accompanying Mrs. Blake to the visits. As Mrs. Blake's symptoms worsened and she had increasing difficulties with home maintenance management, Marjorie invited her mother into her home and took over responsibility for paying bills, scheduling appointments, preparing meals and doing laundry for Mrs. Blake. This soon was followed by having to assist Mrs. Blake with dressing, bathing, and transferring.

The mother and daughter grew into this new relationship naturally, without fanfare, and as needs arose. This parallels the experience of many families.

Caregiving is far from an easy task for families. In addition to the often exerting physical demands of bathing, toileting, feeding, lifting, and turning, there are a host of psychosocial challenges faced by family caregivers (Box 3-5). Families need to consider these possibilities and be helped to plan measures to minimize the physical, psychological, emotional, social, and economic costs of caregiving. Many of the same educational and counseling approaches for families discussed earlier are applicable to the caregiving situation. The clinician can guide the family in realistically preparing for and evaluating their potential for caregiving by presenting specific descriptions of care requirements. For instance, the family of a person with advanced Alzheimer's disease may need to be told that they will need to toilet the client at intervals, bathe her, supervise her wandering, guide her in eating or feed her, and adjust the environment to prevent injuries. If possible, it can be very beneficial to arrange for the family to meet other caregivers who have had a similar experience. Because many individuals want to assist their loved ones and, consequently, may assume responsibilities that exceed their capabilities or impose considerable hardships, the clinician may need to introduce issues for caregivers to consider; for example, it can be helpful to ask specific questions, such as:

- How will you arrange food shopping and cooking?
- If you are awake a good part of the night caring for your spouse, will you have enough energy to maintain your outside job?
- What adjustments and sacrifices will your children face, if you care for their ill grandfather in your home?
- Have you discussed the care needs of this disabled child with his siblings, and if so, how do they feel about performing the tasks that you expect them to do?
- What is your plan to provide the care for the client in the event that you are ill or need to go away for a brief period?
- Have you made plans for private time with your spouse and children?

The clinician can suggest and perhaps lead a family meeting in which caregiving issues are addressed and responsibilities are discussed and assigned. It can be difficult for a caregiving spouse to ask children, grandchildren, and other family members for help; however, if the reality of this need is introduced by the clinician in a family meeting, assistance may be offered. Also, this forum can serve the purpose of establishing from the start the commitments family members can and cannot make to caregiving. The same relatives who adamantly insist that the client be cared for at home by loved ones rather than "by strangers" may become more open to home care or nursing home care when they realize that they will need to assist with caregiving responsibilities. Likewise, other family members may have more sensitivity and patience with the caregiving relative, and be more willing to offer a helping hand, support, and financial assistance, if they have a realistic understanding of the requirements and impact of caregiving.

When family resources are limited, a wonderful source of support and assistance sometimes can be found in neighbors and friends. In her book *Carepooling* (1993), Paula Lowe describes the exchange of practical help between caregivers and suggests that one needn't enjoy a close or long-term relationship with someone else to exchange caregiving help. Carepooling can occur between friends, neighbors, coworkers, church members, and other individuals. For example, the wife of a

BOX 3-5   Potential Costs of Caregiving

Physical
Inadequate rest and sleep
Poor eating habits
Fatigue
Muscle and joint strain
Inattention to personal grooming
Postponement of attention to personal
    health problems
Ineffective coping via use of drugs,
    alcohol, smoking
Lack of time, energy, privacy for sex-
    ual relationship

Psychological/Emotional
Depression
Anxiety
Frustration
Anger
Guilt
Powerlessness
Low morale
Helplessness
Lack of patience
Forgetfulness
Reduction in personal and physical
    space
Preoccupation
Altered parenting, grandparenting role
Abusive behaviors

Social
Limited opportunities to participate in
    events outside home
Lack of ability to be away from client
Insufficient time, energy or money for
    social activities
Decreased shared interests with friends
Withdrawal of friends
Feelings of isolation

Economic
Missed time from work
Need to cease employment
Care-related costs of client
Home modifications to accommodate
    client
Cost of respite care
Increased use of paid services (e.g.,
    carry-out, laundry, housekeeping)

homebound man may be willing to baby-sit a neighbor's child every Saturday evening in exchange for the child's mother staying with the disabled husband every Wednesday afternoon so that the wife can shop and visit friends. Prospective care-poolers can be found by word of mouth, and advertising on bulletin boards, in newsletters, and community newspapers. The success of these carepooling arrangements can be enhanced by being specific about care that will be provided (ideally, putting responsibilities in writing), setting limitations, and developing schedules.

Caregivers should learn some healthy selfishness. They need to learn to ask for help and to free themselves of stress-inducing "shoulds" and "should nots" (e.g., "You shouldn't leave a sick child with a sitter in order to get a weekend away with your husband." "A good daughter should care for her mother at home rather than place her in a nursing home."). They need to consider the balance of their personal needs against the needs of the person for whom they provide care (Figure 3-2), appreciating the fact that they have rights as caregivers (Box 3-6). Caregivers' rights to enjoy family, friends, employment, school, earnings, and participation in social and religious organizations must be encouraged. An unhealthy caregiver will be less able to create a positive caregiving experience.

Respite options must be introduced to caregivers. Such options could include stays with other relatives, home care, adult day care, group homes, and short-term nursing home care. The clinician can help caregivers understand that although respite care arrangements may not be ideal and could even be disliked by the client, the long-term benefits of respite have a therapeutic value that outweighs the negatives. Local information and referral services and social workers can aid in locating various respite services in the specific community. General resources to assist caregivers are provided at the end of this chapter (Box 3-7).

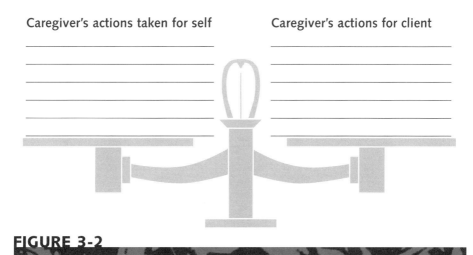

Caregiver's actions taken for self

Caregiver's actions for client

FIGURE 3-2

Balancing the Needs of the Caregiver and Client. A tool such as this can be used to help caregivers consider their own needs with the needs of the client and to identify areas for change.

BOX 3-6	Caregivers' Rights and Responsibilities

Caregivers are responsible to:
- become knowledgeable of the disease and its effects, complications, risks, and treatments
- know the correct administration, use, dosage, expected effects, adverse effects, and interactions of the medications the client uses
- demonstrate competency in performing required caregiving tasks
- understand the client's reactions and displaced feelings
- communicate with health care professionals and other persons involved in the client's care
- respect and protect the privacy and confidentiality of the client
- manage the client's finances responsibly
- engage in good personal health care practices
- communicate assertively
- be open to constructive feedback and insights
- recognize their own limitations and ask for assistance as needed

Caregivers have the right to:
- respect and meet their personal care needs
- obtain periodic respite from caregiving
- request and expect help
- express feelings
- be free from guilt or the "shoulds" and "should nots" imposed by others
- feel valued and appreciated for the help provided
- set limits and say no
- enjoy time and experiences with family and friends
- be forgiven for less than perfect behavior
- preserve their own physical, emotional, socioeconomic, and sexual well-being
- balance the needs of the client against the needs of themselves and their other family members

Trends That Will Affect Family Caregiving

Family caregiving will be a reality of the future. In fact, with the increased number of persons reaching advanced ages and the increased survival of individuals who possess chronic illnesses, caregiving demands on families could significantly increase. The ability of families to meet these demands is an issue, considering that:

- family size is decreasing, leaving fewer numbers of children to care for older relatives.
- postponement of having children causes parents to face child-care and parent-care responsibilities during the same period.
- more people are living alone and without caregivers available in the same household.
- divorces and remarriages increase the number of step-families, and subsequently, parents, in-laws, and grandparents who may be in need of assistance.
- women will continue to increase their employment outside the home, thereby reducing the availability of homemakers to serve in caregiving roles.

Clinicians will sometimes need a little creativity to identify significant others and community resources to assist with caregiving.

Joys of Caregiving

Although most of the discussion has centered on the demands and stresses of caregiving, there is another side of the coin: the joys associated with helping an ill loved one. The intimacy of a caregiving relationship enables family members to gain insight into each other as individuals and strengthen bonds. Satisfaction can be gained by adult children being able to help a parent who provided and sacrificed for them. The parents of a developmentally disabled child can experience immeasurable rewards in watching the unexpected achievements of their child as a result of their efforts. A husband can live with a sense of peace knowing that he cared for his wife prior to her death. Children can learn valuable lessons in values and intergenerational solidarity by observing and participating with their parents in the care of other relatives. One can become a richer individual by offering himself or herself in a caregiving experience. And for those with a strong faith, caregiving is consistent with God's will (in virtually all religions) that people take care of their families and attempt to repay parents and grandparents.

> "...should learn first of all to put their religion into practice by caring for their own family and so repaying their parents and grandparents, for this is pleasing to God."
>
> 1 Timothy 5:4

BOX 3-7

Resources for Information About Organizations to Assist Caregivers

(Resources pertaining to specific chronic diseases are listed in the sections of the book reviewing each specific disease.)

Association of Birth Defect Children, Inc.
827 Irma St.
Orlando, FL 32803
(800) 313-2232
www.birthdefects.org
Family Resource Coalition
200 South Michigan Ave.
Suite 1520
Chicago, IL 60604
(312) 341-0900
chtop.com/frc.htm
MUMS (Mothers United for Moral Support)
150 Cluster Court
Green Bay, WI 54301
(414) 336-5333
National Council on Family Relations
3989 Central Ave. NE
Suite 550
Minneapolis, MN 55420
(612) 781-9331
www.ncfr.com/
National Information Center for Children and Youth with Disabilities
PO Box 1492
Washington, DC 20013
(800) 999-5599
www.nichcy.org

National Information Center for Handicapped
PO Box 1492
Washington, DC 20013
(202) 522-3332
National Parent Network on Disabilities
1600 Prince St.
Suite 115
Alexandria, VA 22314
(703) 684-6763
www.npnd.org
Step-Family Association of America
215 Centennial Mall South
Suite 212
Lincoln, NE 68508
(402) 477-STEP
www.stepfam.org
Work and Family Resource Kit
U.S. Dept. of Labor
200 Constitution Ave., NW
Room S-331
Washington, DC 20210
www.dol.gov
The Families and Work Institute
330 Seventh Ave., 14th Floor
New York, NY 10001
(212) 465-8637
www.familiesandworkinst.org

References

Eliopoulos C: Family assessment. In Eliopoulos C (ed.): *Health assessment of the older adult*, ed 2, Menlo Park, CA, 1990, Addison-Wesley.

Lowe PC: *Carepooling: How to get the help you need to care for the ones you love*, San Francisco, 1993, Berrett-Koehler Publishers.

Shallenbarger S: Care-giver duties make generation Xers anything but slackers, *Wall Street Journal*, May 22, 1996, p. B1.

Recommended Readings

Allert G, Sponholz G, and Baitsch H: Chronic disease and the meaning of old age, *The Hastings Center Report* 24(5):11, 1994.

Beer WR: *American Stepfamilies*, New Brunswick, NJ, 1992, Transaction Publishers.

Benet A: A portrait of chronic illness: inspecting the canvas, reframing the issues, *American Behavioral Scientist* 39(6):767-777, 1996.

Bowe F: *Equal Rights for Americans with Disabilities*, New York, 1992, Franklin Watts.

Brazelton TB: Overcoming crisis, *Advances, The Journal for Mind-Body Health* 6(40):31-32, 1989.

Burman B and Margolin G: Marriage and health, *Advances, The Journal for Mind-Body Health* 6(40):51-58, 1989.

Czerwiec M: When a loved one is dying: families talk about nursing care, *Amer J Nurs* 96(5):32-36, 1996.

Doherty WJ and Campbell TL: The family health and illness cycle, *Advances, The Journal for Mind-Body Health* 6(40):35-41, 1989.

Erdal KJ and Zautra AJ: Psychological impact of illness downturns: a comparison of new and chronic conditions, *Psychology and Aging* 10(4):570, 1995.

Finn KL: A family affair: coping with heart disease and other chronic illnesses, *USA Today* 123(2592):63-65, September 1994.

Frieman BB and Settel J: What the classroom teacher needs to know about children with chronic medical problems, *Childhood Education* 70(4):196-202, 1994.

Giger J and Davidhizar R: *Transcultural Nursing: Assessment and Intervention*, ed 2, St Louis, MO, 1995, Mosby.

Growald ER: The power of love, *Advances, The Journal for Mind-Body Health* 6(40):26-30, 1989.

Heartquist J: A well-spouse perspective: the (inter)changing role of caregiver, *Real Living with Multiple Sclerosis* 1(4):6-8, 1994.

Hirshorn B: Family caregiving as an intergenerational transfer. In: Young RF and Olson EA (eds): *Health, Illness, and Disability in Later Life: Practice Issues and Interventions*, Newbury Park, CA, 1991, SAGE Publications.

Kahanaa E and Kinney J: Understanding caregiving interventions in the context of the stress model. In: Young RF and Olson EA (eds): *Health, Illness, and Disability in Later Life: Practice Issues and Interventions*, Newbury Park, CA, 1991, SAGE Publications.

Kelleher KJ and Wolraich ML: Diagnosing psychosocial problems, *Pediatrics* 97(6):899-92, 1996.

Kutner L: Getting children with chronic diseases involved in their care helps them cope with adolescence, *New York Times* 142: B5, C12, February 25, 1993.

Lewise S, Izraeli D, and Hootsman H (eds): *Dual-earner families: international perspectives*, Newbury Park, CA, 1992, SAGE Publications.

Lubkin IM: *Chronic Illness. Impact and Interventions*, ed 3, Boston, 1995, Jones and Bartlett Publishers.

Mace N: *The 36-hour day: A family guide to caring for persons with Alzheimer's disease, related dementia illness and memory loss at later life*, Baltimore, MD, 1991, Johns Hopkins University Press.

Mandelker J: Managing chronic disease, *Business and Health* 12(11): 45-48, 1994.

Mechanic D: Sociological dimensions of illness behavior, *Social Science and Medicine* 41(9): 1207-1217, 1995.

Michaels B and McCarty E: *Solving the work/family puzzle*, Homewood, IL, 1992, Business One Irwin.

Miller JF: *Coping with chronic illness: overcoming powerlessness*, ed 2, Philadelphia, 1992, F.A. Davis Co..

Roberto KA (ed): *The elderly caregiver: caring for adults with developmental disabilities*, Newbury Park, CA, 1993, SAGE Publications.

Roberts, DJ: *Taking care of caregivers*, Palo Alto, CA, 1991, Bull Publishing.

Robinson AR: Causal attributions about mental illness: relationship to family functioning, *America Journal of Orthopsychiatry* 66(2):282-296, 1996.

Ruppert RA: Caring for the lay caregiver, *American Journal of Nursing* 96(3): 40-45, 1996.

Schrauben L: Intervention strategies: support services for family caregivers. In: Young RF and Olson EA (eds): *Health, illness, and disability in later life: practice issues and interventions,* Newbury Park, CA, 1991, SAGE Publications.

Smith DM: *Kin care and the American corporation*, Homewood, IL, 1991, Business One Irwin.

Spacapan S and Oskamp S (eds): *Helping and being helped*, Newbury Park, CA, 1992, SAGE Publications.

Starer, D: *Who to call: the parents source book*. New York, 1992, William Morrow.

Stocker S: Six tips for caring for aging parents, *American Journal of Nursing* 96(9): 32-33, 1996.

Stolman MD: *A guide to legal rights for people with disabilities*, New York, 1994, Demos Publications.

Thara R: A family burden, *World Health* 47(2):10-12, 1994.

Thompson SC and Pitts JS: In sickness and in health: chronic illness, marriage and spousal caregiving. In: Spacapan S and Oskamp S (eds): *Helping and being helped*, Newbury Park, CA, 1992, SAGE Publications.

Time Books: *Helping Yourself Help Others*, New York, 1994, Random House.

Trad PV: Stress and child development, *Advances, The Journal for Mind-Body Health* 6(40):42-50, 1989.

Turner DC: The role of culture in chronic illness, *American Behavioral Scientist* 39(6): 717-729, 1996.

Maximizing
Conventional Care

*C*onventional treatments are those that are accepted and proven effective by our society's traditional or allopathic medical establishment. Tremendous advances in the conventional care of chronic diseases have enabled these patients to live longer and higher quality lives than previous generations. Effective chronic care helps clients maximize the benefits of conventional care.

Assessing Chronic Care Needs

Assessment is the foundation for all care activities. The basic process of assessment is no different for the chronically ill than for other groups of clients; although those basics will not be presented here, it may be helpful to reinforce some aspects of assessment that particularly apply to chronically ill clients. First, a comprehensive assessment is crucial. Although comprehensive assessment is always encouraged, in some chronic care situations the consequences of not considering all components of the assessment can be more damaging than it would be for other patients. For instance, in most circumstances omitting a review of family dynamics, spiritual beliefs, or financial concerns would have minimal impact when assessing a client having cataract surgery in an outpatient center to which he will not return. On the other hand, the ongoing nature of chronic care and the interrelationship of physical, emotional, social, and spiritual dynamics warrant a thorough evaluation of all aspects of the individual when case or care management is established.

Regular re-assessment is essential. As clients' health status, relationships, and lives change, so will their service needs. An exacerbation of symptoms could affect self-care capacity, an unexpected decline in status could cause depression, and increased family expenses could cause noncompliance with the treatment plan. Treatment and service plans that were appropriate in the past may have become ineffective. Likewise, the health, motivation, and circumstances of caregivers can change. Clients' and caregivers' status and needs should be evaluated during every encounter.

Clients need to actively participate in the assessment process. The active participation of clients is essential to a meaningful assessment. In the care of chronic conditions, there are many subjective evaluations that are best made by clients, such as pain, dizziness, mood, and appetite. One means of tracking changes in these symptoms over time is to use various scales for clients to self-rate symptoms; an example is shown in Figure 4-1.

Some of the factors to consider when assessing clients with chronic illnesses are listed in Box 4-1.

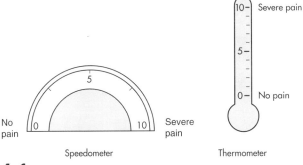

FIGURE 4-1

Tools to Use In Helping Clients Self-Assess Symptoms.

BOX 4-1	Factors to Consider in Assessing the Chronically Ill Individual

Health Perception/Health Management

- Understanding of health management and self-care practices
- Physical, mental, and socioeconomic abilities to engage in health management and self-care practices
- Motivation to engage in health management and self-care practices
- Knowledge base to engage in health management and self-care practices
- Ability and motivation to learn
- History of compliance with health care requirements
- Use of alternative therapies
- Availability of safe, clean, appropriate housing
- Ability to maintain safe, clean environment
- Health care provider
- Health and social resources utilized
- Amount, type and frequency of assistance required
- Date of last comprehensive examination
- Date and reason for last visit to health professional

- Illnesses: status and requirements
- Previous illnesses and hospitalizations
- Risk factors

Nutritional/Metabolic

- Appetite
- Weight, height; recent changes
- Condition of teeth, gums
- Presence and condition of dentures
- Ability to purchase, prepare, and ingest adequate diet
- Ability to eat independently
- Knowledge of dietary needs
- Ability to obtain and drink fluids
- Ability to resist/control infection
- Food preferences, intolerances, allergies
- Need for special diet; compliance
- Average daily caffeine consumption
- Use of dietary supplements, herbs
- Skin status
- Menstrual history and status

Elimination

- Frequency and characteristics of urinary elimination
- Frequency and characteristics of bowel elimination

- Ability to sense urge to void, defecate
- Ability to toilet independently
- Recent changes in bowel or urinary elimination
- Skin status

Activity/Exercise

- Vital signs
- Status of peripheral pulses, vessels
- Breath sounds
- Sputum characteristics
- Ability to engage in activities of daily living
- Mobility
- Exercise pattern and frequency
- Ability to ambulate, transfer
- Use of cane, walker, wheelchair
- Breathing pattern
- Energy
- Diversional activities, recreation
- Ability to engage in diversional activities, recreation

Sleep/Rest

- Sleep/rest pattern and characteristics
- Sleep inducers

Cognitive/Perceptual

- Cognitive function
- Level of consciousness
- Mood
- Educational level
- Ability to articulate, understand and use language
- Ability to read, write
- Visual capacity
- Use of eyeglasses
- Date of last eye examination
- Hearing capacity
- Use of hearing aid
- Date of last hearing examination
- Ability to taste and smell
- Pain, unusual sensations

Self-Perception and Self-Control

- Mood
- Self-concept

- Perception of self
- Sense of power
- Sense of hope

Role/Relationship

- Roles and responsibilities fulfilled
- Forfeited roles and responsibilities secondary to illness
- Marital status
- Family composition, roles, and responsibilities
- Availability and quality of friendships, support system
- Connectiveness with community
- Employment status, issues
- Opportunities for and frequency of socialization

Sexuality/Reproductive Pattern

- Self-image as sexual being
- Availability and health status of partner
- Ability to engage in satisfying sexual activity

Coping/Stress Tolerance

- Significant or unusual stresses
- Recent stressful life events
- Stress management techniques and their effectiveness
- Usual problem-solving techniques
- Use of and opportunities for humor
- Caregiving responsibilities for others
- Dependency on others

Value/Belief System

- Spiritual beliefs, religious preferences
- Opportunities to fulfill spiritual needs, engage in religious practices
- Important religious practices
- Compatibility of prescribed treatments with belief systems
- Personal goals
- Level of optimism

Providing Care

As discussed in Chapter 1, measures involved in caring for the chronically ill generally focus on the goals of helping clients to:

- effectively manage the disease
- develop and stimulate the body's own healing abilities
- prevent complications
- achieve the highest possible quantity and quality of life, and
- die with peace, comfort, and dignity.

A variety of resources can help clients to achieve the goals of chronic care, and the most important of these is the selection of a multidisciplinary caring team to assist in addressing the wide range of possible needs. No single health care provider will possess all of the resources and expertise to meet all of the often complex, multidimensional needs typically presented by a chronically ill individual; therefore, the talents of various disciplines are useful. There is no standard ideal team that can be universally effective for every chronically ill person; the mix of talent depends on the needs of the individual and could include physicians, nurses, social workers, dieticians, psychologists, pharmacists, speech pathologists, ophthalmologists, audiologists, dentists, and other specialists. Typically, a single professional or core team has the most frequent contact with the client and assumes responsibility for the coordination of care efforts. The educational preparation, expertise, and holistic orientation of nurses make them ideal leaders of the caring team.

The core providers who comprise the chronic care team can be expected to have a long-term relationship with the client. Therefore, it is important that the providers are appropriate for the client in terms of expertise and style. If the client's sole medical provider is a general practitioner, consideration should be given to consulting with a specialist. Realistically, few general practitioners can possess the knowledge and skill in managing a specific disease at the same level as a specialist, who dedicates a career to that one pathology. (When one considers the amount of knowledge that exists and the almost daily introduction of new approaches and research findings in a given specialty, it is enough of a challenge for a specialist to stay abreast of his or her specialty area alone.) Nurses and other clinicians may advocate for the client by discussing with the physician and client the value of consulting a specialist.

If the client is under the care of a specialist, consulting with another specialist can provide a second opinion and perhaps offer new perspectives. Clients need to be assured that most physicians are not threatened by second opinions and that clients needn't be apologetic or secretive about seeking this consultation. The right and responsibility of clients to obtain the best possible care for themselves should be reinforced.

In addition to feeling confident with their health care providers' expertise, clients must feel at ease with their providers; i.e., the chemistry should be right. Clients should trust and feel comfortable communicating with their providers. Since the provider-client relationship is a partnership that could last a lifetime, clients will do best if they are in agreement with the style, approaches, and values of their providers. Regardless of the fine reputation possessed, a health care provider who is inaccessible, abrupt, insensitive, or patronizing can cause unnecessary stress and frustration to a client. Some of the expectations that clients should have of their health care providers are listed in Box 4-2.

It is reasonable for clients to expect their health care providers to explain, in layman's terms, the meaning of the diagnosis, the expected course of the disease, anticipated outcomes and possible risks of diagnostic and treatment procedures, and the pros and cons of various treatment and care options. Equipped with these facts, clients have a right to accept or refuse procedures and care. Health care providers must respect clients' informed decisions and not attempt to coerce clients into complying with professional recommendations. The initial experiences in the manner in which a health care provider offers explanations, responds to questions, and senses concerns will most likely indicate what clients can expect in the future. If warning lights go off from the start, clients may be wise to consider other providers.

BOX 4-2   Positive Characteristics to be Expected in a Health Care Provider

- Possesses competency and credentials in clinical specialty
- Speaks on a level the client understands
- Values the client's contributed subjective data
- Respects the role of the family in the client's caregiving process
- Shares similar values regarding care and quality of life
- Demonstrates desire for client to be informed and involved in care
- Affords the client opportunities to make decisions concerning care and accepts informed decisions by the client
- Ensures that client's needs and concerns have been addressed prior to terminating visit
- Makes client feel at ease and unrushed
- Communicates in a sympathetic, nonintimidating, noncondescending manner
- Fully explains diagnoses and treatments
- Is open to suggestions, feedback, and second opinions
- Demonstrates interest in learning about the client as a person
- Orders all essential tests and procedures but not those that are unnecessary
- Conveys confidence in treatment and care measures
- Is respected by other health care professionals
- Is accessible and able to arrange a timely office/home visit when necessary
- Responds to telephone calls in the same day
- Charges competitive fees
- Demonstrates optimism and hope
- Conveys appreciation and concern for all aspects of the client: body, mind, and spirit

Most health care providers are busy and have many demands; therefore, clients have the responsibility to use providers' time wisely. Prior to the visit, clients should prepare by writing questions, concerns, and suggestions to review. During the visit it is helpful for notes to be taken and for important instructions and facts to be restated by clients to ensure a proper understanding. Clients should be advised to keep their own file or notebook of notes, laboratory results, and other relevant medical information for future reference.

Many clients pressure their health care providers for a prognosis. *How long will I live? Can I expect to suffer? Will I become bedridden and dependent?* It is reasonable for clients to want a realistic view of expectations so that they can prepare accordingly. Health care providers can offer some generalities about prognosis, but clients must understand that the key word is *generalities*: the course of an illness is unique for each individual. Age, general health status, attitude, motivation, and lifestyle practices are among the factors that cause differences among people in the progression of the disease and response to treatment. Certainly it is helpful to know whether the disease will progressively worsen or remain stable with proper care, and whether people typically live a full lifetime with the disease or seldom survive more than two years. Major life decisions can hinge on such appraisals. But clients should be advised to use these predictions as broad estimates and not engrave them in stone as absolutes. They may be helped by learning of examples of people who have beat the odds and lived a quality and quantity of life that no one expected.

While being realistic and honest, it is important for health care providers to demonstrate hope and optimism. For instance, a client who has early stage Alzheimer's disease may be experiencing a worsening of memory. A health care provider who reacts to this with the statement, *"Well, this is what can be expected"*, conveys a different level of hope and optimism than one who responds, *"Let's try this new medication and build memory exercises into your daily routine."* The latter professional is not giving false hope that the Alzheimer's disease can be reversed or cured, but instead is demonstrating a willingness to try every reasonable means to help the client slow the progression of symptoms, feel a sense of control, and live the highest quality life possible.

Clinicians need to appreciate the power to influence outcomes by their attitudes, comments, and behaviors. Health care professionals have known for some time of the placebo effect, in which a harmless drug or treatment of no therapeutic value produces some beneficial effect in an individual. Now we are being told of the inversion of the placebo effect, coined by Deepak Chopra as the *nocebo effect*, in which a person experiences negative effects as a result of the health care professional's hopelessness or lack of faith in the treatment (Chopra, 1990). Conventional physicians' statements along the line that *"You have three months to live at best"* and *"There is nothing more we can do"* have been compared to medical hexing in shamanistic cultures (Weil, 1995). Despair can result when clients believe their health care providers lack faith in their ability to recover. A more therapeutic approach is for health care providers to demonstrate hope and optimism in their ability to help clients live the most comfortable, highest quality life possible despite the inability to stop the progression of the disease. Perhaps this is where the value of alternative therapies can be realized. Certainly, a clinician would be remiss to knowingly allow a client to engage in quackery or a hazardous treatment without advising the client of the realities; however, some alternative therapies could benefit the client, even if just through a placebo effect, without producing adverse effects, and these should not be discouraged. The fact that reams of research do not exist supporting the alternative measure does not mean the therapy isn't useful or effective. A clinician needn't promote or condone the use of an alternative therapy, but unless there is proof that the measure is harmful, the clinician should accept the client's decision to try anything that could potentially be beneficial.

Recruiting a Chronic Care Coach

Many chronic conditions necessitate a change in diet, activity, and lifestyle practices. For example, a person with diabetes may need to consume a designated amount of certain nutrients at specific times of the day; an individual with emphysema may practice breathing exercises several times daily to promote effective air exchange, and someone with hypertension may attempt to control the disease by joining a smoking cessation program and finding new outlets for stress. Anyone who has engaged in a weight reduction program recognizes that possessing the best intentions and knowing that weight loss is in one's best interest doesn't mean that there aren't difficulties adhering to a new diet as time progresses. Likewise, sticking to lifestyle modifications or administering medications or treatments day after day, month after month, year after year, as is necessary with a chronic condition, can be a tremendous challenge. Clients become discouraged, frustrated, and even bored with treatment regimens; sometimes, because they feel good and their conditions are under control, they may believe that they needn't follow their prescribed treatments any longer. Such ups and downs in caring for chronic conditions are perfectly normal.

There also are many times when people with chronic illnesses need extra support in coping with their feelings about their conditions. Adjusting to and living with chronic illness entails adjustments, and in many situations, losses. For example, one can lose an unrestricted lifestyle, function, normal appearance, and independence. As with any loss, the client experiencing the losses associated with chronic illness may experience grief, similar to that associated with death and dying.

Although it is understandable that chronically ill individuals occasionally could "slip off the treatment wagon" or experience reactions that interfere with compliance to the treatment plan, the reality is that consistent attention and care of the illness are essential to optimal health and the prevention of complications. An aid to staying focused and encouraged to comply with care demands of chronic conditions is for the client to recruit and use a coach. Some of the functions of a chronic care coach are listed in Box 4-3.

A coach can be a spouse, parent, child, friend, another client with a similar condition, or anyone else who cares about and has regular contact with the client. The coach needs to become knowledgeable about the disease and treatment plan. When the client is complying and coping without difficulty, the coach recognizes this accomplishment and offers positive reinforcement, such as praise, a small gift, or a card. On the other hand, when the coach detects or the client expresses that there

BOX 4-3   Functions of a Chronic Care Coach

- Maintain regular contact with the client
- Learn about the condition; keep abreast of new information about the condition and share this with the client
- Help client develop effective self-care practices
- Remind client of caregiving activities, appointments, etc.
- Listen to concerns and feelings without judgment
- Offer feedback about self-care practices
- Recognize and praise small and large accomplishments
- Understand and accept displaced feelings
- Identify and help client review causes of noncompliance, regression
- Encourage client to discuss questions and concerns with health care provider
- Assist client in locating resources to help with health and social needs
- Challenge client to consider new approaches, life changes
- Accompany client to appointments with health care provider and other care-related activities as necessary
- Be available for support, comfort, assistance

have been "slips" in compliance or that discouragement is brewing, the coach helps the client explore reasons for this and offers support and assistance in re-establishing care practices. Giving a "pep talk", offering a shoulder to cry on, pointing out observed behaviors, and being present are among the strategies the coach can use to assist the client. The client needs to feel secure that he or she can trust the coach, confide problems and concerns, and freely ask for help when needed. The coach needs to be committed to being available to offer time, energy, and assistance to the client when needed on a long-term basis, recognizing that the client may not be appreciative or pleasant all the time, and that there is a real possibility that the coach will observe the client's condition worsening. It can be beneficial for the coach to identify a means of support for himself or herself.

Becoming Informed

Knowledge is basic to the effective management of a chronic illness. Feelings of helplessness and powerlessness can be alleviated when diseases and treatments are demystified.

Clinicians can provide significant information about chronic care issues; however, there are many other valuable educational sources, most of which are free of charge. A listing of some associations for specific conditions is offered in Box 4-4. Contact with these organizations can help clients learn about lectures and support groups for people with specific conditions. Local newspapers regularly publicize schedules of lectures and group meetings for persons interested in specific conditions. Public libraries not only possess books, magazines, pamphlets, and audiovisual materials pertaining to various health problems, but also, many are equipped

BOX 4-4
Resources for Information About Specific Health Conditions

AIDS/HIV POSITIVE
National Association of People with AIDS
1413 K Street NW
Suite 7
Washington, DC 20005
(202) 898-0414
www.thecure.org
ALZHEIMER'S DISEASE
Alzheimer's Disease and Related Disorders Association
919 North Michigan Avenue
Suite 1000
Chicago, IL 60611
(800) 272-3900
Respite Programs for Caregivers of Alzheimer's Disease Patients (Hotline)
(800) 648-COPE
ARTHRITIS
Arthritis Foundation
P.O. Box 19000
Atlanta, GA 30326
(800) 283-7800
ASTHMA/ALLERGY
Asthma and Allergy Foundation of America
1125 15th Street NW
Suite 502
Washington, DC 20005
(800) 7-ASTHMA
www.aafa.org
CANCER
American Cancer Society
777 Third Avenue
New York, NY 10017
(212) 371-2900
www.cancer.org
Leukemia Society of America
600 Third Avenue
New York, NY 10016
(212) 573-8484
www.leukemia.org
Make Today Count
PO Box 303
Burlington, IA 52601
(319) 753-6251
userpages.itis.com/lemoll/index.html
National Cancer Institute
Office of Cancer Communications
Building 31, Room 10A18
Bethesda, MD 20205
(800) 492-6600
www.nci.nih.gov

National Coalition for Cancer Survivorship
1010 Wayne Avenue
Silver Spring, MD 20910
(301) 650-8868
www.cansearch.com
National Hospice Organization
301 Tower
Suite 506
301 Maple Avenue
Vienna, VA 22181
(804) 243-5900
www.nho.org
CARDIOVASCULAR CONDITIONS
American Heart Association
7320 Greenville Avenue
Dallas, TX 75231
(214) 750-5551
www.amhrt.com
CHASER (Congenital Heart Anomalies Support, Education, Resource)
2112 N. Wilkens Road
Swanton, OH 43558
(419) 825-5575
www.csun.edu/(hfmth006/chaser
Coronary Club, Inc.
9500 Euclid Avenue
Mail Code E37
Cleveland, OH 44106
(216) 444-3690
www.heartline-news.org
High Blood Pressure Information Center
120/80 National Institutes of Health
Bethesda, MD 20205
(301) 496-1809
www.nih.gov
International Association of Pacemaker Patients
PO Box 54305
Atlanta, GA 30308
(800) 241-6993
Mended Hearts
7272 Greenville Avenue
Dallas, TX 75231
(214) 706-1442
www.mendedhearts.org
National Amputation Foundation
12-45 150th Street
Whitestone, NY 11357
(212) 767-0596
www.social.com/health/nhic/data/hr0300/hr03
59.html

National Heart, Lung, and Blood Institute
Office of Information
Bethesda, MD 20205
www.nhlbi.nih.gov/nhlbi/nhlbi.htm

DIABETES
American Diabetes Association
1660 Duke Street
Alexandria, VA 22314
(800) 232-3472
www.diabetes.org

Diabetics Anonymous
PO Box 60905
Sunnyvale, CA 94088
(408) 746-2022

Diabetes Education Center
4959 Excelsior Boulevard
Minneapolis, MN 55416
(612) 927-3393

EPILEPSY
Epilepsy Foundation of America
4351 Garden City Drive
Landover, MD 20785
(301) 459-3700
Patient Info Hotline: (800) 332-1000
www.efa.org

GASTROINTESTINAL CONDITIONS
National Foundation for Ileitis and Colitis
295 Madison Avenue
New York, NY 10017
(212) 685-3440

Pediatric Support Group for Ostomy and Colon
Disease
11385 Cedarbrook Road
Roscoe, IL 61073
(815) 623-8034

United Ostomy Association
36 Executive Park #120
Irvine, CA 92714
(800) 826-0826
www.uoa.org

HEARING IMPAIRMENT
Alexander Graham Bell Association for the
Deaf
3417 Volta Place NW
Washington, DC 20007
(202) 337-5220

American Humane Association Hearing Dog
Program
1500 West Tufts Avenue
Englewood, CO 80110
(303) 762-0342

National Association of the Deaf
814 Thayer Avenue
Silver Spring, MD 20910
(301) 587-1788
www.nad.org/

National Center for Law and the Deaf
7th Street and Florida Avenue NE
Washington, DC 20002
(202) 651-5454

Self-Help for Hard of Hearing People
PO Box 34889
Washington, DC 20034
www.shh.com

INCONTINENCE
Help for Incontinent People
Box 544
Union, SC 29389
(803) 585-8789

Kimberly Clark Corporation
2001 Marathon Avenue
Neenah, WI 54946
(414) 721-2000
www.Kimberly-clark.com

Procter and Gamble
Procter and Gamble Plaza
Cincinnati, OH 45202
(800) 428-8363
www.pg.com

Simon Foundation for Continence
PO Box 835
Wilmette, IL 60091
(800) 23-SIMON
www.aacp.org/welcome/WHP/simon.html

MENTAL HEALTH AND ILLNESS
Alcoholics Anonymous
PO Box 459
Grand Central Station
New York, NY 10017
(212) 686-1100
www.alcoholics-anonymous.org

Depressed Anonymous
1013 Wagner Avenue
Louisville, KY 40217
(502) 569-1989

Mental Health Association
1800 North Kent Street
Arlington, VA 22209
(703) 528-6405

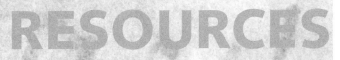

National Depressive and Manic-Depressive Association
730 North Franklin Street
Suite 501
Chicago, IL 60610
(800) 826-3632
www.ndmda.org

Neurotics Anonymous
PO Box 12
Casa, AR 72012

Obsessive-Compulsive Anonymous
PO Box 215
New Hyde Park, NY 11040
(516) 741-4901

Schizophrenics Anonymous
15920 West 12 Mile
Southfeld, MI 48076
(313) 557-6777

MULTIPLE SCLEROSIS

Multiple Sclerosis Association of America
601 White Horse Pike
Oaklyn, NJ 08107
(800) 833-4MSA

National Multiple Sclerosis Society
Information Resource Center
733 Third Avenue
New York, NY 10017
(800) 344-4867
www.nmss.org/

MUSCULOSKELETAL CONDITIONS

Arthritis Foundation
3400 Peachtree Road
Suite 1101
Atlanta, GA 30326
(404) 266-0795

Arthritis Information Clearinghouse
PO Box 34427
Bethesda, MD 20034
(301) 881-9411

National Osteoporosis Foundation
1150 17th Street NW
Suite 500
Washington, DC 20036
(202) 223-2226

PARKINSON'S DISEASE

American Parkinson's Disease Association
60 Bay Street
Suite 401
Staten Island, NY 10301
(800) 223-2732
www.the-health-pages.com/
resources/apda/intex.html

National Parkinson Foundation
1501 NW 9th Avenue
Miami, FL 33136
(305) 547-6666
www.parkinson.org/

Parkinson's Disease Foundation
William Black Medical Research Building
650 West 168th Street
New York, NY 10032
(800) 457-6676

Parkinson's Support Groups of America
11376 Cherry Hill Road
Suite 204
Beltsville, MD 20705
(301) 937-1545

United Parkinson Foundation
220 South State Street
Chicago, IL 60604
(312) 922-9734
www.stepstn.com/nord/org_sum/102.htm

PULMONARY CONDITIONS

American Lung Association
1740 Broadway
New York, NY 10019
(212) 245-8000
www.lung.usa.org/

Asthma and Allergy Foundation of America
1125 15th Street NW
Suite 502
Washington, DC 20005
(800) 7-ASTHMA
www.aafa.org/

Emphysema Anonymous
PO Box 66
Fort Myers, FL 33902
(813) 334-4226

VISUAL IMPAIRMENT

American Council of the Blind
1155 15th Street, NW
Suite 720
Washington, DC 20005
(202) 467-5081, (800) 424-8666
www.acb.org

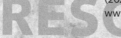

Blinded Veterans Association
477 H Street, NW
Washington, DC 20001-2694
(202) 371-8880
www.bva.org
Guide Dogs for the Blind, Inc.
PO Box 151200
San Rafael, CA 94915-1200
(415) 499-4000, (800) 295-4050
www.guidedogs.com
Guiding Eyes for the Blind
250 East Hartsdale Avenue
Hartsdale, NY 10530
(914) 723-2223
www.guiding-eyes.org
Leader Dogs for the Blind
PO Box 5000
Rochester, MI 48307
(810) 651-9011, (800) 777-5332
www.leaderdog.org
National Association for the Visually Handicapped
305 East 24th Street
New York, NY 10010
(212) 899-3141

National Eye Institute
Building 31, Room 6A-32
Bethesda, MD 20892
(301) 496-5248
www.nei.nih.gov
National Federation of the Blind
1800 Johnson Street
Baltimore, MD 21230
(410) 659-9314
National Library Service for the Blind and Physically Handicapped
Library of Congress
1291 Taylor Street NW
Washington, DC 20542
(202) 707-5100, (800) 424-8567
Recorded Periodicals
919 Walnut Street
Philadelphia, PA 19107
(215) 627-0600
Recordings for the Blind
215 West 58th Street
New York, NY 10022
(212) 751-0860

Local chapters of the above associations can be located through telephone directories for specific communities

to locate and obtain materials nationally and internationally via their computer networks. Popular magazines and newspapers publish articles on medical advancements and can be a significant source of information about new treatment approaches and insights into diseases. (Often, newspapers publish the information within days of its appearing in the *New England Journal of Medicine* and other leading medical journals.)

Finally, in a mobile society clients need to be sufficiently informed to be able to explain their conditions and treatments to new health care providers in the event that they require medical attention while traveling or staying in another state. Clients can be advised to carry small medical fact sheets in their wallets that provide a brief summary of relevant health histories for quick reference (Figure 4-2). For a nominal fee, there are groups that will store and provide medical information on a 24-hour basis, such as Medic Alert (800-825-3785) and Life-Fax (800-715-4334).

Linking with Support Groups

Although many people think of support groups as people who get together for help in coping with an illness, these groups provide much more. Group members possess rich experiences in various aspects of the disease and its management, and they usually are willing to share with others who are journeying down the same path.

```
┌─────────────────────────────────────────────────────────────┐
│  Name                              D.O.B.                     │
│  Address                                                      │
│  Phone SS#                                                    │
│  Medical Insurance Type   #                                   │
│                                                               │
│  Contact Person                        Phone                  │
│  Health Provider(s)                    Phone                  │
│                                                               │
│  Diagnoses/ Health Conditions                                 │
│                                                               │
│  Medications Used                                             │
│                                                               │
│  Allergies                                                    │
│  Advance Directive Available       Location                   │
└─────────────────────────────────────────────────────────────┘
```

FIGURE 4-2

Health Facts Summary.

Members can share practical tips ranging from where to get the best prices for supplies to recipes for making special diets more palatable. They may be able to recommend books that they've found particularly helpful and provide information that they've learned regarding new treatments.

In addition to sharing information about the disease and its management, support groups offer the unique aspect of being able to explain the realities of living with the disease from the client's perspective. Hearing these realities from someone in a similar circumstance has special meaning. The client may be more willing to ask questions and express concerns to a peer than to a health care professional. The associations listed in Box 4-4 can be a source of information regarding the location of a support group in a given community; they also can give guidance on forming support groups if these do not exist in the area.

Making Smart Lifestyle Choices

After seeking expert medical advice and locating health care providers who possess all the desired attributes, the client has the responsibility of complying with the recommended treatment plan and engaging in positive practices that promote health and healing. When clinicians detect that clients are noncompliant, they need to analyze the underlying reasons. Does the client not comply with the special diet because she is 85 years old and feels that eating an unrestricted diet is one of the few pleasures she has left? Is the client not exercising because he is unable to find the time to attend a fitness center? Has the client failed to stop smoking because withdrawal symptoms are so unbearable? By discussing the reason for noncompliance, the client may be helped to discover measures that can increase adherence to treatment plans and healthy living practices. For example, perhaps a compromise can be reached in which a few food items from the "forbidden" list of the diet can be eaten; literature can be provided describing exercises that can be done at home without special equipment; and a referral can be made to a smoking cessation clinic. Rather than forfeit the plan altogether, alternative or compromised approaches should be considered.

Diet

A sound diet is basic to good health for anyone, but it is vital to someone with a chronic illness who may need an extra boost to fight infections, stimulate healing, and maintain adequate energy to carry on activities of daily living. Adjustments may need to be made based on the client's diagnosis and medications. For instance, dietary restriction of sodium may be required of someone with hypertension, and foods high in vitamin K (e.g., dark leafy green vegetables and beef liver) may need to be avoided by someone using an anticoagulant. Specific dietary recommendations should be sought from physicians and nutritionists; the pharmacist should be consulted about food restrictions when taking certain medications and the potential impact of drugs on nutritional status. Nutritionists can provide useful information on substitutes and recipes that can make restricted diets more appealing.

A fuller discussion of nutritional needs is provided in Chapter 7.

Exercise

Exercise is another essential ingredient to a healthy lifestyle. Immunity is enhanced through regular physical activity and vigorous exercise is known to raise the levels of endorphins that produce a sense of well-being. Exercise can take various forms (Box 4-5).

Restrictions to exercise may be imposed by certain illnesses. For instance, high-impact aerobics may be contraindicated for someone with osteoporosis. Prior to launching any exercise program, the client should obtain a complete physical examination and advice from the physician. Physical therapists are excellent resources for instructions on exercises for specific needs and outcomes. (More information on traditional and nontraditional forms of exercise will be discussed later in this book.)

Environment

Our environment influences our health and sense of well-being. Colors, scents, noise levels, and objects in the environment affect mood, function, and health status. Modifications in the environment can be made to improve physical and mental function, including noise control, the selection of room colors to achieve therapeutic effects, the use of scents to create certain moods, and renovations to accommodate specific disabilities. A fuller discussion of the various aspects of creating a therapeutic environment is provided in Chapter 6.

BOX 4-5   **Various Types of Exercise**

Flexibility: Consists of gentle stretching; advisable to do daily.

Strengthening: Includes weight training, calisthenics, sports, and any physical labor that develops and strengthens muscles; can be performed approximately every other day.

Aerobic: Involves activities such as brisk walking, swimming, bicycling, rowing, and rope jumping; helpful to do at least three times a week.

Assertiveness

Assertiveness is a skill that should be mastered to live effectively with a chronic disease. Studies have shown assertive clients function better, have fewer health problems, and lose less time from work than nonassertive individuals (McCall, 1995). Clients must be able to challenge medical decisions with which they are uncomfortable, refuse care when they have cause, request that they be afforded the time and attention they need, and defend their treatment decisions. In addition to assertiveness with health care providers, chronically ill persons must learn to apply assertiveness skills to their daily lives. For instance, families and friends of chronically ill individuals may:

- insist the client could do better if he or she only tried harder
- interpret *looking* normal as *feeling* normal
- impose demands that the client cannot fulfill
- unnecessarily take responsibilities from the client or attempt to take control of the client's life

  Clients need to politely, but firmly, let their feelings, needs, and concerns be known in order to maintain control of their lives. Helpful responses that assist in this effort include:

- "I believe I am doing the best I can."
- "There are times when the disease plays havoc inside me, although my exterior appears normal."
- "I feel too tired to _____ (work, baby-sit, cook dinner) and will not be able to do it."
- "I appreciate your concern, but I can _____ (make my own decision, do that myself)."

A statement of fact without apology or beating around the bush is all that is necessary for an assertive response. Examples of assertive and nonassertive responses to situations are described in Box 4-6.

BOX 4-6	Assertive and Nonassertive Approaches to Situations

Situation: Mrs. J, who has hypertension, is about 30 pounds overweight. Her efforts at dieting have been unsuccessful. Her husband of 20 years continually reminds Mrs. J of her weight problem, teases her in the presence of friends, and points out the "great figures" of thinner women that he sees in public.

Nonassertive approach: Mrs. J apologizes to her husband for her weight and that she "is not attractive for him." Although she is embarrassed by her husband's comments to others, she says nothing.

Assertive approach: Mrs. J speaks to her husband when they are alone and tells him that although she appreciates that he is concerned about her health, she does not like the comments he makes, and in fact, the stress caused by these comments leads her to eat more. She asks him to stop making the comments and for his support as she attempts to diet.

Situation: Mr. B, who is hemiplegic and wheelchair-bound, accompanies his family to a restaurant for dinner. The waiter repeatedly asks Mrs. B what her husband would like rather than addressing Mr. B directly.

Nonassertive approach: Mr. B angrily shouts at the waiter, "My wife's not my ventriloquist. If you ignore me one more time, we're leaving this place."

Assertive approach: Mr. B says, "I have no problem hearing or answering you, so please feel free to speak to me directly."

Situation: Ms. Y is a healthy-looking woman who has a problem with asthma. At a banquet, a man seated at the same table lights up and smokes one cigarette after another.

Nonassertive approach: Ms. Y attempts to shield herself from the smoke and leaves the table whenever she can. As the smoke triggers an asthma attack, she retreats to the ladies' room to use her inhaler.

Assertive approach: Ms. Y politely but firmly tells the smoker that his smoking is bothersome to her and asks that he refrain from smoking at the table.

Situation: Mr. H is attending a dinner party at a friend's home when the hostess approaches and introduces him to another guest by stating, "Mary S, this is Tim H. You'd never know by looking at him that he is an MS patient, would you?"

Nonassertive approach: Mr. H is embarrassed and angry at being labeled as an MS patient and having this information shared with a stranger. He smiles, excuses himself from the guest, and keeps to himself the remainder of the evening.

Assertive approach: After being introduced, Mr. H responds, "It is a pleasure to meet you, Mary. Let me clarify that I am a pretty normal guy who happens to have MS, but I don't consider myself an MS patient, and you really needn't think of me in that way either." Later Mr. H privately tells the hostess that he would prefer not being introduced as an MS patient.

Healing Mindset

Last, but not least, people with chronic illnesses can enhance their health and sense of well-being by developing a healing attitude and making the decision to live positively with their illnesses (Box 4-7). This does not imply that people should be pleased that they have been diagnosed with chronic health problems, but rather, that they have accepted the cards they've been dealt and are choosing to live the best possible quality of life that they can achieve with their diagnoses. Clients should be helped to understand that they have the power to:

- develop a lifestyle that accommodates an illness rather than living a life controlled by it,
- be as active as possible rather than use the illness as an excuse to withdraw from activity, and
- define themselves as people who happen to have an illness (diabetes, Parkinson's disease, or asthma) rather than being defined by their illness (diabetic, Parkinson's disease patient, asthmatic).

BOX 4-7   Behaviors Consistent with a Healing Attitude

- Identifies self as person with a health condition rather than being defined by the condition (e.g., a person with diabetes rather than a diabetic).
- Recognizes and accepts self and realities of condition.
- Maintains maximum control of life and decisions affecting care and life.
- Engages in good health practices.
- Develops meaningful lifestyle which accepts and includes care of, and any limitations imposed by, health condition without being controlled by condition.
- Builds on capabilities rather than limitations to achieve fullest potential.
- Accepts responsibility for one's care to the fullest extent possible.
- Reaches out to others for help and support when necessary.
- Participates actively in care and as a partner with physician or other health care professional.
- Has confidence in health care professionals involved in care.
- Learns and uses coping mechanisms to deal with uncertainty of condition.
- Looks at problems realistically.
- Maintains meaningful roles, relationships, and activities; modifies these as necessary.
- Remains emotionally involved with significant others.
- Practices stress reduction techniques.
- Feels a connection with the universe.
- Appreciates and lives in harmony with nature.
- Refuses to be unnecessarily limited by disease or condition.
- Discovers joy in little accomplishments and the ordinary events of daily living.
- Clarifies values; determines that which is important to life.
- Develops balance among physical, mental, and spiritual components of self.
- Demonstrates hope and optimism in ability to live a satisfying lifestyle despite health condition.

Clients become victims of their illnesses when they unnecessarily allow their conditions to interfere with a normal lifestyle and inhibit their life experiences (e.g., *I'd love to go on a trip, but I'm afraid my arthritis will flare up; I don't think it is a good idea that I be around all the children at my grandson's birthday since I have a weak heart*). Persons with chronic illnesses have the capacity to be in charge of their illnesses and their direction, and to live satisfying, productive lives (Box 4-8).

Affirmations promote a healing mindset. Affirmations are *strong, positive statements acknowledging that something is already so* (Dossey et al., 1989). This form of self-talk aids a person in believing positive thoughts and changing outlook and views of self. Affirmations can enable the chronically ill individual to develop a new mindset toward self, commit to goals and actions to meet goals, and increase the sense of power over circumstances. Simply put, affirmations can promote the self-fulfilling prophecy in that when people believe enough in their ability to behave in a specific manner, they may actually demonstrate that behavior. Examples of affirmations are provided in Box 4-9.

A cheerful heart is good medicine, but a crushed spirit dries up the bones (Proverbs 17:22) is an ancient yet relevant perspective on the role of humor in our lives. Humor and optimism have a positive impact on health and healing. Nurse humorist Patty Wooten describes humor as "a quality of perception that enables us to experience joy even when faced with adversity" (Wooten, 1996). Humor can assist people in coping with difficult situations and the stresses of living with

---

BOX 4-8	Famous People with Chronic Conditions

Individuals who feel their lives are limited due to their chronic health problems need to be reminded of famous people who lived productive, satisfying lives despite their chronic conditions; examples include:

Ludwig van Beethoven Composed wonderful masterpieces although he was totally deaf

Louis Braille Invented the Braille reading system after having lived with blindness since early childhood

Emily Dickinson Produced great poetry while living in seclusion due to poor health

Joni Eareckson Tada Creates beautiful greeting cards and art without the ability to use her limbs

Helen Keller Became a great communicator despite being blind and deaf

Henri Matisse Picked up a paintbrush to occupy himself while recovering from an illness and realized a hidden talent that lead him to become a renowned artist

Mary Tyler Moore Manages a busy acting career while living with diabetes

Franklin Delano Roosevelt Polio survivor who became president

Paul Tsongas Ran for president despite a history of cancer

Robert Louis Stevenson Produced *Treasure Island*, *Dr. Jekyll and Mr. Hyde*, and other classics while living with a severe respiratory disorder

Vincent van Gogh Produced hundreds of highly-acclaimed paintings and drawings while living with serious mental illness

chronic conditions. Play and laughter produce many physiological and psychological effects (Box 4-10). For instance, laughter is believed to stimulate the release of endorphins that can help to improve mood and reduce pain perception, and reduce anxiety and muscle tension. In his book *Anatomy of an Illness as Perceived by the Patient*, Norman Cousins (1991) described his experience with humor in which he was relieved of pain for several hours and had a reduction in sedimentation rate following laughter from watching classic comedies or reading humorous material. Clinicians should encourage clients to take advantage of the health-promoting benefits of humor and laughter by sharing jokes, watching comedy shows, listening to humorous audiotapes, engaging in playful activities, and spending time with funny people. Most of us appreciate from personal experiences the effect of humor on our mood. Chronically ill individuals can learn to use humor to reduce the tension associated with their condition (e.g., in breaking the ice in new relationships or in the discussion of difficult issues).

Most human beings need a sense of purpose to give direction to their lives and a reason for living. A sense of purpose is particularly important to persons with chronic illnesses. Victor Frankl (1984), a psychiatrist who was a concentration camp survivor, in his observations of concentration camp survivors concluded that those prisoners with a sense of purpose were able to survive, whereas those who felt depressed and hopeless became victims and fared less well. He concluded that in the midst of misfortune and chaos, one must set new goals and create new purpose.

BOX 4-9   Examples of Affirmations for Persons with Chronic Conditions

- I follow my special diet.
- I engage in 10 minutes of exercise every morning.
- I do not smoke cigarettes.
- I limit my caffeine consumption to two cups of coffee daily.
- I take my medications as prescribed daily.
- I engage in relaxation exercises daily.
- I keep my appointments with my health care provider.
- I recognize and report symptoms promptly to my health care provider.
- I believe my treatments are having a positive result.
- I invest in personal private time daily.
- I prioritize my activities and schedule my time effectively.

- I talk with my coach/spouse/friend when I feel the need for support.
- I protect my rights.
- I express my feelings appropriately.
- I establish and maintain positive relationships.
- I have a right to be treated as an adult.
- I find something joyful in each day.
- I can be healed.
- I believe in a power greater than myself.
- I believe God is watching over me.
- I believe life has meaning.
- I am a worthwhile individual.
- I know my life has meaning.
- I am not controlled or limited by my illness.

BOX 4-10	Physiological Effects of Laughter

Increased oxygenation
Increased heart rate
Rise (temporary) in pulse and blood pressure
Exercise of thoracic and abdominal muscles
Release of endorphins
Stimulation of immune system

This challenge is particularly relevant for the chronically ill. Goals help to give a sense of hope for the future, provide activity, and structure time. Goals can be as simple as planning a trip to a friend's home or spending an afternoon at the library, or as ambitious as taking a long-desired trip to another country; the important aspect is that there be something planned for which one can take action.

To view a chronic illness as a gift can be a difficult concept to accept. In reality, most people would choose a disease-free, unimpaired life over one that must be lived with the inconveniences, self-care demands, discomforts, and limitations imposed by a disease. However, possessing a chronic disease can alter our views of ourselves and life in general, and provide the stimulus for many positive changes. A chronic illness can shatter the fallacy that many of us have that we are invincible and immortal. In sometimes subtle and sometimes profound ways, we realize that there are forces beyond our control that change our lives and disrupt the best laid plans. That which was important yesterday can seem irrelevant today. Persons who possess chronic illnesses can find benefit in clarifying their values in terms of that which is truly important to their lives. Recognizing how precious and uncertain life is can cause chronically ill people to journey down life paths more mindfully and avoid the wasteful detours of those unaffected by illness. Joy can be found in the small pleasures and little victories of daily life, enabling individuals to see the special in the ordinary. For this reason, being affected by a chronic illness can cause one to live a more meaningful life that takes full advantage of what each new day offers.

Many people affected by serious illnesses find considerable comfort in strengthening the spiritual foundations of their lives. A healed spirit can provide a quality of life that far compensates for the body's frailties. Spiritual well-being can be found through a variety of means, including active participation in a church or synagogue, meditating in a garden, or praying with a loved one. Spiritual beliefs provide the strength to accept the uncertainty and finiteness of our physical existence on earth. Faith, belief, and purpose can help us cope more effectively with whatever physical, emotional, or socioeconomic challenges we face. Bonding with a superior being or power can provide nourishment for the soul that is essential for healing and health promotion. (More on spirituality is discussed in Chapter 16.)

References

Chopra D: *Quantum healing: exploring the frontiers of mind/body medicine,* New York, 1990, Bantam Books.

Cousins N: *Anatomy of an illness as perceived by the patient,* New York, 1991, Bantam Books.

Dossey BM, et al.: *Holistic health promotion: a guide for practice,* Rockville, MD, 1989, Aspen.

Frankl V: *Man's search for meaning,* ed 3, New York, 1984, Simon and Schuster.

McCall TB: *Examining your doctor,* New York, 1995, Carol Publishing Group.

Weil A: *Spontaneous healing,* New York, 1995, Alfred A. Knopf.

Wooten P: Humor, an antidote for stress, *Holistic Nursing Practice* 10(2):49, 1996.

Recommended Readings

Amsterdam EA, et al.: Following the patient with stable chronic disease, *Patient Care* 29(15):22-36, 1995.

Benet A: A portrait of chronic illness: inspecting the canvas, reframing the issues, *American Behavioral Scientist* 39(6):767-777, 1996.

Budd MA: New possibilities for the practice of medicine, *Advances, The Journal of Mind-Body Health* 8(1):7-16, 1992.

Consumers Union: Working out chronic illness, *Consumer Reports on Health* 7(10):113, 1995.

Davidson D: Partners in change are ready to roll, *Hospitals and Health Networks* 69(8):58, 1995.

Dreher H: Proven mind/body medicine: scientific approaches provide hope for those suffering from chronic conditions, *Natural Health* 23(3):86-96, 1993.

Dunkin MA: Managing multiple health problems: a balancing act, *Arthritis Today* 7(3):24-30, 1993.

Edwards S: *Sally Edwards' heart zone training: exercise smart, stay fit and live longer,* Holbrook, MA, 1996, Adams Media Corp.

Eliopoulos C: Chronic care coaches: helping people to help people, *Home Healthcare Nurse* 15(3):185-188, 1997.

Gallager W: *The power of place: how our surroundings shape our thoughts, emotions, and actions,* New York, 1993, Poseidon.

Hawkins AH: *Reconstructing illness: studies in pathography,* West Lafayette, IN, 1993, Purdue University Press.

Hawkins AH: Reforming the biomedical model: finding a successor model or going beyond paradigms? *Advances, The Journal of Mind-Body Health* 10(1):55-56, 1994.

Hester LE: Coordinating a successful discharge plan, *American Journal of Nursing* 96(6):35-37, 1996.

Hornbrook MC and Goodman MJ: Chronic disease, functional health status, and demographics: a multi-dimensional approach to risk adjustment, *Health Services Research* 31(3):283-308, 1996.

Lorig K, et al.: *Living a healthy life with chronic conditions,* Palo Alto, CA, 1994, Bull Publishing Co.

Mandelker J: Managing chronic disease, *Business and Health* 12(11):45-48, 1994.

Marwick C: Another health care idea: disease management, *Journal of the American Medical Association* 274(18):1416-18, 1995.

Michael SR: Integrating chronic illness into one's life, *Journal of Holistic Nursing* 14(3):251-267, 1996.

Miller JF: *Coping with chronic illness, overcoming powerlessness,* ed 2, Philadelphia, 1992, F.A. Davis Co.

Mosby's Patient Teaching Guides, St Louis, MO, 1995, Mosby.

Murray RH and Rubel AJ: Physicians and healers, unwitting partners in health care, *New England Journal of Medicine* 326:61-64, 1992.

Olfson M, Weissman MM, Leon AC, et al.: Psychological management by family physicians, *Journal of Family Practice* 41(6):543-51, 1995.

Partners in Caregiving: *Life after diagnosis,* Winston-Salem, NC, 1995, Wake Forest University.

Perrin EC, et al.: Issues involved in the definition and classification of chronic health conditions, *Pediatrics* 91(4):787, 1993.

Rew L: *Awareness in healing*, Albany, NY, 1995, Delmar Publishers.

Rood RP: Patient and physician responsibility in the treatment of chronic illness: the case of diabetes, *American Behavioral Scientist* 39(6):729-52, 1996.

Shoor R: Looking to manage care more closely, *Business and Health* 11(10):46-52, 1993.

Spitzer RL, et al.: Health-related quality of life in primary care patients with mental disorders: results from the PRIME-MD 1000 study, *Journal of the American Medical Association* 274(19):1511-18, 1995.

Suber R: Chronic care in ambulatory settings: components of an integrated care system, *American Behavioral Scientist* 39(6):665-676, 1996.

Turner DC: The role of culture in chronic illness, *American Behavioral Scientist* 39(6):717-729, 1996.

Wichramaekera IE: Diagnosis by inclusion: the perspective of a behavioral medicine practitioner, *Advances, The Journal of Mind-Body Health* 8(1):17-30, 1992.

Woog P, editor: *The chronic illness trajectory framework—the Corbin and Strauss nursing model*, New York, 1992, Springer Publishing Co.

Zauszniewski JA: Self-help and help-seeking behavioral patterns in healthy elders, *Journal of Holistic Nursing* 14(3):223-236, 1996.

Using Alternative/ Complementary Therapies to Enhance Conventional Treatments

As mentioned earlier, growing numbers of Americans are using alternative/complementary healing measures to maintain health and manage illness, and more and more health care professionals are adding alternative/complementary practices to their conventional treatment plans. One study of persons with Alzheimer's disease showed 55% of their caregivers tried at least one alternative/complementary therapy to help improve their clients' memories, and 20% used three or more alternative measures (Coleman et al., 1995). A survey of HIV-positive people in Philadelphia revealed that 40% used alternative/complementary therapies (Anderson et al., 1993). It would be difficult to identify any chronic condition for which some alternative/complementary therapy has not been recommended or used.

Although the use of alternative/complementary therapies is relatively new to health care practices in the United States, many of these therapies have been widely used and accepted for a very long time in other parts of the world. For example, for thousands of years, acupuncture and herbal medicines have been used in China for mainstream care, and in India, Ayurvedic medicine, a personalized system of restoring balance to the body, mind, and spirit, has been an acceptable approach to preventing and treating disease. In many ways, the United States is lagging behind other countries in its use of comprehensive health care approaches.

This chapter will examine issues related to the use of alternative/complementary therapies and provide descriptions of the more common therapies available. The term alternative/complementary therapy will be used throughout this book to represent therapies that are considered by mainstream Western medicine to be nontraditional measures used as complements to conventional medical treatments.

Past Resistance to Alternatives

Why aren't alternative/complementary therapies more widely used in this country? Historically, medicine had a limited view of disease prevention and management and the role of the client in this process. Diseases were attributed to forces exterior to the person that invaded or injured the body. The client assumed the role of victim, passively accepting his or her health fate. The physician was the master of the client's health care destiny, using scientific skills to battle the forces that threatened the body. Little credence was given to the realities that (1) people had the power to influence their own states of health and illness, (2) diseases could arise from disharmony within the individual, and (3) clients had a role as important as their physicians in their healing process.

Medical schools perpetuated their traditional thinking about health and illness from one generation to the next by their approaches to medical education. Rather than viewing the client as a unique network of physical, emotional, and spiritual variables, the client was approached as an organ or disease entity. Hard sciences predominated while minimal time was allocated to teaching the healing arts. Although they have been refined over the years, the approaches to treatment that were taught were, for the most part, limited to drugs, surgery, and radiation. Many medical schools continue to place little emphasis on nutrition, exercise, biofeedback, relaxation techniques, and other alternative/complementary measures that are known to affect health and healing. Since the educational models of other health care professionals frequently mirrored that of medical schools, this view of health and medicine permeated the entire health care system. Finally, this system was reinforced as health care insurers continually reimbursed consumers only for traditional diagnostic and treatment measures while disallowing equally effective alternative/complementary healing approaches.

Unproven Does Not Mean Ineffective

Besides adherence to tradition, alternative/complementary therapies have not been incorporated into the mainstream because they are regarded by the medical establishment as "unproven" and therefore ineffective. True, many alternative/complementary approaches to healing lack the volumes of scientific research that exist for conventional practices; however, unproven does not necessarily mean ineffective. Many alternative/complementary therapies have lacked research funds to demonstrate their effectiveness. Government support for alternative/complementary medicine research has been minimal at best. A large university stands a better chance of receiving funds to test and retest conventional therapies than isolated alternative/complementary practitioners have of obtaining grants to demonstrate the effectiveness of their methods. In addition, researchers who have a history of receiving funding to test their approaches are more likely to receive future funds than a newcomer who wants to test alternatives. And finally, in most circumstances, the professionals who review grant applications represent conventional science. Thus, they may have a bias toward and better understanding of grant applications that are within the mainstream.

Likewise, private funds for research and development are more likely to be invested in projects that have the potential for the funder to capitalize and generate profit from the research findings. For example, drug manufacturers may be willing to spend the millions of dollars that are required to test and bring a new drug to the market because they know that a patent to a drug can yield many times their investment. However, what incentive would a company have to invest millions in testing an alternative/complementary healing approach, such as the use of herbs or acupuncture, when there is no product that can be patented and exclusively sold? Health care providers and consumers must take these factors into consideration and not expect the same level of scientific evidence for alternative/complementary treatments as exists to validate the heavily funded conventional treatments.

When mainstream practitioners criticize today's alternative/complementary health practices as being without merit, they should be reminded that initially Lister and Semmelweis were viewed as outrageous for suggesting that doctors wash their hands between patients to prevent the spread of infection, and Roentgen's x-rays were once considered quackery. Today's unorthodox treatment could be tomorrow's innovative breakthrough!

Principles Underlying Alternative/Complementary Treatments

Interestingly, for all the thousands of years they have been used and in all the different cultures, there have been some common beliefs woven through alternative/complementary therapies. Some of these are as follows:

The body has the ability to heal itself

Unlike conventional medicine that has worked from the premise that treatment involves doing something to the body to rid it of disease (e.g., medicate, operate, radiate), alternative/complementary therapies strengthen the body's abilities to heal itself. Self-healing is not so farfetched a thought when you consider that it is quite common and natural for broken bones to mend, cuts to close, and invading bacteria to be destroyed by antibodies produced by the body.

Health and healing are related to a harmony of mind, body, and spirit

A healthy state is dependent upon a balance within the body. The mind, body, and spirit are inseparable and influenced by each other. Anyone who has experienced a change in appetite, sleep habits, energy level, and sexual interest as a result of feeling depressed can attest to the interconnectiveness of mind, body, and spirit. To treat the physical symptom without addressing the emotional and spiritual aspects of the client is an incomplete response. Illness must be viewed by taking into perspective all aspects of the individual, and healing measures must address the dynamics of the entire person as a functional system, rather than a single system or part of the person, as in the conventional health care system.

Basic, good health practices build the foundation for healing

Of course, it sounds very basic to say that to be healthy and to heal, people need good nutrition, exercise, rest, and avoidance of harmful practices (such as cigarette smoking and excessive alcohol consumption). However, many people fail to meet these requirements on a regular basis. People will try one pain relief medication after another to rid themselves of headaches while continuing to be sedentary at their desks, drinking endless cups of coffee, eating junk foods, and lighting cigarette after cigarette. To compound this, they may visit physicians who treat their symptoms with prescription drugs without assessing lifestyle practices that contribute to their health problems.

Alternative/complementary medicine does not view symptoms in isolation, but rather looks at the total health practices and promotes healthful practices and a balanced lifestyle. Alternative/complementary therapies include preventive practices to maintain health in addition to therapeutic measures to treat illnesses.

Healing practices are individualized

Each person is an individual, possessing his or her own dynamics and needs. The symptoms of illness manifested may look alike on the surface in several people, but the cause of the symptoms can vastly differ. Alternative/complementary therapies explore the root of the problem and utilize practices that address the unique characteristics and imbalances.

Clients are responsible for their own healing

Clients can use a wide range of conventional and alternative/complementary therapies to treat their illnesses, but ultimately, they are responsible for their own healing. A sense of power over their bodies and destinies instills the hope and motivation that strengthens clients' abilities to overcome losses, frustrations, and discomforts imposed by illness. Perhaps Albert Schweitzer said it best: "Each patient carries his own doctor inside him. They come to us not knowing that cure. We are at our best when we give the doctor who resides within each patient a chance to go to work."

Alternative/Complementary Health Practitioners

Practitioners of alternative/complementary therapies come from a wide range of backgrounds with vastly different educational preparation and experiences based on their specific alternative/complementary specialty areas. Some, such as chiropractors and doctors of naturopathy, have completed college degrees in their fields and received clinical supervision. Others, such as acupuncturists and some massage therapists, have been trained, clinically supervised, and certified in the therapy. Still others may have gained expertise through experience, self-study, mail-order programs, or courses. There do tend to be some characteristics similar to most alternative/complementary therapists in their approaches toward healing and their relationships with clients (Box 5-1). Clinicians should become familiar with the requirements of practitioners in various alternative/complementary therapies and help clients ensure that they are in the hands of safe, competent practitioners; associations that can assist in this effort are provided later in this chapter with the discussion of the specific therapy.

Customizing Treatment

Some alternative/complementary treatments—like acupuncture, herbal medicine and meditation—have received recognition and even popularity in this country, while others are more obscure. Some are relatively simple to incorporate into a daily routine, while others require a significant change in lifestyle. Clients should survey the various treatments and explore those which seem appropriate. Factors to consider in making this decision are listed in Box 5-2. Because healing is influenced by mindset, clients must feel committed to the alternative/complementary therapies they select.

It is advisable for clients to discuss the alternative/complementary therapies they plan to use with their conventional health care practitioners to ensure that all therapies complement rather than interfere with one another. For example, herbs such as ephedra and licorice should be avoided in persons with hypertension, and hyperthermia is not a wise choice of therapy for persons with cardiovascular disease. Because many conventional health care practitioners are not knowledgeable about alternative/complementary therapies, clients may find it beneficial to do their own

BOX 5-1	Common Characteristics of Alternative/ Complementary Practitioners

- View the client as a whole composed of the body, mind, and spirit, and consequently, address all aspects of the individual when treating an illness rather than a symptom or body part; interested in the total person
- Favor interventions that address physical, mental, and spiritual concerns
- Build up the client's general health status and promote healthy practices
- Tailor treatment to the needs of the individual
- View the client as being an active participant in the treatment plan and in control of self
- Promote self-care by client
- View healing as an ongoing process
- Encourage inner development and a balanced life
- Use touch, empathy, good communication skills
- Spend more time with clients than conventional practitioners
- Demonstrate openness and creativity in healing approaches
- Respect nature and a higher power

BOX 5-2	Factors to Consider in Selecting an Alternative/ Complementary Therapy

- Use, benefit, and effectiveness for the given condition
- Personal comfort with and confidence in the treatment
- Consistency of therapy with values and spiritual and cultural belief systems
- Ability and willingness to incorporate the practice into one's lifestyle
- Cost
- Availability

research and share information about the alternative/complementary measure with medical personnel to enable them to have a better understanding.

Best of Both Worlds

Conventional medicine has many highly effective treatments available to help in the management of chronic illnesses, and clients would be cheating themselves if they didn't take advantage of everything modern medicine has to offer. Alternative/complementary therapies should serve to *complement, not replace* conventional treatments. Clients may discover that some alternative/complementary treatments may be able to eliminate the need for medications and other conventional treatments; for example, meditation, exercise, and herbs can often maintain blood pressure within a normal range without the need for antihypertensive drugs. In some circumstances, clients may attempt to manage the condition with use of simple and safe alternative/complementary measures and, if these prove ineffective, move to conventional therapies. However, clients shouldn't be tempted to reject all conventional medical treatments because they have discovered an alternative/complementary therapy that holds promise. Decisions to discontinue any conventional treatment should be the result of careful consideration and discussion with the physician. Ideally, the integration of alternative/complementary therapies should enable the client to derive more benefit than would have been otherwise achieved; in other words, one plus one could equal three or more!

Incorporating alternative/complementary therapies into practice is a detour from the main road of medical treatments. As with any deviation from the main highway, the unfamiliar new territory of alternative/complementary therapies can be resisted and criticized as inappropriate, inefficient, ineffective, and incorrect by those who have known only the popular route. However, some of the most special and fruitful destinations are those not found on the beaten path.

Common Alternative/Complementary Treatments

There are dozens of alternative/complementary therapies that can be used in promoting health and managing chronic diseases. Some are fairly well known and relatively easy for lay people to incorporate into their care plans, while others are obscure, complicated, or require special training or assistance. The Office of Complementary and Alternative Medicine at the National Institutes on Health has categorized alternative/complementary therapies into seven fields of practice (National Institute on Health, 1994):

- Mind/Body (biobehavioral) interventions
- Alternative (nonbiomedical) systems of healing
- Manual healing methods
- Pharmacological and biologic treatments
- Herbal medicine
- Bioelectromagnetic applications
- Diet and nutrition in prevention of chronic disease

The section below reviews some of the more common alternative/complementary therapies, followed by a brief description of some of the less common ones. Some of these alternative/complementary practices require that the treatment be given by a skilled practitioner, whereas others can be used independently by the client after some instruction. Laws vary from state to state in regard to the requirements for practitioners of alternative/complementary therapies. It is essential that clinicians be familiar with their state laws in regard to these therapies to protect clients and ensure compliance with their practice acts.

None of the alternative/complementary therapies discussed are intended to substitute for good conventional medical care.

Mind/Body (Biobehavioral) Interventions

Biofeedback

Biofeedback is a process of teaching individuals to bring certain bodily functions (e.g., respiratory and heart rate, blood pressure, skin temperature) under conscious, voluntary control. Biofeedback training enables clients to identify changes associated with targeted symptoms and develop measures to alter those changes. Ultimately, this process enables clients to relax at will, but rather than general relaxation, biofeedback teaches clients to focus on a specific response (e.g., slowing the respiratory rate).

Initially, electronic equipment is used to assist clients in acquiring sensitivity to internal changes as they use this modality. This equipment can include electroencephalogram to monitor brain waves (used when problems such as insomnia, chronic pain, and anxiety exist), electromyogram to measure muscle relaxation (used with bruxism and spasticity), galvanometer to measure galvanic skin response (used with unconscious emotional states), and thermistor to measure skin temperature (used with migraines when clients need to learn to shift blood volume from central to peripheral regions). As clients become familiar with their symptoms and ways to elicit the relaxation response on their own, they needn't use this equipment.

Biofeedback has been found helpful in the treatment of irritable bowel syndrome, PMS, Raynaud's syndrome, neck and back pain, attention deficit disorder, epilepsy, urinary and fecal incontinence, temporal mandibular jaw syndrome, cardiac arrhythmias, anxiety, and stress (Anselmo, 1994). Studies have found that persons who have suffered a stroke were able to improve their gait, grasp, and grip with the use of biofeedback training (Schleenbaker and Mainous, 1993)

Qualified biofeedback practitioners are certified by the Biofeedback Certification Institute of America. For information on biofeedback and its practitioners, the organizations found in Box 5-3 can be contacted.

BOX 5-3
Resources for Information About Biofeedback and Its Practitioners

Association for Applied Psychophysiology and Biofeedback
10200 West 44th Avenue
Suite 304
Wheat Ridge, CO 80033
(303) 422-8436
www.aapb.org
Biofeedback Certification Institute of America
10200 West 44th Avenue
Suite 304
Wheat Ridge, CO 80033
(303) 420-2902

Center for Applied Psychophysiology
Menninger Clinic
PO Box 829
Topeka, KS 66601
(913) 273-7500
www.menninger.edu

RESOURCES

Hypnosis

Hypnosis refers to an induced trancelike state in which the individual has increased receptivity to suggestion. The use of suggestion and trancelike states in healing is hardly new: anthropologists indicate that all known primitive cultures have used some form of hypnotic process or trance state as part of religious and healing practices (Shames, 1996). Hypnotherapy was approved as a valid medical treatment by the British Medical Association in 1955 and the American Medical Association in 1958. Over 15,000 physicians combine hypnosis with conventional treatments of medical conditions, and 94% of persons receiving these treatments report benefits (Findlay et al., 1991).

A hypnotic state is achieved by first guiding the body into a relaxed state. The client then follows suggestions that narrow the focus of attention toward a specific area. In a superficial state of hypnosis the client will attain a relaxed state and accept suggestions but not necessarily follow them, whereas in the deepest state, somnambulism, the client will follow post-hypnotic suggestions. A hypnotherapy session usually lasts from 60 to 90 minutes. Most people are able to be hypnotized. Success of hypnotherapy can depend on the willingness of the client to engage in this therapy, the amount of trust the client has toward the therapist, and the control of environmental distractions.

Hypnotherapy can benefit a wide range of physical and psychological conditions, including chronic pain, migraines, asthma and other respiratory conditions, ulcers, nausea, irritable bowel syndrome (Whorwell, 1991), and behavioral disorders. It has been popular and effective for use in smoking cessation and weight reduction programs (Barabasz and Spiegel, 1989).

The World Health Organization advises against the use of hypnotherapy in persons with psychosis, antisocial personality disorders, and organic psychiatric conditions. Clients should be advised to use only those hypnotherapists who have been properly trained and certified. Reputable hypnotherapists and additional information can be obtained by contacting the organizations found in Box 5-4.

BOX 5-4
Resources for Information on Hypnotherapy and Hypnotherapists

American Institute of Hypnotherapy
1805 East Garry Avenue
Suite 100
Santa Ana, CA 92705
(714) 261-6400
www.hypnosis.com/aih

American Society of Clinical Hypnosis
2200 East Devon Avenue
Suite 291
Des Plaines, IL 60018
(708) 297-3317
www.asch.net

International Medical and Dental Hypno-therapy Association
4110 Edgeland
Suite 800
Royal Oak, MI 48073
(800) 257-5467
www.infinityinst.com/aboutim.htm

National Guild of Hypnotists
P.O. Box 308
Merrimack, NH 03054
(603) 429-9438
www.hollys.com/ngh

Imagery

Imagery has been a rapidly rising star in the universe of mind-body medicine. It is based on the principle that images in the mind can create specific responses in the body. Although imagery is used in hypnosis, imagery differs from hypnosis in that in hypnosis an image and suggestion is offered to the client, whereas in imagery, the client uses his or her own images.

Images can be receptive or active. Receptive images are those that just seem to appear in the conscious mind. For instance, some people may feel certain sensations (feelings of warmth, scent, taste, or sound) or receive images in a dream prior to the exacerbation of an illness. With active images, there is a conscious formation of an image, such as imagining a headache as a fire in one's head and creating a counter image of water to throw on the fire. Images also can be concrete or symbolic. Concrete images offer an accurate description of the situation; for example, a realistic description of a clogged vessel might include images of the medication dissolving the particles. A symbolic image might picture the vessel as having a closed gate that one must try to open. Affirmations can be coupled with imagery.

Imagery begins by establishing a goal or identifying a problem. The client can be aided by being educated as to the physiology involved in the normal healing. The client then works toward achieving a state of relaxation; this can be promoted by using the technique for progressive relaxation described later in this chapter. When fully relaxed, the client then develops an image that depicts the desired state of healing. For example:

- to achieve relaxation, the client can imagine being in a peaceful, beautiful place (either one that has been visited or a vision created in the mind);
- to facilitate the healing from cancer, the client can view the cancer cells as dark spots that are swallowed by "PAC Man" type creatures or whited out with the stroke of a brush;
- to promote circulation, the client can visualize blood gushing through every part of the body and creating a feeling of warmth as it does;
- to cope with a diagnostic test, the client can mentally travel to another activity while the procedure is taking place.

Imagery has been shown to be an effective method for use in pain control and is believed to have usefulness in stimulating healing responses in the body.

Mastering imagery requires practice. Libraries and book and health food stores have books and audiotapes that can assist people in learning guided imagery. (There may be problems in packaged programs in that they do not address individual differences.) There also are practitioners, some certified in guided imagery, who can provide assistance. Information can be obtained from organizations found in Box 5-5.

BOX 5-5

Resources for Information About Guided Imagery and Its Practitioners

Academy for Guided Imagery
P.O. Box 2070
Mill Valley, CA 94942
(800) 726-2070
www.healthy.net/agi

Simonton Cancer Center
P.O. Box 890
Pacific Palisades, CA 90272
(310) 459-4434
www2.lainet.com/(simonton

Resources specific to the use of guided imagery
for people with cancer include:

Exceptional Cancer Patients
1302 Chapel Street
New Haven, CT 06511
(203) 865-8392
www.hmt.com/cyp/nonprof/ecap

RESOURCES

Meditation

Although meditation has been used in other parts of the world for thousands of years, it has been just in the past three decades that meditation has had a role in health promotion in the United States.

Meditation basically is an activity that calms the mind and focuses it on the present. There are several approaches to meditation, including:

Concentrative meditation: Attention is focused on breathing, an image, or a sound (e.g., a mantra or chant); this calms and promotes a sharp awareness and clarity of the mind.

Mindfulness meditation: Attention is given to the sensations, sounds, smells, thoughts, and feelings that are being experienced; one is aware without becoming involved in the experiences; this promotes a calm, nonreactive state of mind.

Transcendental meditation: This form of meditation was introduced by Maharishi Mahesh Yogi and involves the body reaching a level of profound relaxation while the mind achieves a more alert state.

Meditation is an excellent means of stress control for all individuals and can be particularly beneficial for clients who have conditions such as high blood pressure and anxiety; use of meditation has been shown to promote improvement in anxiety disorders and depression (Kabat-Zinn et al., 1992). Studies have shown that relaxation and meditation can reduce the frequency of seizures (Deepak et al., 1994; Whitman et al., 1990). Meditation can boost immune functioning, thereby helping clients who have cancer, AIDS, and other conditions that compromise the immune system. Some clients have been able to achieve reductions in pain with the practice of meditation. Nearly anyone who meditates can experience higher levels of mental function, creativity, and improved self-esteem.

Many libraries and book and health food stores carry books and tapes on meditation. Additional information can be obtained by contacting organizations listed in Box 5-6.

BOX 5-6

Resources for Information on Meditation

Maharishi University of Management
1000 North 4th Street
Fairfield, IA 52556
(515) 472-5031
www.mum.edu

Mind/Body Health Sciences, Inc.
393 Dixon Road
Boulder, CO 80302
(303) 440-8460
www.healthy.net/wellness/mindbody.htm

Progressive Relaxation

Progressive relaxation is another approach to achieve a state of deep relaxation. The individual learns to guide himself or herself through a series of steps that relaxes the entire body. Initially an audiotape can be used that talks the listener through the process. Box 5-7 outlines a typical progressive relaxation exercise, although there can be minor variations.

This exercise can be practiced whenever one feels stressed. After some practice, people find that they can quickly enter the state of total relaxation without going through each step and in any location where they can close their eyes.

Research has shown relaxation exercises to have similar benefits as meditation. Persons with insomnia who used the relaxation response were found to fall asleep four times more rapidly that those who did not (Jacobs et al., 1993). The relaxation response has been shown to lower blood pressure by 5 to 10 mm/Hg in individuals with hypertension and reduce physician visits in persons with chronic pain (Caudill, 1991).

Yoga

Yoga is a 5000-year-old discipline that combines breathing exercises, meditation, and asanas, or postures, to achieve a sense of balance and health. In fact, the word *yoga* means union and appropriately describes the connection of mind, body and spirit that is achieved through this practice. Various studies have proven that many bodily functions can be controlled by persons who practice yoga on a regular basis. Yoga has been found to be helpful for persons with pain, anxiety, stress, fatigue, poor circulation, high blood pressure, tachycardia, and digestive and respiratory system problems.

The breathing exercises focus on the regulation of respiration, a process called pranayama. It is based on the belief that interrupted flow of life forces results in disease. Yogic breathing is calm, smooth, and controlled, with equal lengths of inspiration and expiration. The breathing exercises are done in preparation for meditation, the state of focused concentration discussed in the previous section of this chapter. It produces a sense of calm, peace and acute awareness.

The various postures used in yoga stimulate the nervous system and endocrine glands to increase circulation. Different postures influence different effects on the body. Some of the common postures are shown in Figure 5-1.

Videotapes and books to assist in learning yoga are available from libraries and book and health food stores. Alternative/complementary practitioners and local telephone directories can be resources for locating classes and guides. Additional information can be obtained from organizations found in Box 5-8.

BOX 5-7   **Sample Relaxation Exercise Script**

- Find a quiet room with soft lighting where you will not be interrupted.
- Sit in a comfortable chair with feet flat on the floor and arms supported at your sides.
- Slowly take in several deep breaths. Focus on your breathing.
- Tense your facial muscles, tightly closing your eyes and holding your mouth closed.
- Relax your face, making the muscles feel as though they are sagging.
- Clench your right fist and tighten the muscles in your right arm.
- Open your right fist and relax the arm muscles, making your arm feel loose and heavy.
- Clench your left fist and tighten the muscles in your left arm.
- Open your left fist and relax the arm muscles, making your arm feel loose and heavy.
- Tighten the muscles in your right leg and squeeze the toes on your right foot.
- Relax your right leg muscles and toes.
- Tighten the muscles in your left leg and squeeze the toes on your left foot.
- Relax your left leg muscles and toes.
- Tighten your buttocks.
- Relax your buttocks.
- Relax your entire body. Allow it to feel free and heavy. You are in a state of total relaxation.
- Stay in this relaxed state for about five minutes. Pay attention to how your body feels in this state.
- Gradually open your eyes and slowly stretch. You should feel relaxed.

FIGURE 5-1

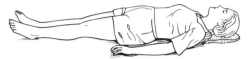

Yoga Postures

Corpse Pose

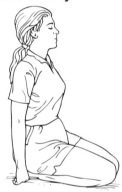

This posture promotes the function of the circulatory and nervous systems and relaxes the body. It is a good initial posture to use before practicing other postures. To achieve this pose:

- Lie on your back with arms straight at your side, about one foot from the body, with palms facing up. A small pillow or rolled towel can be used to support the head and neck if the flat position is uncomfortable.
- Close your eyes and breathe.
- Continue this exercise for five to ten minutes.

Child or Baby Pose

This posture is effective for relieving lower back discomforts. It is not advised when knee problems exist.

- Sit on your heels with the top of your feet flat on the floor.
- Keep the upper extremity straight.
- Exhale as you slowly bend forward until your forehead touches the floor.
- Position your arms at your sides so that your elbows are resting on the floor and your palms face upward.
- Breathe normally and relax.
- If the position is uncomfortable, try extending your arms above your head, keeping palms up, or cross your arms and rest your head on your arms.
- Remain in the pose for no more than five minutes.
- Inhale as you slowly raise the upper extremity and end in a kneeling position.

Posterior Stretch

This position stimulates the abdominal area and assists in the relief of indigestion, constipation, and anorexia (poor appetite). It stimulates organs in the abdominal cavity, such as the spleen, pancreas, kidneys, liver, and stomach.

- Sit on the floor with the legs extended in front of the body.
- Keep the upper extremity straight.
- Inhale and extend your straight arms over your head.
- Exhale as you bend forward to try to touch your toes.
- Place your hands on your legs and relax.
- Relax and breathe deeply, smoothly and evenly.

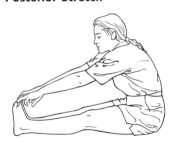

Cobra

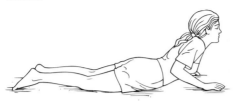

This posture has many benefits to the spinal column. In addition to helping back pain, it can relieve gas, stomach discomforts, and constipation, and promote improved respiratory function.

- Lie on your stomach with the legs together.
- Extend the body with arms at your side, head on the floor.
- Position your arms as though you are going to do push-ups.
- As you inhale, slowly begin to raise your head, then your shoulders and chest. Do not use the hands or arms to raise yourself. Bend as far back as possible.
- Hold the pose for five seconds as you breathe smoothly and evenly.
- As you exhale, lower the chest, shoulders, and head to resume the original position.

Locust Pose

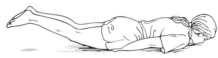

This exercise is primarily used for lower back problems.

- Lie on your stomach with legs together and arms straight at your sides.
- Put your chin on the floor with your head straight.
- Make fists and slip your hands under your thighs with the thumb-side of your hands on the floor.
- As you inhale, raise both legs as high as possible while keeping your upper extremity on the floor.
- Hold your breath for five seconds and let down your legs.

Half Spinal Twist

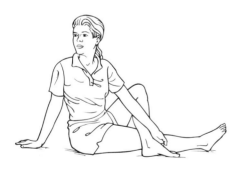

In addition to promoting flexibility of the back muscles, this exercise places pressure on the abdominal cavity, which improves the function of the organs in that region and facilitates good digestion and elimination.

- Sit on the floor with the legs extended in front of you and your upper extremity straight.
- Bend the left leg and position the left foot along the outside of the right knee.
- Place the left hand flat on the floor about six inches from the body with fingers pointing away from the body.
- Reach on the outside of the left leg and grab the left foot.
- Twist the entire spine toward the left and look over your left shoulder.
- Inhale and hold the pose for five seconds.
- Resume the original position and repeat the exercise on the opposite side.

Shoulder Stand Pose

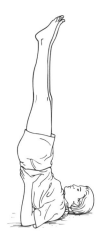

This position has multiple benefits including: increasing circulation, improving thyroid function, enhancing diaphragmatic breathing, and strengthening back, chest, and abdominal muscles. Persons with hypertension should avoid this exercise as it causes an increase in blood pressure.

- Lie flat on your back with legs together.
- Keep your elbows on the floor as you place your hands on the small of your back.
- Raise both legs and your hips so that your toes are pointing toward the ceiling.
- Press your sternum (breastbone) toward your chin.
- Support your back with your hands as your elbows stay bent at your sides.
- Breathe smoothly and evenly.
- Hold the pose for twenty seconds during your first practice of this pose; gradually increase the time you hold the pose to one minute.
- Slowly return your legs to the floor.

Half Fish Pose

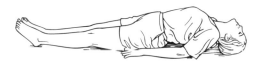

This exercise should follow the shoulder stand as it will relax muscles that could feel slightly stiff from that exercise. This pose helps to increase lung capacity and benefits people with respiratory disease.

- Sit on the floor with your upper extremity straight and your legs extended in front of your body.
- Lean back so that you are lying on the floor.
- Keep your arms at your sides with palms facing downward.
- Arch your back and pull your head as far as possible toward your back. Keep your mouth closed.
- Hold the pose for twenty seconds as your breath smoothly and evenly.
- Gently lower the body to the original position.
  After completing all poses that you care to use, resume the corpse pose for about ten minutes.

BOX 5-8

Resources for Information About Yoga

Himalayan Institute of Yoga, Science and Philosophy
RR1, Box 400
Honesdale, PA 18431
(800) 822-4547
www.geocities.com/Athens/Acropolis/6602/hi mausa.html

International Association of Yoga Therapists
109 Hillside Avenue
Mill Valley, CA 94941
(415) 383-4587

Alternative (Nonbiomedical) Systems of Healing

Acupuncture

Acupuncture is a therapeutic technique used in traditional Chinese medicine (Box 5-9). Although it originated in China over two thousand years ago and was introduced in America by Chinese immigrants in the middle of the 19th century, acupuncture was given little notice in this country until the 1970s.

Most people think of acupuncture as helpful for pain relief; however, this is but one use of this treatment. Acupuncture is being used to treat addictions, asthma, sciatica, osteoarthritis, Meniere's disease, depression, AIDS (as an immune system booster), and other disorders.

Simply put, acupuncture is a treatment performed by a trained acupuncturist in which special needles are placed under the skin at acupoints along meridians (Figure 5-2) to stimulate the energy flow of qi (see Box 5-9). Not only is the site at which the needles are placed important, but also the angle and depth of the needle insertion. The goal is to restore or promote the balance of qi.

The acupuncturist will assess the patient during the first visit by interviewing, observing, examining the tongue, and evaluating the twelve radial pulses. Based on assessment findings, a diagnosis is made that will dictate the placement of the needles. There may appear to be little relationship between the area of the body that is diseased and the placement of the needles. The needles are sterilized stainless steel, extremely thin, and of different lengths and gauges. For infection control purposes, most acupuncturists use disposable needles. Usually, less than a dozen needles are used in a treatment, and with the exception of a slight pricking sensation as the needles are inserted, there is no pain associated with the treatment. Some treatments consist of a quick insertion and removal of needles, while others can take nearly one hour to complete; the average time for most needles to be in place is twenty minutes.

Sometimes heat is applied to the acupoints. The heat is supplied by burning the dried herb mugwort (*Artemesia vulgaris*) and placing it at the acupoint. This procedure is called *moxibustion*.

Food can be eaten prior to the treatment, although large heavy meals are not advised. It is not unusual to feel weak and dizzy after an acupuncture treatment. Many people report an increased sense of well-being after a treatment.

Adverse reactions and complications from acupuncture are rare. Since 1965 only ten incidents of injury to internal organs have been reported (National Commission for the Certification of Acupuncturists, 1993). A review of the literature for the past 30 years indicated 165 complications of all types from acupuncture, including pneumothorax, spinal cord injury, hepatitis, and contact dermatitis (Lao, 1996a). There is a risk of infection if needles are reused; for this reason, most acupuncturists use disposable needles. It is advised that acupuncture in the abdominal and lumbar-sacral region not be used on pregnant women and that persons suffering from conditions that could lead to syncope (e.g., anxiety, hunger, and exhaustion) not be treated (Lao, 1996b).

BOX 5-9   Chinese Medicine

Chinese medicine has been practiced for thousands of years and incorporates measures such as acupuncture, acupressure, herbal medicine, massage, and therapeutic exercise. It is based on the principle that the body must have balance and harmony to maintain health; therefore, illness indicates an imbalance and disharmony of the person's internal environment. One of the theories that explains the body's balance and harmony is the principle of *yin and yang*. *Yin*, the negative female energy, refers to that which is soft, dark, cold, and wet, and *yang*, the positive male energy, is represented by that which is hard, bright, hot, and dry. Different body parts are ascribed more yin or yang qualities. For example, yin organs include the lungs, kidneys, liver, heart, and spleen; yang organs include the gallbladder, small intestine, stomach, colon, and bladder. Daytime activity is considered more of a *yang* state, whereas sleep is more of a *yin* state.

The body depends on a total system of balance of *yin* and *yang*. Illness is viewed as an imbalance of *yin* and *yang*. Chinese medicine involves restoring this balance when one is ill.

Chinese medicine also considers the body's balance in relation to the five phases or elements which are categorized by *wood* (spring), *fire* (summer), *earth* (long summer), *metal* (autumn), and *water* (winter). Each element has an influence on the other and influences what happens in the natural world. The human organs and functions of the body correspond to each of the *five elements*.

Qi is the life force within an individual that encompasses all physical, spiritual, emotional, and mental activities that are vital. Invisible pathways or channels, called meridians (Figure 5-2), circulate *qi* on the body surface. *Qi* ensures a balance of *yin* and *yang* that helps to keep the body functioning and protects it from external forces that could be harmful. A deficiency or blockage of *qi* can cause discomfort and illness. There are points on the various meridians that can affect the flow of *qi* when stimulated; these points are used as acupuncture and acupressure points.

Traditional Chinese medicine also uses herbs to achieve a state of harmonious balance. Each of the five elements is associated with specific tastes by which plants are evaluated. *Wood* is associated with sourness, *fire* with bitterness, *earth* with sweetness, *metal* with acidity, and *water* with saltiness. Certain therapeutic actions are attributed to each taste: sour herbs nourish the *yin* and prevent the undesired loss of *qi*, bitter herbs dry and drain, sweet herbs tonify and ease pain, acidic herbs disperse, and salty herbs nourish the kidneys. Herbs with no distinct taste are considered bland and have a diuretic effect. Temperatures are ascribed to each herb, also.

T'ai chi is a therapeutic exercise that looks like a slow, graceful dance. It releases energy, allows a free flow of qi, and is another means to achieve balance and harmony.

Many people with chronic pain obtain relief from acupuncture, validated by scientific research (Pomeranz, 1996). Studies have shown acupuncture to reduce back and neck pain (Coan et al., 1980; 1982), migraine headaches (Vincent, 1989), and postoperative pain (Christensen et al., 1989). Nausea and vomiting have been shown to be improved by acupuncture (Yang et al., 1993; Parfitt, 1996). Acupuncture has shown evidence of being efficacious in the management of asthma and

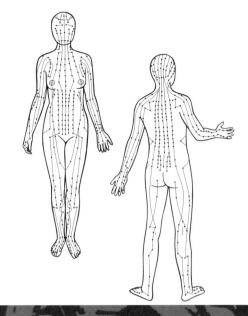

FIGURE 5-2

Acupuncture Meridians.

chronic obstructive pulmonary disease (Jobst, 1996), and some researchers believe that acupuncture can increase bone metabolism and facilitate the healing of fractures (Kunor and Cerquerira, 1995). Although research on the efficacy is in an early stage, there is some evidence that acupuncture can be useful in substance abuse treatment (Culliton and Kiresuk, 1996).

Increasingly, insurers are covering acupuncture treatments. Clients should check with their individual insurer as to the terms of reimbursement.

When selecting an acupuncturist, make sure that he or she has trained in an approved school (there are currently over 50 schools of acupuncture in the United States). Some states require that acupuncturists graduate from an approved school and pass a licensing examination; state health departments can be contacted for information on qualifications within individual states. Further information can be obtained by contacting the organizations found in Box 5-10.

BOX 5-10
Resources for Information About Acupuncture and Acupuncturists

American Academy of Medical Acupuncture
5820 Wilshire Boulevard
Los Angeles, CA 90036
(213) 937-5514
www.medicalacupuncture.org/aama.htm
American Association of Oriental Medicine
433 Front Street
Catasauqua, PA 18032
(610) 266-1433
www.aaom.org

National Commission for the Certification of Acupuncturists
P.O. Box 97075
Washington, DC 20090
(202) 232-1404
acupuncture.com/TCMSchools/NCAA.htm

Ayurvedic Medicine

Ayurveda is Sanskrit for *the science of life* and is a form of medicine that has been practiced in India for thousands of years. Ayurvedic medicine places equal emphasis on the body, mind, and spirit and uses herbs, yoga, diet, meditation, massage, exposure to the sun, and breathing exercises to restore balance to the body. In recent years, this branch of medicine has gained visibility and popularity through the writing and lectures of Deepak Chopra (1990, 1991, 1993).

In Ayurvedic medicine, individuals are viewed as having metabolic body types or *doshas*; these doshas are *vata, pitta,* and *kapha* (Box 5-11). The doshas are centered in specific areas, although they are present in varying degrees in every cell of the body:

Vata is responsible for movement and facilitates breathing and circulation. It is centered in the large intestine, pelvic region, thighs, bones, skin, and ears.

Pitta is responsible for metabolism and stimulating enymatic activities. It is centered in the small intestine, stomach, sweat glands, blood, skin, and eyes.

Kapha cements the body together and is responsible for nourishment and protection. It is centered in the chest, lungs, and spinal fluid.

When the delicate balance of the doshas is disturbed, the body is vulnerable to external stressors and shows signs of illness. The body's balance, according to Ayurveda, can be disrupted by any of seven factors: genetic, congenital, internal, external trauma, seasonal, natural habits, or magnetic and electrical influences. Ayurvedic physicians primarily rely on observation to diagnose, although some contemporary Ayurvedic physicians are utilizing conventional diagnostic tests, also. The methods of treatment include:

- cleansing and detoxifying (shodan).
- palliation (shaman).
- rejuvenation through special herbs and minerals (rasayana).
- mental hygiene and spiritual healing (satvajaya).

The body type will determine the mix of measures used to restore balance; the season and time of day are factors that are considered in prescribing treatments. A discussion of the use and effectiveness of the herbal therapies and yoga used in Ayurveda are offered under the discussions of those modalities.

Further information on this branch of medicine and its practitioners can be gained by contacting the organizations found in Box 5-12.

BOX 5-11	Characteristics of Ayurvedic Metabolic Body Types

Vata
   Changeable, unpredictable, moody
   Vivacious, hyperactive
   Imaginative, enthusiastic, intuitive, impulsive
   Fluctuating energy level
   Tendency toward starting but not completing projects
   Eats and sleeps at varying times throughout day
   Slender
   Cool, dry skin
   Prominent features and joints
   Prone to insomnia, PMS, cramps, constipation

Pitta
   Predictable, orderly, efficient, perfectionist
   Articulate, intense, passionate, short-tempered
   Maintains routines, eats and sleeps at consistent times
   Medium build, well-proportioned
   Warm, ruddy skin
   Prone to heavy perspiration, thirst, acne, ulcers, hemorrhoids, stomach problems

Kapha
   Relaxed, slow, graceful
   Tendency toward procrastination
   Affectionate, forgiving, tolerant, compassionate
   Sleeps long and deeply
   Cool, thick, pale, oily skin
   Eats slowly
   Prone to high cholesterol, obesity, allergies, sinusitis

BOX 5-12

Resources for Information About Ayurveda and Its Practitioners

American School of Ayurvedic Sciences
10025 NE 4th Street
Bellevue, WA 98004
(206) 453-8022

Ayurvedic Institute
11311 Menaul NE
Suite A
Albuquerque, NM 87112
(505) 291-9698
www.ayurveda.com

College of Maharishi Ayur-Veda Health Center
PO Box 282
Fairfield, IA 52556
(515) 472-586
www.maharishi_medical.com

RESOURCES

Homeopathy

Homeopathy comes from the Greek words *homoios*, meaning similar, and *pathos*, meaning suffering. Those words explain the foundation of homeopathy, which is that suffering is helped by that which is similar, or "like cures like." Remedies are prescribed in a unique manner for each individual, i.e., two people with similar symptoms may receive different prescriptions.

Homeopathic treatments are dilute forms of a biological material (plant, animal, mineral) that produce symptoms similar to that caused by the client's disease. An extract of the substance is made by soaking it in alcohol to form a "mother" tincture. The mother tincture is then diluted many times to achieve different levels of potency. In homeopathic remedies, the more dilute a substance is, the higher its potency. The final solution can be added to sugar tablets or a powder for consumption (usually by dissolving them on or under the tongue). Some homeopathic remedies are prescribed in lotions and ointments for external use. The homeopathic remedy stimulates the body to fight the disease. The more closely the effects of the remedy match the client's symptoms, the more effective the remedy will be. A classic example would be the use of belladonna for the treatment of headaches. Belladonna, a poison in its natural form, causes a headache (among other serious symptoms), but when given in a diluted form can cure a headache.

Giving the client small doses of the substance that was causing his or her disease as a means to treat the disease is not as farfetched as some may believe. Many people suffering from allergies are given injections of the suspected allergens to increase tolerance to the allergen, and trace amounts of the disease-causing pathogen, given through a vaccine, aid in immunizing against the disease.

Homeopaths, the practitioners of homeopathic medicine, observe the client's symptoms and reactions and prescribe accordingly. Homeopaths assess the healing of the client using the Law of Cure, which is based on the principles that symptoms:

- move from vital organs to less vital parts of the body.
- move from within the body outward.
- disappear in reverse order of appearance.

If the symptoms are responding according to the Law of Cure, the remedy is judged as effective; if symptoms fail to change, additional treatment of either repeating the first remedy or using a new one may be necessary. Sometimes persons with chronic illnesses may experience a worsening of symptoms after homeopathic remedies are started; this is viewed as part of the healing process.

When homeopathic remedies are used, it is advisable to avoid caffeine, mint, and menthol products because they can act as antidotes to some remedies.

Homeopathy has been shown to be effective for many conditions. Hay fever sufferers have been shown to have a reduction in symptoms and decrease their use of antihistamines when taking homeopathic remedies (Reilly et al., 1994). Studies have shown homeopathic remedies to reduce symptoms of rheumatoid arthritis, influenza, and fibrositis (Jacobs, 1996).

Homeopathic remedies are regulated by the Food and Drug Administration.

The names of practicing homeopaths and information on educational programs for lay and professional persons can be obtained from the organizations listed in Box 5-13.

BOX 5-13

Resources for Information About Homeopathy and Homeopaths

International Foundation for Homeopathy (IFH)
2366 Eastlake Avenue East
Suite 325
Seattle, WA 98102-3366
(206) 324-8230
www.healthy.net/pan/pa/homeopathic/ifh/
  index.html

National Center for Homeopathy
801 North Fairfax
Suite 306
Alexandria, VA 22314
(703) 548-7790
www.healthy.net/nch

Naturopathy

For centuries, among practitioners of the healing arts there has been the belief that healing occurred naturally in the body if proper nutrition, pure water, fresh air, exercise, rest, and sunlight were provided. In the late 19th century, people who developed practices upon the foundation that "nature cures" became formally known as naturopaths.

Naturopathy emphasizes good health practices to prevent disease. When disease occurs, a naturopath will attempt to find and eliminate the cause by helping the client establish an internal and external environment that facilitates healing. A symptom is evaluated in perspective to the whole person—body, mind, and spirit—rather than in isolation. Traditional naturopaths are less interested in diagnosing and treating a disease than in educating clients about healthy choices that foster good health and healing. They may treat earaches, allergies and many other problems seen by primary physicians, only they rely on nutrition, herbs, and other natural remedies to correct these disorders.

Traditional naturopaths do not believe in the use of drugs because drugs are seen as harmful substances that can be toxic to the body. Invasive procedures are not performed by traditional naturopaths either.

Practitioners have become naturopaths in a variety of ways, ranging from formal educational programs that resemble that of allopathic physicians, to correspondence courses, to hanging out a shingle and calling themselves a naturopathic doctor. There is movement afoot by the American Association of Naturopathic Physicians to institute licensure of naturopaths and require graduation from one of the three schools of naturopathy in the country (Bastyr University, National College, or Southwest College). Most traditional naturopaths have not received their education from those schools and could be ineligible to be licensed; therefore, there is resistance to licensure by traditional naturopaths.

Growing numbers of insurance companies are covering naturopathic services. Directories of qualified naturopaths can be obtained from the organization listed in Box 5-14.

BOX 5-14

Resources for Information About Naturopathic Physicians

American Association of Naturopathic Physicians
2366 Eastlake Avenue E
Suite 322
Seattle, WA 98102
www.naturopathic.org

Naturopathic Association of America
109 Holiday Court #A-2
Franklin, TN 37067
(615) 591-9445
www.tnaa.com

Manual Healing Methods

Chiropractic Therapy

Chiropractic therapy, a specialty developed in the United States in the latter part of the 19th century, is the use of manipulation or adjustment of the spine and joints to restore proper alignment. Misalignments of the spine, known as subluxations, can cause pressure on nerves which can lead to interference with bodily functions and pain. For instance, respiratory symptoms can be a result of subluxation of the spine; realigning the spine is believed to do more to correct the respiratory symptoms than drugs that act directly on the lungs.

Chiropractic services are among the better understood alternative/complementary therapies in this country, supported by the fact that ten percent of the population has used this service (Eisenberg et al., 1993). Although most people who visit trained professional chiropractors do so for back problems (according to Eisenberg et al., one fifth of back pain sufferers have had this therapy), chiropractic therapy can benefit other conditions, including asthma, arthritis, depression, cardiac disease, addictions, menstrual problems, and gastrointestinal disorders. Studies have shown that people with work-related back disorders who received chiropractic care missed less time from work and cost their employers less than employees who received only conventional medical care (Moore, 1993). The Federal Agency for Health Care Policy and Research has endorsed and published guidelines related to the use of chiropractic care for acute back pain (Bigos et al., 1994).

Chiropractors make their diagnosis from a physical examination, history, and palpation of the spine. They also may take x-rays. Reputable chiropractors will not treat conditions in which spinal manipulation is inappropriate.

Adjustments during the chiropractic treatment can include:

- *active motion*, in which the client independently moves or stretches;
- *passive motion*, in which the chiropractor assists the client in moving or stretching;
- *palpation*, in which the chiropractor touches the spine.

Chiropractic techniques can be forceful or nonforceful. A forceful technique is an adjustment in which the joint is gently stretched slightly beyond its normal range of motion; sometimes an audible click is heard during this maneuver. A non-forceful technique involves the application of gentle pressure or touching along the spine, skull, and pelvis. Spinal adjustments vary depending on the characteristics of the client and assessed problem.

Some chiropractors limit their therapy to the identification and relief of subluxations, while others combine additional approaches with their treatments.

Chiropractic therapy should be obtained only from health care professionals trained in this specialty. Manipulation of the spine by unskilled hands can create new problems. Some conventional practitioners work closely with chiropractors and will refer clients to them. If conventional practitioners cannot provide the names of chiropractors, clients usually can find them listed in telephone directories or learn about them through word of mouth. Many health insurers are reimbursing for chiropractic therapy.

Additional information on chiropractic therapy can be obtained from the organizations listed in Box 5-15.

Massage and Bodywork

Therapeutic massage is a means of manipulating soft tissue by using rubbing, kneading, rolling, pressing, slapping, and tapping movements. Bodywork is the term applied to the combination of massage with deep tissue manipulation, movement awareness, and energy balancing. There are four major categories of massage and bodywork:

European: long strokes, kneading, and friction (e.g., Swedish)

Deep tissue: deep manipulations of fascia (e.g., rolfing, Hellerwork)

Pressure-point: application of pressure to unblock meridians (e.g., shiatsu, acupressure, Reiki, jin shin do, reflexology)

Movement integration: rebalancing and teaching new ways to move the body (e.g., Feldenkrais, Alexander)

A brief description of some massage techniques is provided in Box 5-16. Depending on the type of technique used, massage is believed to benefit people by promoting relaxation, or unblocking life forces or energy channels.

Massage has been used for a variety of conditions, including stress, edema, respiratory congestion, and constipation. Studies have found massage to be useful in reducing anxiety and depression (Field et al., 1992) and pain (Ferrell-Torry and Glick, 1993). European style massages can cause temporary changes in pulse and blood pressure, although different effects were found in various studies (Yates, 1990). An anticoagulant effect has been achieved through massage (Ernst et al., 1987).

Although therapeutic touch is a form of bodywork, it is discussed separately later in this section.

More information can be obtained by contacting the organizations listed in Box 5-17.

BOX 5-15

Resources for Information About Chiropracty and Chiropractors

American Chiropractic Association
1701 Clarendon Boulevard
Arlington, VA 22209
(703) 276-8800
www.amerchiro.org
International Chiropractors Association
1110 North Glebe Road
Suite 1000
Arlington, VA 22201
(703) 528-5000
www.chiropractic.org

World Chiropractic Alliance
2950 North Dobson Road
Suite 1
Chandler, AZ 85224
(800) 347-1011
www.choicemall.com/worldchiropractic

BOX 5-16   Types of Massage and Bodywork

Alexander Technique: Rebalances the body by teaching new awareness and images of body postures and using movement and touch.

Feldenkrais Method: Improves movement and self-image by guiding (through instruction and touch) people to replace old patterns with new ones; believes each person has an individualized optimum style of movement.

Rolfing (Structural integration): Reestablishes balance through manual manipulation and stretching of body's fascial tissues (thin, elastic membrane that encases muscles); uses pressure applied with fingers, knuckles and elbows to release fascial adhesions.

Hellerwork: Improves body alignment and flexibility by using some of the same manual manipulations of Rolfing with dialogue to increase awareness of emotions and attitudes that affect body alignment and movement.

Trager Approach: Uses gentle, rhythmic touch combined with series of movement exercises to increase awareness of patterns, release tension, and change movement; movements learned promote deep relaxation, also.

Reflexology: Stimulates reflex points by applying finger pressure to specific areas on hands and feet that correspond to various parts of body. Used to relieve stress, promote deep relaxation, increase circulation, unblock nerve impulses and balance body.

Swedish: Promotes relaxation by using long strokes, friction, and kneading of muscles; most prevalent type of massage.

BOX 5-17

Resources for Information About Massage and Bodywork

American Massage Therapy Association
820 Davis Street
Suite 100
Evanston, IL 60201
(312) 761-2682
www.amtamassage.org
American Reflexology Certification Board and Information Service
PO Box 246654
Sacramento, CA 95824
(916) 455-5381
Body of Knowledge/Hellerwork International, LLC
406 Berry Street
Mt. Shasta, CA 96067
(916) 926-2500
www.hellerwork.com

Feldenkrais Guild
PO Box 489
Albany, OR 97321
(503) 926-0981
www.feldenkrais.com
International Institute of Reflexology
PO Box 12462
St. Petersburg, FL 33733
International Rolf Institute
P.O. Box 1868
Boulder, CO 80306
(303) 449-5903
North American Society of Teachers of the Alexander Technique
(800) 473-0620
Trager Institute
33 Millwood
Mill Valley, CA 94941
(415) 388-2688

Therapeutic Touch

As mentioned earlier, therapeutic touch is a type of bodywork; however, its widespread use and popularity in the nursing community support a separate discussion of this modality.

Although the use of laying on of hands for healing has been practiced since ancient times, this technique gained popularity in the 1970s with the work and research of Delores Krieger (1979). Therapeutic touch is based on the principle that people are energy fields who can transfer energy to one another to potentiate healing. The Rogerian conceptual framework has been the foundation for most therapeutic touch practice and research. At the core of therapeutic touch is the intent of the practitioner to help, which has promoted this therapy being labeled *healing meditation* (Krieger et al., 1979).

One of the assumptions underlying therapeutic touch is that people who are sick have closed down physically, emotionally or spiritually and need to have their channels reopened. The clinician draws upon the universal field of energy and focuses the energy on the client, to enable the client to mobilize his or her own inner resources for healing. The flowing energy of the clinician unblocks the client's obstructed energy. The touch is not just haphazard but conscious and purposeful, and the effects achieved are greater than would be obtained through casual touch.

In addition to the caring and compassion exchanged between the clinician and client during therapeutic touch, there are other benefits. Studies have shown therapeutic touch to decrease anxiety in hospitalized patients (Kramer, 1990), speed wound healing (Wirth, 1990), relieve pain (Meehan, 1993), and enhance immunologic function (Quinn and Strelkauskas, 1993).

A multilevel educational and certification program is offered by the Colorado Center for Healing Touch (address below). Healing Touch educational programs are provided throughout the country and provide training in interventions that surpass the basic therapeutic touch techniques developed by Delores Krieger.

Clinicians need to be sensitive to the fact that not all clients or health care professionals respond positively to the use of therapeutic touch. Some members of the Christian community link this intervention to occult practices and advise Christians "to avoid TT, even if we thereby miss an opportunity to feel a little better" (O'Mathuna, 1998). Although therapeutic touch is not taught or promoted as an occult practice and virtually any modality, alternative or conventional, could be misused in the hands of misguided practitioners, clinicians should be aware that some clients and professionals could be opposed to its use. Organizations to obtain information about touch therapy and its practitioners are listed in Box 5-18.

Herbal Medicine

For centuries and in all cultures, herbs have been used in healing remedies. The use of the plant kingdom for healing has long been viewed as a natural means to promote health and conquer disease. In fact, many of today's medications are derived from plants, such as digoxin (from foxglove, *Digitalis purpurea*), reserpine (from Indian snakeroot, *Rauwolfia serpentina*), morphine (from the opium poppy, *Papaver somniafera*), and colchicine (from autumn crocus, *Colchicum autumnale*).

Decades ago, the growth of modern medicine in America had threatened to move herbal medicine into extinction. The quick fixes promised by commercial drugs made the use of plants grown in our grandmothers' gardens somehow appear crude and backward. But that attitude is changing as growing numbers of people are demanding more natural medicines with fewer side effects than that offered by synthetic drugs. Further, the increased emphasis on holistic health care has also reignited interest in herbal medicine.

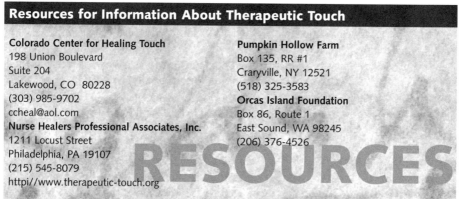

BOX 5-18

Resources for Information About Therapeutic Touch

Colorado Center for Healing Touch
198 Union Boulevard
Suite 204
Lakewood, CO 80228
(303) 985-9702
ccheal@aol.com
Nurse Healers Professional Associates, Inc.
1211 Locust Street
Philadelphia, PA 19107
(215) 545-8079
httpi//www.therapeutic-touch.org

Pumpkin Hollow Farm
Box 135, RR #1
Craryville, NY 12521
(518) 325-3583
Orcas Island Foundation
Box 86, Route 1
East Sound, WA 98245
(206) 376-4526

Different parts of plants are used for medicinal purposes. For example:

Medicinal herb:	Part of plant for therapeutic use:
Garlic	Bulb
Chamomile	Flower
Comfrey	Leaf
Echinacea	Root
Slippery elm	Bark
Celery	Seed
Cayenne	Fruit/berry
Nettle	Entire above-ground portion

Different parts of the same plant can yield different therapeutic actions. For instance, the leaf of the dandelion plant can have a diuretic effect while the root of the plant can act as a laxative. Herbs are categorized according to their actions (Box 5-19). Each individual will require different types of herbs based on their unique body system and health state.

Herbs can be consumed in various forms:

Internally

Teas: Teas can take the form of infusions or decoctions. They can be consumed hot or cold, and sweetened to taste. An infusion is used for leaves, stems and flowers of herbs. One teaspoon of the herb is placed in one cup of boiling water and allowed to seep for about five to ten minutes. Since fresh herbs contain a higher water content, two to three teaspoons may be needed. A decoction is used for bark, roots, and certain seeds and requires longer boiling for the flavor of the herb to be released. The herb should be broken into small pieces prior to boiling. One teaspoon of the dried herb (or three teaspoons if fresh) is placed into a pot containing one cup of water. The mixture is boiled for ten to fifteen minutes. Many herbs are available in tea bag form for ease in use.

Capsules and Tablets: These easy-to-consume forms allow the herb to be ingested without having to taste it or go through any special preparation. Another advantage is that one knows exactly the amount of the herb that is consumed. Most companies that market these products have good quality control standards and ensure that they are herbicide- and pesticide-free.

Tincture: Tinctures are much stronger per volume than infusions and decoctions. Most are alcohol based. Depending on the herb, the dosage will range from 5 to 15 drops at a time. They can be taken undiluted or mixed with a small amount of water. One way of making a tincture is to put about 120 grams of a ground or finely chopped herb (twice that amount if fresh herbs are used) into a half liter of vodka or wine, allow it to sit in a warm place for two weeks (shaking it twice daily), strain, and store in a tightly closed dark bottle. Many herbs can be purchased in tincture form.

Syrup: Bitter-tasting herbs can be made more palatable by mixing them in a syrup. A syrup can be made by boiling two pounds of sugar with one quart of water; an alternative is to add sugar to an infusion or decoction as it is being prepared. Because sugar is not the healthiest product to consume, syrups should be used occasionally and only when absolutely necessary, as in cough syrups.

BOX 5-19   Actions of Selected Herbs

Adaptogen: Increases resistance to stress by improving body's adaptability. Examples: ginseng, hawthorn, lobelia, blue cohosh.

Alternative: Formerly called "blood cleansers"; gradually restores proper function of body, increases health and vitality. Examples: burdock, cleavers, nettles.

Antiemetic: Relieves nausea, prevents vomiting. Examples: ginger, black horehound.

Antihelminthic: Destroys or expels worms. Examples: aloe, garlic, pomegranate, wormwood.

Antimicrobial: Prevents infections, destroys microorganisms by strengthening body's own resistance. Examples: Echinacea, myrrh.

Antispasmodic: Prevents or relieves muscle spasms and cramps; some relieve nervous tension. Examples: crampbark, blackhaw, valerian, skullcap.

Astringent: Exerts binding action on mucous membrane, skin, and other tissue to reduce skin irritation and inflammation and protect against infection. Examples: oak bark, Comfrey, periwinkle.

Bitter: Bitter taste triggers sensory response in central nervous system, which causes appetite stimulation, increased flow of digestive juices, increased bile flow, improved liver detoxification, and stimulation of self-repair mechanisms for damaged gut. Examples: wormwood, gentian root, rue, mugwort.

Cardiac tonic: Increases efficiency of heart muscles without increasing their need for oxygen. Examples: foxglove, lily of the valley, motherwort.

Carminative: Improves digestive function, soothes and settles gut wall, aids in removal of gas; rich in volatile oils. Examples: fennel, ginger, caraway.

Demulcent: Soothes and protects irritated or inflamed internal tissue, prevents diarrhea, and eases bronchial and bladder spasms; contains mucilage that has direct action on intestinal lining. Examples: Comfrey, marshmallow, slippery elm bark.

Diuretic: Increases production and elimination of urine, aids in inner cleansing and ridding body of wastes. Examples: dandelion leaf, yarrow, lily of the valley, elder, parsley.

Emetic: Causes vomiting. Examples: ipecacuanha, lobelia, snake root.

Emmenagogue: Stimulates menstrual flow and activity, normalizes and tones female reproductive system. Examples: black cohosh, goldenseal.

Emollient: Softens, smooths, and protects skin. Examples: balm of gilead, coltsfoot, Comfrey, fenugreek, slippery elm.

Expectorant: Stimulates removal of mucus from lungs. Examples: white horehound, coltsfoot, mullein, aniseed, elderflowers.

Hepatic: Aids function of liver. Examples: dandelion root or leaf, boldo, milk thistle.

Hypnotic/Sedative: Induces sleep and deep relaxation. Examples: hops, skullcap, valerian, passion flower, lavender.

> **Hypotensive:** Lowers blood pressure. Examples: hawthorn berries, lime blossom, mistletoe.
>
> **Laxative:** Stimulates bowel elimination. Examples: senna, cascara sagrada, dandelion root, butternut.
>
> **Nervine:** Has beneficial effect on nervous system; includes nervine tonics that strengthen nervous system function, nervine stimulants that increase nerve activity, and nervine relaxants that tranquilize. Examples: nervine tonics: skullcap, oats, St John's wort, vervain; nervine stimulants: coffee, tea, kola; nervine relaxants: black cohosh, chamomile, Jamaican dogwood, lime blossom, lady's slipper, mistletoe, skullcap, motherwort, St John's wort.
>
> **Tonic:** Strengthens and enlivens specific organ or entire body. Examples: goldenseal, black cohosh, ginseng.

Externally

Bath: Herbs can be absorbed through the skin by bathing. Usually a quart infusion or decoction of the herb is added to the bath water. Foot soaks can be used for herbs that cause discoloration of the skin.

Compress, Poultice: A compress is a clean cloth that has been soaked in an infusion or decoction of the herb. A poultice is a paste made from the herb and warm water that is placed on the body in the same manner as a compress.

Ointment: Ointments are semi-solid preparations that can be applied to the skin. They can be prepared by simmering two tablespoons of an herb in 220 grams of a petroleum-based jelly for about ten minutes. These can be purchased in prepared form also.

Oil: Many herbs are rich in essential oils. Herbal oils can be made through a careful process of distillation, but it is easier to buy them already prepared. Herbal oils can be used for massages or aromatherapy.

Regardless of the form consumed, herbs should be fresh (meaning not old) when used. It is advisable to buy herbs from reputable sources or, better still, have clients grow their own if possible.

Although herbs are natural nutritional products, they can produce adverse effects. Clinicians should ensure that clients understand these risks and use herbs wisely (Box 5-20). Some herbalists can assist in recommending and preparing herbal medicines for an individual's unique needs. Because herbalists are not licensed professionals, there can be variation in their capabilities; it is useful to request the names of clients who have used the herbalist's services who can be consulted for references. More information on herbal therapies can be obtained from the organizations listed in Box 5-21.

BOX 5-20   Selected Herbs and Their Adverse Effects

Alfalfa: Can cause stomach upset and diarrhea.

Aloe: Can cause allergic dermatitis; aloe latex used as a laxative is powerful in large doses.

Angelica: Can cause rash when person is exposed to sunlight.

Anise: Estrogenic action.

Balm: Can interfere with thyroid-stimulating hormone and create problems for persons with thyroid disorders.

Barberry: Large doses can cause drastic drops in blood pressure, heart rate, and respirations; contraindicated in pregnancy due to stimulant effect on uterus.

Bayberry: Can cause elevated blood pressure and edema; contraindicated with history of cancer.

Black cohosh: Can depress cardiac function; estrogen-like properties can lead to abnormal coagulation and liver dysfunction.

Burdock: Can stimulate uterus; contraindicated if pregnant.

Cascara sagrada: Can cause severe intestinal cramps.

Celery: Long-term use can cause hypokalemia.

Chaparral: Can cause liver damage.

Comfrey: Highly toxic to liver; recommended for external use only.

Dandelion: Long-term use can cause hypokalemia.

Ephedra (ma huang): Elevates blood pressure and heart rate. Contraindicated with pregnancy, heart disease, diabetes, glaucoma, and hyperthyroidism.

Fenugreek: Estrogenic action can cause uterine contractions; contraindicated in pregnancy.

Feverfew: When the raw leaves are ingested orally on regular basis, can cause mouth ulcers, loss of taste sensation, and swelling of mouth, lips or tongue. (This risk reduced when taken in capsule form.) Can stimulate uterine contractions; contraindicated in pregnancy. Can interfere with blood clotting.

Garlic: Has an anticoagulation effect; persons using prescribed anticoagulants need to be cautioned. Can cause allergic reaction. Not advised for women who are breast-feeding as it can pass to breast milk and cause colic.

Germander: Can cause liver damage.

Ginkgo: Can cause irritability, restlessness, nausea, vomiting, diarrhea. Contraindicated for children, pregnant women, nursing mothers, and persons with clotting disorders.

Ginseng: Can elevate blood pressure, which is of concern to hypertensive clients. Can cause insomnia if taken near bedtime. Has an estrogenic effect, which can lead to bleeding in some post-menopausal women.

Goldenseal: Can cause uterine contractions; contraindicated for pregnant women.

Hawthorne: Can cause dramatic drop in blood pressure with large doses.

Juniper: Long-term use can cause hypokalemia.

Licorice: Long-term use can cause edema, hypertension, headache, hypokalemia, and hormonal imbalance (pseudoaldosteronism).

Mistletoe: Can cause bradycardia and blood pressure alterations. Is potentially fatal.

Parsley: Long-term use can cause hypokalemia.

Pennyroyal: Highly toxic internally. Can stimulate uterine contractions.

Red clover: Estrogen-like; contraindicated in pregnancy, estrogen-dependent cancer, or history of heart disease, thrombophlebitis, and stroke.

Rhubarb: Can cause severe intestinal cramps, diarrhea.

St. John's wort: Acts as MAO inhibitor. Can cause photosensitivity, hypertension, nausea, vomiting. Can interact with amphetamines, asthma inhalants, coffee, beer, wine, fava beans, salami, smoked or pickled foods, narcotics, nasal decongestants.

Shepherd's purse: Can cause strong uterine contractions.

BOX 5-21

Resources for Information About Herbal Medicine and Herbalists

American Botanical Council
P.O. Box 201660
Austin, TX 78720
(512) 331-8868
www.herbalgram.org/index.html

American Herbalist Guild
P.O. Box 1683
Sequel, CA 95073
www.healthworld.com/associations/pa/herbal
medicine/ahg/index.html

Herb Research Foundation
1007 Pearl Street
Suite 200
Boulder, CO 80302
(303) 449-2265
www.herbs.org/index.html

Bioelectromagnetic Applications

Magnets and related electrical devices to generate controlled magnetic fields have been used in the treatment of a variety of conditions including rheumatoid disease, post-polio syndrome, headaches, sleep disorders, circulatory problems, pain and stress. Magnetic therapy has been used for some time in Japan and Germany, but it is the recent use by professional athletes that has increased popularity of this modality in the United States (Ruibal, 1997).

Theories suggest that magnetic therapy accelerates healing by attracting and repelling charged particles in the blood, thereby stimulating activity and heat which dilates blood vessels and increases circulation. Magnets are believed to relieve pain by creating a slight electrical current that stimulates the nervous system, thereby blocking pain sensations.

A variety of devices are used for magnetic therapy including blankets, pads, coin-sized disks, shoe insoles, wristpads, and face masks.

There are some precautions when using magnets. They should not be applied to the abdomen within 90 minutes after a meal if wearing a pacemaker or during pregnancy. Because research on the benefits and risks of magnetic therapy is in an elementary stage, there still is much to learn about the safe use of these products. Clients should be encouraged to consult with a professional prior to using magnetic therapy; more information can be obtained from the organization listed in Box 5-22.

BOX 5-22

Resources for Information About Bioelectromagnetic Therapy

Bio-Electro-Magnetics Institute
2490 West Moana Lane
Reno, NV 89509
(702) 827-9099

RESOURCES

Other Alternative/Complementary Therapies

A description of additional alternative/complementary therapies is provided below. As mentioned with the alternative/complementary therapies previously discussed, further information on specific therapies can be found by consulting with alternative/complementary practitioners, exploring the telephone directory, and seeking resource material from libraries and book and health food stores. An extensive listing of alternative/complementary practitioners throughout the country is provided in the book *Alternative Medicine Yellow Pages* published by Future Medicine Publishing, Inc., (800) 249-8800.

Aromatherapy: Branch of herbal medicine that uses scents from the essential oils of various plants to achieve physiological and emotional effects.

Biological Dentistry: Dental practice based on belief that many chronic illnesses result from dental problems or substances used to treat dental problems (c.g., materials used in fillings that can have toxic effects in body).

Cell Therapy: Injection of cellular material to repair damaged organs and stimulate healing.

Colon Therapy: Uses colon irrigations to cleanse and release toxins from the body, boost immune functioning, and restore body's pH.

Detoxification Therapy: Use of fasting, special diets, vitamin therapy, colon therapy, hyperthermia and other measures to rid body of toxic chemicals and pollutants.

Energy Medicine: Use of special devices based on acupuncture meridian system that measures various electromagnetic frequencies generated from the body in order to identify energy imbalances. Electromagnetic treatment devices are then used to restore balance to body.

Enzyme Therapy: Based on principle that enzymes stimulate every chemical reaction in body, suggesting that illness stems from enzyme deficiency. Enzyme supplements are used to restore and maintain health.

Feng Shui: Ancient Asian art of determining effect of energy and how it can be positively utilized in our home and work environments.

Hydrotherapy: Therapeutic use of all forms and temperatures of water to treat conditions.

Hyperthermia: Based on principle that fever is important defense against disease. Induces elevation in body temperature above normal level to treat health problems.

Juice Therapy: Use of vegetable and fruit juices to cleanse body, promote health, and achieve specific medicinal outcomes.

Light Therapy: Use of different shades and intensity of light to promote health and correct certain disorders.

Osteopathy: Branch of physical medicine that uses physical therapy, joint manipulation, and postural correction to improve the total health of the person so that healing can take place and health is promoted.

Oxygen Therapy: The use of various forms of oxygen (e.g., hyperbaric chambers, hydrogen peroxide, ozone therapy) to kill pathogens and promote healing.

Qigong: Ancient Chinese exercise that stimulates and balances qi (vital life energy) by using movement, meditation, and breathing exercises.

Sound Therapy: Use of music and other sounds to stimulate certain physiologic and psychologic responses.

Vitamin/Mineral Supplementation: Based on belief that body needs intake of vitamins and minerals that surpass RDA levels in order to remain healthy and heal, and that specific nutrients can promote certain therapeutic results.

References

Anselmo J: *Biofeedback. At the heart of healing: experiencing holistic nursing*, Woodstock, NY, 1994, Holistic Nursing Associates and Kineholistics Foundation.

Anderson W, et al.: Patient use and assessment of conventional and alternative therapies for HIV infection and AIDS, *AIDS* 7:561-66, 1993.

Barabasz M and Speigel D: Hypnotizability and weight loss in obese subjects, *International Journal of Eating Disorders* 8(3):335-41, 1989.

Bigos SJ, et al.: Acute low back problems in adults: clinical practice guidelines #14, Rockville, MD, 1994, U.S. Department of Health and Human Services, PHS Agency for Health Care Policy.

Caudill M: Decreased clinic use by chronic pain patients' response to behavioral medicine intervention, *Clinical Journal of Pain* 7:305-10, 1991.

Chopra D: *Ageless body, timeless mind*, New York, 1993, Harmony Books.

Chopra D: *Perfect health*, New York, 1991, Harmony Books.

Chopra D: *Quantum healing*, New York, 1990, Bantam Books.

Chopra D, Manchanda SK, and Maheshwari MC: Meditation improves clinicoelectroencephalographic measures in drug-resistant epileptics, *Biofeedback and Self-Regulation* 19(1):25-40, 1994.

Coan RM, Wong G, Coan PL: The acupuncture treatment of low back pain: a randomized controlled study, *American Journal of Chinese Medicine* 8:181-89, 1980.

Coan RM, Wong G, Coan PL: The acupuncture treatment of neck pain: a randomized controlled study, *American Journal of Chinese Medicine* 9:326-32, 1982.

Coleman LM, Fowler LL, and Williams ME: Use of unproven therapies by people with Alzheimer's disease, *Journal of the American Geriatrics Society* 43:747-50, 1995.

Culliton PD and Kiresuk TJ: Overview of substance abuse acupuncture treatment research, *Journal of Alternative and Complementary Medicine* 2(1):149-159, 1996.

Eisenberg DM, et al.: Unconventional medicine in the United States: Prevalence, costs, and patterns of use, *New England Journal of Medicine* 328:246-52, 1993.

Ernst E, et al.: Massages cause changes in blood fluidity, *Physiotherapy* 73(1):43-45, 1987.

Ferrell-Torry AT and Glick OJ: The use of therapeutic massage as a nursing intervention to modify anxiety and the perception of cancer pain, *Cancer Nursing* 16(2):93-101, 1993.

Field T, et al.: Massage reduces anxiety in child and adolescent psychiatric patients, *Journal of the American Academy of Child and Adolescent Psychiatry* 31(1):125-31, 1992.

Findlay S, Podolsky D, and Silberner J: Wonder cures from the fringe, *U.S. News and World Report* 3(13):68-74, 1991.

Jacob GP, et al.: Multifactor treatment of chronic sleep-onset insomnia using stimulus control and the relaxation response, *Behavioral Modification* 17:498-508, 1993.

Jacobs J: Homeopathy. In Micozzi MS, ed: *Fundamentals of complementary and alternative medicine*, New York, 1996, Churchill-Livingstone.

Jobst KA: Acupuncture in asthma and pulmonary disease: an analysis of efficacy and safety, *Journal of Alternative and Complementary Medicine* 2(1):179-206, 1996.

Kabat-Zinn J, et al.: Effectiveness of a meditation-based stress reduction program in treatment of anxiety disorders, *American Journal of Psychiatry* 149(7):936-43, 1992.

Kramer NA: Comparison of therapeutic touch and casual touch in stress-reduction of hospitalized children, *Pediatric Nursing* 16(5):483-85, 1990.

Krieger D: *Therapeutic touch: how to use your hands to help or heal*, Englewood Cliffs, NJ, 1979, Prentice-Hall.

Krieger D, Peper E, Ancoli S: Physiologic indices of therapeutic touch, *American Journal of Nursing* 4:660-662, 1979.

Kuno RC and Cerqueira MD: Enhanced bone metabolism induced by acupuncture, *Journal of Nuclear Medicine* 36(12):2246-47, 1995.

Lao L: Safety issues in acupuncture, *Journal of Alternative and Complementary Medicine* 6(2)(1); a: 29, b: 27, 1996.

Meehan TC: Therapeutic touch and postoperative pain: a Rogerian research study, *Nursing Science Quarterly* 6(2):69-78, 1993.

Moore JS: *Chiropractic in America*, Baltimore, MD, 1993, Johns Hopkins University Press.

National Commission for the Certification of Acupuncturists: Safety record of acupuncture, Washington, DC, 1993, National Commission for the Certification of Acupuncturists.

Christensen PA, et al.: Electroacupuncture and postoperative pain, *British Journal of Anesthesia* 62:258-62, 1989.

National Institute on Health: *Alternative medicine: expanding medical horizons*, Chantilly, VA, 1994, NIH Report No. 94-066.

O'Mathuna DP: The subtle allure of therapeutic touch, *Journal of Christian Nursing* 15(1):12, 1998.

Parfitt A: Acupuncture as an antiemetic treatment, *Journal of Alternative and Complementary Medicine* 2(1):167-173, 1996.

Pomeranz B: Scientific research into acupuncture for the relief of pain, *Journal of Alternative and Complementary Medicine* 2(1):53, 1996.

Quinn JF and Strelkauskas AJ: Psychoimmunologic effects of therapeutic touch on practitioners and recently bereaved recipients: a pilot study, *Advances of Nursing Science* 15(4):13-26, 1993.

Reilly D, Taylor MA, Beattie NGM: Is evidence for homeopathy reproducible? *Lancet* 344: 1601-06, 1994.

Ruibal S: Ironclad cures for pain? Athletes put their faith in power of magnets, *USA Today*, Wednesday, 3C, August 3, 1997.

Schleenbaker RE and Mainous AG: Electromyographic biofeedback for neuromuscular reeducation in the hemiplegic stroke patient: a meta-analysis, *Archives of Physical Medicine and Rehabilitation* 74(12):11301-04, 1993.

Shames KH: *Creative imagery in nursing*, Albany, 1996, Delmar Publishers.

Vincent CA: A controlled trial of the treatment of migraine by acupuncture, *Clinical Journal of Pain* 5(4):305-12, 1989.

Whitman S, et al.: Progressive relaxation for seizure reduction, *Journal of Epilepsy* 3:17-22, 1990.

Whorwell PJ: Use of hypnotherapy in gastrointestinal disease, *British Journal of Hospital Medicine* 45:27-29, 1991.

Wirth DP: The effect of non-contact therapeutic touch on the healing rate of full thickness dermal wounds, *Subtle Energies* 1(1):1-20, 1990.

Yang LC, et al.: Comparison of P6 acupoint injection with 50% glucose in water and intravenous droperidol for prevention of vomiting after gynecological laparoscopy, *Acta Anaesthesioloica Scandanavica* 37(2):192-94, 1993.

Yates J: *A physician's guide to therapeutic massage: its physiological effects and their application to treatment*, Vancouver, B.C., Canada, 1990, Massage Therapists Association of British Columbia.

Recommended Readings

General and Miscellaneous Topics

Avery C: Native American medicine: traditional healing, *Journal of the American Medical Association* 265:2271, 2273, 1991.

Beinfield HL and Korngold EL: *Between heaven and earth: a guide to Chinese medicine*, New York, 1991, Ballantine Books.

Benes P, ed: *Medicine and healing: The Dublin seminar for New England folklife*, Boston, 1992, Boston University Press.

Burros M: Federal regulators say that herbal remedies pose their most difficult challenge, *New York Times* 142:B7, C8, June 16, 1993.

Butler K: *A consumer's guide to "alternative medicine"*, Buffalo, NY, 1992, Prometheus Books.

Chaitow L: *Osteopathic self-treatment*, San Francisco, CA, 1990, Thorsons.

Chee VE: Medicine men, *Journal of the American Medical Association* 265:2276, 1991.

Chen Ze-lin and Chen Mei-fang: Eight guiding principles of traditional Chinese medicine, *Health News and Review* 3(3):A2, 1993.

Cornacchia HJ and Barrett S: *Consumer health: a guide to intelligent decisions*, ed 5 St. Louis, 1993, Mosby Year Book.

DeSmet PA: Is there any danger in using traditional remedies? *Journal of Ethnopharmacology* 32:43-50, 1991.

Dreher H: Proven mind/body medicine: scientific approaches provide hope for those suffering from chronic conditions, *Natural Health* 23(3):86-96, 1993.

Eisenberg DM, et al.: Unconventional medicine in the United States: prevalence, costs, and patterns of use, *New England Journal of Medicine* 328:246-52, 1993.

Frandzel S: The sound of healing: the role of music, *Alternative and Complementary Therapies* 2(4):225-29, 1996.

Frazer K, ed: *The hundredth monkey and other paradigms of the paranormal*, Buffalo, 1991, Promethus Books.

Fugh-Berman A: *Alternative medicine: what works*, Tucson, 1996, Odonian Press.

George M: *Art for health's sake*, Community Care 1102(2):26, 1996.

Hafner AW, Carson JG, and Zwicky JF: *Guide to the American Medical Association historical health fraud and alternative medicine collection*, Chicago, 1992, American Medical Association.

Kalweit H: *Shamans, healers, and medicine men*, Boston, 1992, Shambhala.

Kuhn CC and Driscoll C: Humor yourself II: more lessons on laughter, *Real Living with Multiple Sclerosis* 1(5):12-15, 1994.

Macnair A: *Self-help and prevention: the alternative to pharmaceuticals?* SCRIP World Pharmaceutical News 1928(9):S16-18, 1994.

Merzer M: Many Americans are seeking relief in alternative and off-the-wall home remedies, *Knight-Ridder/Tribune News Service*, October 29, 1993, p. 11029.

Motz J: Healing hopes: alternative medicine emerges in the nation's capital, *Advances, Journal of Mind-Body Health* 10(1):68-74, 1994.

Murray M and Pizzorno J: *Encyclopedia of Natural Medicine*, Rocklin, CA, 1991, Prima Publishing.

Murray RH and Rubel AJ: Physicians and healers, unwitting partners in health care, *New England Journal of Medicine* 326:61-64, 1992.

O'Regan B and Hirschberg C: *Spontaneous remission: an annotated bibliography*, Sausalito, 1993, Institute of Noetic Sciences.

Strohecker J, ed: *Alternative medicine: the definitive guide*, Puyallup, WA, 1994, Future Medicine Publishing, Inc.

Young JH: *American health quackery*, Princeton, NJ, 1992, Princeton University Press.

Zwicky JF, et al.: *Reader's guide to alternative health methods*, Chicago, 1993, American Medical Association.

Acupuncture

Brewington V, Smith M, and Lipton D: Acupuncture as a detoxification treatment: an analysis of controlled research, *Journal of Substance Abuse Treatment* 11(4):289-307, 1994.

Ehrlich D and Haber P: Influence of acupuncture on physical performance capacity and hemodynamic parameters, *International Journal of Sports Medicine* 13:486-91, 1992.

Hung VC and Mines JS: Eschars and scarring from hot needle acupuncture treatment, *Journal of the American Academy of Dermatology* 24:148-149, 1991.

Kaptchuk T: *The web that has no weaver: understanding Chinese medicine*, New York, 1992, Congdon and Weed.

Lao L: Acupuncture techniques and devices, *Journal of Alternative and Complementary Medicine* 2(1):27-32, 1996.

Lytle CD: History of the Food and Drug Administration's regulation of acupuncture devices, *Journal of Alternative and Complementary Medicine* 2(1):253-256, 1996.

Mitchell BB: Educational and licensing requirements for acupuncturists, *Journal of Alternative and Complementary Medicine* 2(1):33-36, 1996.

Morris MM: Overview of acupuncture in chronic pain clinical research, *Journal of Alternative and Complementary Medicine* 2(1):125-128, 1996.

Moffet H: Acupuncture and Oriental medicine update, *Alternative and Complementary Therapies* 2(2):115-117, 1996.

Wu JN: A short history of acupuncture, *Journal of Alternative and Complementary Medicine* 2(1):19-22, 1996.

Ayurvedic Medicine

Chopra D: *Ageless body, timeless mind*, New York, 1993, Harmony Books.

Chopra D: *Perfect health*, New York, 1991, Harmony Books.

Chopra D: *Quantum healing*, New York, 1990, Bantam Books.

Dash VB: *Fundamentals of Ayurvedic medicine*, ed 7, Delhi, India, 1992, Konaark Publishers Pvt. Ltd.

Frawley D: *Ayurvedic healing*, Salt Lake City, 1990, Morson Publishing.

Sharma HM, et al.: Ayur-Veda: modern insights into ancient medicine, *Journal of the American Medical Association* 265:2633-37, 1991.

Chiropractic

Barrett S: Views of a chiropractic critic: your real enemy is yourself! *ACA Journal of Chiropractic* 27(11):61-64, 1990.

Coplan-Griffiths M: *Dynamic chiropractic today: the complete and authoritative guide to this major therapy*, San Francisco, CA, 1991, Harper Collins.

Fultz O: Chiropractic: what can it do for you? *American Health* 11(4):41-44, 1992.

Haldeman S, ed: *Principles and practice of chiropractic*, New York, 1992, Appleton and Lange.

Martin RT: *Today's health alternative*, Tehachapi, CA, 1992, America West Publishers.

Palmer DD: *The chiropractor's adjuster*, Davenport, IA, 1992, Palmer College Press.

Sweere JJ, ed: *Chiropractic family practice: a clinical manual*, Gaithersburg, MD, 1992, Aspen Publishers.

Wardwell WI: *Chiropractic: history and evolution of a new profession*, St Louis, 1992, Mosby Year Book.

White K: Manual therapies: advances in osteopathy, chiropractic, massage, and other techniques, *Alternative and Complementary Therapies* 2(1):9-15, 1996.

Herbal Medicine

Adams R: Pouring over herbal teas, *Better Nutrition for Today's Living* 57(2):76-80, 1995.

Atchison SD: A few herbs, a prayer and often a cure, *Business Week* 3330:16a-18a, 1993.

Bates CD: Herbs: tonic or toxic, *Shape* 16(2):104-110, 1996.

Bergner P: How much of an herb is enough? Rules for effective self-care, *Natural Health* 23(3):66-70, 1993.

Bergner P: Herbs that calm your nerves, *Natural Health* 23(4):56-59, 1993.

Bird C: Shamans and the scientists: a future for traditional medicine, *SCRIP World Pharmaceutical News*, September 2, 1994, p. S17.

Blevi V and Sween G: *Aromatherapy*, New York, 1993, Avon Books.

Brooke E: *Herbal therapy for women*, London, 1992, Thorsons Publishing.

Brown DJ: Herbal Rx for the immune system: Echinacea can help fight off a myriad of ills, *Vegetarian Times* 229(9):92-95, 1996.

Candee A: So you're going to an herbalist, *Health News and Review* 3(2):14, 1993.

Castleman M: *The healing herbs*, Emmaus, PA, 1991, Rodale Press.

Christopher JR: *School of natural healing: the reference volume on herbal therapy for the teacher, student, or practitioner*, Springville, UT, 1996, Christopher Publications.

Dawson AG: *Herbs: partners in life*, Rochester, VT, 1991, Healing Arts Press.

Foster S: Milk thistle: herbal seeds, medicinal seeds, *Better Nutrition for Today's Living* 57(4):64-67, 1995.

Foster S: Ginseng: get to the root of health, *Better Nutrition for Today's Living* 57(3):66-69, 1995.

Foster S and Duke JA: *Eastern/central medicinal plants*, New York, 1990, Houghton Mifflin Co.

Godlee F: The power in a flower, *The Guardian*, August 13, 1996, p. T8-10.

Gordon DW, et al.: Chaparral ingestion: the broadening spectrum of liver injury caused by herbal medications, *Journal of the American Medical Association* 273(6):489-91, 1995.

Gotzkowsky S and McMahon G: Can garlic reduce levels of serum lipids? A controlled clinical study, *American Journal of Medicine* 94(6):632-36, 1993.

Guiness A, ed: Family guide to natural medicine, Pleasantville, NY, 1993, *Reader's Digest* Association.

Hobbs C: St John's wort: a magical herb, *Let's Live* 63(5):52-55, 1995.

Kloss J: *Back to Eden: a herbal guide*, Loma Linda, CA, 1991, Gordon Press.

Lawless J: *The encyclopedia of essential oils*, Rockport, MA, 1992, Element, Inc.

Lustgarden S: Rx for pharmacists, *Vegetarian Times* 201(5):20, 1994.

Mars B: Improve your digestion with bitter herbs: the sharp taste of pungent herbs peps up the digestive system, *Natural Health* 23(1):43-45, 1993.

Mars B: Increase energy with herbs and other natural remedies, *Let's Live* 62(5):38-41, 1994.

Mayer R: The problem with herbal remedies, *Parenting* 10(4):56-58, 1996.

McCaleb R: Chamomile: the world's most soothing herb, *Better Nutrition for Today's Living* 55(9):48-51, 1993.

McCaleb R: Herbs for long-term mental and physical stimulation, *Better Nutrition for Today's Living* 56(2):50-54, 1994.

McCaleb R: Milk thistle: herbal detoxifier, *Better Nutrition for Today's Living* 55(3):50-55, 1993.

Mowrey DB: Tonics can tone up your liver, eliminate toxins, boost health, *Health News and Review* 4(2):18, 1994.

Natelson EJ: Beating stress naturally, *Vegetarian Times* 198(2):86-89, 1994.

Picker L and McHugh J: Herbal medicine goes mainstream, *American Health* 15(4):70-76, 1996.

Rodgers K: Back to our roots: searching for new drugs in the rain forest, *Drug Topics* 139(1):57-62, 1995.

Ryman D: *Aromatherapy: the complete guide to plant and flower essences for health and beauty*, New York, 1993, Bantam Books.

Schulick P: The healing power of ginger, *Vegetarian Times* 225(5):78-82, 1996.

Shook EE: *Advanced treatise in herbology*, Banning, CA, 1992, Enos Publishing Co.

Snider S: Beware the unknown brew, herbal teas and toxicity, *FDA Consumer* 25(5):30-33, 1991.

Snyder K: What do pharmacists think of herbal remedies? *Drug Topics* 140(15):101, 1996.

Stashower ME, et al.: Chaparral and liver toxicity, *Journal of the American Medical Association* 274(11):871-73, 1995.

Tyler VE: *The honest herbal*, ed 3, Binghamton, NY, 1992, Haworth Press.

Vukovic L: Introducing the superherbs, *Natural Health* 26(5):104-128, 1996.

Vukovic L: Your A-Z guide to making natural remedies, *Natural Health* 25(5):110-124, 1995.

Wilson R: *A complete guide to understanding and using aromatherapy*, Garden City Park, NY, 1995, Avery Publishing Group.

Winship KA: Toxicity of comfrey, *Adverse Drug Reactions and Toxicological Reviews* 101:47-59, 1991.

Wolfe J: Natural-born healers, *Men's Health* 11(3):68-70, 1996.

Homeopathy

Boericke W: *Pocket manual of homeopathic materia medica and repertory*, New Delhi, India, 1996, B. Jain Publishers Pvt. Ltd.

Cummings S and Ullman D: *Everybody's guide to homeopathic medicines*, Los Angeles, 1991, Jeremy P. Tarcher, Inc.

Kent JT: *Repertory of the homeopathic materia medica and a word index*, New Delhi, India, 1994, B. Jain Publishers Pvt. Ltd.

Kleijen J, Knipschild P, ter Riet G: Clinical trials of homeopathy, *British Medical Journal* 302:316-323, 1991.

Lockie AA: *The family guide to homeopathy: symptoms and natural solutions*, New York, 1993, Prentice Hall Press.

Ullman D: *Discovering homeopathy: your introduction to the science and art of homeopathic medicine*, Berkeley, CA, 1991, North Atlantic Books.

Ullman D: *Homeopathic medicine for children and infants*, Los Angeles, 1992, Jeremy P. Tarcher.

Wright-Hubbard E: *A brief study course in homeopathy*, St. Louis, 1992, Formur Inc., Publisher.

Imagery

Achterberg J: *Imagery in healing*, Boston, 1986, New Science Library.

Bresler D: *Free yourself from pain*, Topanga, CA, 1992, The Bresler Center.

Goleman D and Gurin J: *Mind/body medicine: how to use your mind for better health*, New York, 1993, Consumer Reports Books.

Peper E and Holt C: *Creating wholeness: a self-healing workbook using dynamic relaxation, images and thoughts*, New York, 1993, Plenum.

Rossman ML: *Healing yourself: a step-by-step program for better health through imagery*, New York, 1989, Pocket Books.

Magnetic Field Therapy

Davis A and Rawls W: *Magnetism and its effects on the living system*, Kansas City, MO, 1993, Acres USA.

Philpott W and Taplin S: *Biomagnetic handbook*, Choctaw, OK, 1990, Enviro-Tech Products.

Whitaker J and Adderly B: *The pain relief breakthrough: the power of magnets*, Boston, 1998, Little, Brown, and Company.

Massage and Bodywork

Barlow W: *The Alexander technique*, New York, 1991, Alfred A. Knopf.

Feldenkrais M and Kimmey M: *The potent self: a guide to spontaneity*, San Francisco, 1992, Harper and Row.

Gach M: *Acupressure's potent points*, New York, 1990, Bantam Books.

Gray J: *The Alexander technique*, New York, 1991, St Martin's Press.

Heller J and Henkin W: *Bodywise*, Berkeley, CA, 1991, Wingbow Press.

Kunz K and Kunz B: *Hand and foot reflexology: a self-help guide*, New York, 1987, Simon and Schuster.

Rolf I: *Rolfing: the integration of human structures*, New York, 1977, Harper and Row.

Seidman M: *A guide to polarity therapy: the gentle art of hands-on healing*, Boulder, CO, 1991, Elan Press.

Thomas S: *Massage for common ailments*, New York, 1989, Fireside.

Trager M and Guadagno C: *Trager mentastics: movement as a way to agelessness*, Barrytown, NY, 1987, Station Hill Press.

White K: Manual therapies: advances in osteopathy, chiropractic, massage, and other techniques, *Alternative and Complementary Therapies* 2(1):9-15, 1996.

Meditation and Relaxation

Benson H: *The relaxation response*, New York, 1993, Outlet Books.

Peper E and Holt CF: *Creating wholeness: a self-healing workbook using dynamic relaxation, images, and thoughts*, New York, 1993, Plenum Press.

Roth R: *Transcendental meditation*, New York, 1988, Donal I. Fine.

Mind-Body Connection

Benson H and Stark M: *Timeless healing: the power and biology of belief*, New York, 1996, Scribner.

Cousins N: *Head first: the biology of hope*, New York, 1991, Thorndike Press.

Dienstfrey H: *Where the mind meets the body*, New York, 1991, Harper Collins.

Family Practice News: Research is showing healthful effects of laughter, *Family Practice News* 15(5):52a-52b, 1992.

Friedman HS and VandenBos GR: Disease-prone and self-healing personalities, *Hospital and Community Psychiatry* 43(12):1177-79, 1992.

Fulford RC: *Dr. Fulford's touch of life: the healing power of natural life force*, New York, 1996, Pocket Books.

Gallager W: *The power of place: how our surroundings shape our thoughts, emotions, and actions*, New York, 1993, Poseidon.

Gaynor ML: *Healing essence: a cancer doctor's practical program for hope and recovery*, New York, 1995, Kodansha International.

Goleman D and Gurin J: *Mind/body medicine: how to use your mind for better health*, New York, 1993, Consumer Reports Books.

Kabat-Zinn J: *Full catastrophic living: using the wisdom of your body and mind to face stress, pain, and illness*, New York, 1990, Delacorte Press.

Kerkvliet GJ: Music therapy may help control cancer pain, *Journal of the National Cancer Institute* 82(5):350-52, 1990.

Moskowitz RC: *Your healing mind*, New York, 1992, William Morrow and Co.

Moyers B: *Healing and the mind*, New York, 1993, Doubleday.

Pennebaker JW: *Opening up: the healing power of confiding in others*, New York, 1991, Avon Books.

Phillips DP, Ruth TE, and Wagner LM: Psychology and survival, *Lancet* 342:1142-45, 1993.

Tunks E and Bellisimo A: *Behavioral medicine: concepts and procedures*, New York, 1990, Pergamon Press.

Wickramasekera IE: Diagnosis by inclusion: the perspective of a behavioral medicine practitioner, *Advances, Journal of Mind-Body Health* 8(1):17-31, 1992.

Naturopathy

Baer HA: The potential rejuvenation of American naturopathy as a consequence of the holistic health movement, *Medical Anthropology* 13:368-383, 1992.

Griffin K: The new doctors of natural medicine, *Health* 10(6):60-68, 1996.

Murray M and Pizzorno J: *Encyclopedia of natural medicine*, Rocklin, CA, 1991, Prima Publishing.

Pizzorno JE and Murray MT: *Textbook of natural medicine, volumes 1 and 2*, Seattle, 1989, John Bastyr College Publications.

Spiritual Healing

Aldridge D: Is there evidence for spiritual healing? *Advances, Journal of Mind-Body Health* 9(4):4-21, 1993.

Barasch I: *The healing path: a soul approach to illness*, New York, 1994, Putnam Book.

Benor DJ: *Healing research: holistic energy medicine and spirituality*, United Kingdom, 1993, Helix Editions.

Benor DJ: Survey of spiritual healing research, *Complementary Medical Research* 4(30):9-33, 1990.

Borysenko J: *Fire in the soul: a new psychology of spiritual optimism*, New York, 1993, Warner Books.

Coulter AH: Tapping the soul's healing potential: an interview with Carlos Warter, MD, PhD, *Alternative and Complementary Therapies* 2(5):283-87, 1996.

Dossey L: *Healing words: the power of prayer and the practice of medicine*, San Francisco, 1993, Harper.

Dossey L: *Meaning and medicine*, New York, 1991, Bantam.

Evans D: *Spirituality and human nature*, Albany, NY, 1993, State University of New York Press.

Foster RJ: *Prayer: finding the heart's true home*, San Francisco, 1992, Harper.

Ingerman S: *Soul retrieval: mending the fragmented self*, San Francisco, 1991, Harper San Francisco.

Ingerman S: *Welcome home: life after healing*, San Francisco, 1993, Harper San Francisco.

Kornfield J: *A path with heart: a guide through the perils and promises of spiritual life*, New York, 1993, Bantam.

Krippner S and Welch P: *Spiritual dimensions of healing: from native shamanism to contemporary health care*, New York, 1992, Irvington Publishers.

Rychlak JF: Struggling to understand spiritual healing, *Advances, Journal of Mind-Body Health* 10(1):63-67, 1994.

Wendt SJ: *The radiant heart: healing the heart, healing the soul*, Munster, IN, 1995, Radiant Heart Press.

Therapeutic Touch

Hover-Kramer D, Mentgen I, and Scandrett-Hibdon S: *Healing touch: a resource for health care professionals*, Albany, NY, 1996, Delmar Publishers.

Hughes PP, Meize-Grochowski R, and Harris CN: Therapeutic touch with adolescent psychiatric patients, *Journal of Holistic Nursing* 14(1):6-23, 1996.

Krieger D: *Accepting your power to heal*, Santa Fe, 1993, Bear and Company Publishing.

Krieger D: *Living the therapeutic touch: healing as a lifestyle*, Wheaton, IL, 1988, Quest Books.

Krieger D: *The therapeutic touch*, Englewood Cliffs, NJ, 1979, Prentice Hall.

McCrae J: *Therapeutic touch: a practical guide*, New York, 1992, Knopf.

Yoga

Ballentine RM: *Joints and glands exercises*, Hunesdale, PA, 1977, The Himalayan International Institute of Yoga Science and Philosophy.

Christensen A: *The American Yoga Association wellness book*, New York, 1996, Kensington Books.

Iyengar B: *Light on Pranayama*, New York, Crossroad Publishing, 1992.

*H*ealth Perception and Health Management

The ability to maintain a healthy state and identify, seek help for, and correct deviations from normal health is influenced by individuals' perception of personal health and their health care behaviors. Ideally, people engage in health behaviors to avoid disease; once a disease has developed, they adhere to practices that manage symptoms and prevent complications. The concepts of primary, secondary, and tertiary prevention (Box 6-1) have been used to describe the various levels of preventive practices in which clients can engage (Stanhope, 1988). In the real world, however, not everyone behaves in an ideal manner. People smoke cigarettes, eat junk food, overbook their calendars, engage in unsafe sexual practices, postpone physical examinations, and stop taking their required medications. Poor health practices can have serious consequences for all individuals and can be particularly threatening to persons who have chronic diseases.

Assessment Considerations

An important part of the assessment of chronically ill persons is a determination of health behaviors and preventive practices. This information is obtained through a combination of observation, a health records review, and a direct description of the client's health practices as reported by family members, caregivers, or by the client's own direct report. The clinician can evaluate the usefulness of these reports by noting the degree of congruence between reported practices and health status.

The identification of deficits is the first level of assessment; the causative or contributing factor associated with the deficit must be explored by reviewing each of the requisites necessary to meet health management demands (as discussed in Chapter 1). For example, a client may be noncompliant due to a variety of factors, including cultural influences, incongruency of the treatment with the client's value system, insufficient economic resources to support desired health practices, misinformation, misunderstanding, poor motivation, lack of confidence in the provider, fatigue, or altered cognition. The clinician must identify the reason(s) for the noncompliance in order to effectively plan and provide care.

Health Perceptions and Behaviors

A variety of factors influence health perception. For instance, an elderly client with significant disability related to arthritic joints may judge herself as being in wonderful condition compared to her close friend who has dementia. On the other hand, a client with a mild heart murmur may exaggerate his health problem to be released from undesired roles and to elicit sympathy. Similarly, a person who has lived with a chronic illness for years may view himself as having good health because he feels well enough to maintain a job, while a health-conscious individual who has been free of maladies may view her health status as seriously threatened because she has entered menopause. A client's health perception can determine motivation to engage in or change health practices, as well as social and familial roles and functions.

BOX 6-1   **Levels of Prevention of Health Problems**

Primary Prevention: to prevent disease
   Safe water and sanitation
   Healthy diet
   Weight control within ideal range
   Regular exercise
   Adequate rest and sleep
   Good hygienic practices
   Regular elimination pattern
   Participation in social and leisure activities
   Maintenance of a clean, safe environment
   Avoidance of tobacco use
   Limitation in exposure to sun
   Effective stress management
   Avoidance of pollutants
   Good judgment to avoid injury

Secondary Prevention: to detect disease early
   Health screening
   Examinations
   Self-assessments

Tertiary Prevention: to manage and improve existing condition
   Compliance with treatment plan
   Adjustment of lifestyle as necessary
   Improvement of knowledge and skill regarding condition and its management

---

Changing clients' perceptions of their condition and their health care behaviors may be necessary to achieve compliance with the treatment plan and promote optimum health. Behavioral change can take the form of (Miller, 1992):
   • removal: eliminating the behavior (e.g., smoking cessation),
   • replacement: substituting a new behavior for the old one (e.g., doing progressive relaxation rather than drinking alcohol), or
   • addition: supplementing or expanding usual behaviors (e.g., administering a daily medication).

Providing knowledge about the importance of the change in health practices and the consequences of not changing often are not sufficient to cause the desired health practice. The likelihood of a health practice being incorporated into the client's routine can be influenced largely by the client:
   • believing there is real benefit to the practice,
   • perceiving outcomes associated with the practice to be attainable,
   • viewing the health behavior as consistent with psychological, social, and

spiritual systems, and

- being unrestricted by obstacles (e.g., lack of knowledge, high cost, inconvenient resources).

Specific practices to promote health will be addressed with the discussion of specific conditions throughout the remainder of this text.

Environmental Influence on Health

The home environment consists of more than a structure and the objects contained within. The surroundings in which we spend our time influence the way we feel and function. Most of us can easily visualize settings that put us in the frame of mind for relaxation, focused work, solitude, or socialization. Likewise, we have visited some homes that bubbled with warmth and friendship and others that conveyed a stuffy formality. Often, we are unaware of the factors that influence the differences among environments; however, an understanding of those factors can enable us to therapeutically use environments to promote health and healing.

Light and Color

Although a recent entry into the arena of popular healing arts, color therapy was used by Pythagoras as far back as 500 years before the birth of Christ. We now increasingly find evidence that light and color influence mental and physical activity.

The eye contains millions of cells called *photoreceptors* that are sensitive to color and light. When light enters the eye, the photoreceptors convert the light into electrical impulses that travel through the optic nerve to the brain. In the brain, the hypothalamus gland is stimulated and sends chemical messengers, *neurotransmitters*, throughout the body to regulate body temperature, blood pressure, respirations, digestion, immune system activity, moods, and other bodily functions.

Natural light helps to maintain the body's rhythms; this in turn influences body temperature, sleep cycles, hormone production, and other functions. The pineal gland is responsible for regulating these biological activities, and external light controls this gland's activities. Exposure to light during the normal 24-hour dark-light cycle keeps the body's biological functions regulated; disruption to the body's internal rhythms occurs when this cycle is interrupted; perhaps the clearest example of this occurs when a person works during the night and sleeps during the daytime.

People who spend a significant amount of time indoors may face problems due to the fact that artificial light lacks the full spectrum of sunlight. Even an environment with plenty of windows has limited value if the windows are never opened because ordinary glass prevents a majority of ultraviolet radiation from entering. (The effects of this can be noted when fruits that are grown behind glass have trouble ripening.) Although overexposure to the sun's rays has proven harmful effects, the body does need some contact with ultraviolet light. Fortunately, there are forms of light therapy that can be used to achieve therapeutic results. Full-spectrum light and sunlight can be used to relieve high blood pressure, depression, SAD (seasonal affective disorder), migraines, depression, and other disorders, and this light is believed to have a role in the prevention of certain cancers (Garland, 1990).

Color is the sensation resulting from stimulation of the retina by light waves of certain lengths. Long waves of the color spectrum include oranges and reds; short waves are represented by yellows, greens, and blues. Colors emit energy that affects muscular activity: muscular activity increases slightly when a person is exposed to blue light, moderately when exposed to green light, and significantly when exposed to yellow light. Many of us have realized the personal effects of colors on our mood and behavior, for example:

- black and gray are depressing,
- white is cheering and stimulating,
- red is exciting,
- blue is calming,
- yellow is cerebral-stimulating,
- violet decreases appetite,
- orange stimulates the appetite,
- brown and earth tones are comforting,
- green, the master healer/color, gives a feeling of well-being.

Many factories and institutions have recognized the impact of color and replaced dull grays and blues with brighter, warmer colors to achieve improved morale and productivity. By the same token, changes can be made in the individual's living and work environment to use light and colors therapeutically. Some suggestions could include:

- paint rooms colors that are consistent with their intended use (e.g., bedroom, a restful blue; office, a stimulating yellow; den, comforting earth tones; recreation room, a cheerful white; meditation area, green);
- dress in colors that will influence mood desired for the occasion (e.g., a bright color to perk up, subdued color to be calm and serious);
- use non-fluorescent lighting. If this is not possible, replace fluorescent tubes with tubes that simulate natural light (available at specialty lighting stores);
- whenever possible, open windows to allow natural light to enter the indoor environment.

Sound

Sounds are audible vibrations that produce specific effects. Sound travels from the source in the form of sound waves, or small vibrations. The qualities of sound are frequency and intensity. *Frequency* refers to the pitch; the faster the speed of vibrations, the higher the pitch. The speed of vibrations is measured in cycles per second called hertz (Hz). The human ear can hear sounds as low as 20 Hz and as high as 20,000 Hz. Most speech falls in a range of 500-4000 Hz. *Intensity* refers to the loudness of a sound and is determined by the strength of the vibration; it is measured in decibels (dB). Normal conversation ranges 30-60 dB. The decibel levels of other common noises are listed in Table 6-1.

If noise-induced hearing loss is suspected, audiology testing should be obtained. A quick and easy telephone screening test is available to help in detecting the need for an examination by calling (800) 222-EARS [in Pennsylvania (800) 345-EARS] between 9 A.M. and 5 P.M., EST; an operator will refer the caller to a local number to telephone for the test. Although this is not a full professional audiometeric screening, this free and easy test could stimulate clients to seek testing that they otherwise would not have considered.

Most people are aware of the irritating effects of loud noises; however, dissonant or inharmonic sounds can be disturbing also. One needn't be consciously aware of a sound for it to have an effect; sound vibrations produce a variety of physiological responses. Noise exposure to 100 dB of white noise (sound containing a blend of all audible frequencies distributed equally over the range of the frequency band) can produce vasoconstriction and an elevation in blood pressure. People with Alzheimer's disease and other confusional states will have increased confusion and wandering when noise levels are high. It is important to control noise exposure to avoid ill consequences. For example, it is wise to ask to have the volume of loud music reduced, repair appliances that produce loud or unusual noise, and wear earplugs to buffer industrial or traffic noise.

The other side of the coin is the positive effects of sound. Music can be used to reduce stress, lessen anxiety, and control pain. Since enjoyable music is a matter of taste (the Bach that relaxes one person can be annoying to someone else), it is advisable to assess a client's preference and reaction to various forms of music and select that which brings about the desired effect.

New Age music is nontraditional music that promotes relaxation and contemplation. It has no melody, rhythm, or harmonic progression, and is designed to have wide appeal despite usual musical preferences. Local libraries usually have audiotapes and compact disks of New Age music for those who wish to sample this style of music before investing in a purchase.

TABLE 6-1

Decibel Levels of Common Noises	
Noise	**Decibels**
Refrigerator	40
Light automobile traffic	50
Clothes dryer	55
Air conditioner	60
Hair dryer	50-80
Vacuum cleaner	62-85
Alarm clock	80
Lawn mower (gas)	87-92
City traffic	90
Chain saw	100
Stereo	up to 120

Permanent hearing loss can occur from chronic exposure to noise levels of 85 decibels or more.

Scents

The aroma of cinnamon buns fresh from the oven or popcorn being popped can cause mouths to water in people who hadn't been at all hungry. This is but one example of the physiological effects of scents.

Although fragrances have been used purposefully for centuries, only recently has interest blossomed in the use of scents to create specific physical and emotional effects. In fact, a unique branch of herbal medicine, *aromatherapy*, has developed that uses the essential oils of various plants in a therapeutic manner. Usually, the oils are either dispersed through the air in a diffuser or simmering pot, or applied to the skin through baths, massages, or compresses. The chemical composition of essential oils has been shown to have diuretic, vasodilating, antispasmodic, antibacterial, antiviral, and other effects. For example:

- the scent of lavender has been shown to elevate mood; persons in rooms scented with lemon reported fewer health problems than on days when the room was unscented (Knasko, 1993),
- people with cancer who received massages with roman chamomile and almond oil reported a decrease in anxiety and physical symptoms and a better quality of life (Wilkinson, 1995),
- persons who were given foot massages with orange oil after cardiac surgery felt less anxiety and were more relaxed than patients who received the foot massages with plain oil (Stevenson, 1995), and
- individuals trying to withdraw from cigarette smoking had improved moods and fewer withdrawal symptoms when the smell of black pepper or mint was delivered to them through a special device (Rose and Behm, 1994).

Box 6-2 lists the effects of some scents. Clients should be advised to purchase only pure essential oils from reputable dealers. Less expensive artificial or diluted oils will not produce intended effects and, consequently, will be a waste of money.

Scents can stimulate psychological and physiological reactions associated with previous experiences involving the fragrance or odor. For instance, if one had positive experiences spending time with a grandfather as he worked in his woodshop, the smell of wood could bring back fond memories; on the other hand, if one disliked but was forced to eat lamb as a child, the scent of lamb cooking could evoke an unfavorable response.

Temperature

It has long been realized that temperature affects mood and function. For instance, visual vigilance performance (alertness) is best at 90° F (32° C), general vigilance performance is best between 85° F (29° C) and 90° F (32° C), tactile sensitivity if best at 85° F (29° C), and psychomotor tasks become impaired below 55° F (13° C) (Kobrick and Fine, 1983). Persons of advanced age or who are emaciated can become hypothermic in environmental temperatures below 70° F. An indoor temperature that ranges between 70° and 75° F (21° to 24° C) is therapeutic.

BOX 6-2	Effects of Selected Essential Oils
Antiinflammatory:	chamomile, cinnamon, clove, eucalyptus, lavender, rosemary
Cold symptom relief:	cinnamon, eucalyptus, orange, peppermint
Energizer:	black spruce, cinnamon, eucalyptus, geranium, lemon-grass, peppermint
Headache relief:	basil, chamomile, lavender, peppermint
Mood elevation:	basil, jasmine, lemongrass, peppermint
Relaxation:	chamomile, jasmine, lavender, mandarin, neroli, sandalwood

Pets

More than one-half of all American homes have one or more pets. Pet lovers have long known that animals can add immense joy, activity, companionship, and pleasure to life. But the sense of connectiveness derived through involvement with pets has very positive effects on health status also. Heart attack victims who owned pets were found to have one-fifth the death rate of petless heart attack victims (Ornstein and Sobel, 1987). Talking to or petting an animal, or watching fish in a tank causes a lowering of blood pressure. It is not the type of pet as much as the relationship with the animal that counts.

Environment Functionality

Many chronic conditions affect self-care independence, mobility, and the ability to function in common environments. An environment that is not user-friendly to persons with chronic conditions can cause more dependency than is necessary and contribute to stress, poor morale, and accidents. Specific impairments and disabilities dictate the type of environmental modifications that can be used to improve function and safety. Some suggestions are listed in Box 6-3.

Occupational and physical therapists are wonderful resources in identifying assistive devices and environmental modifications that can promote independent function. Medical supply stores sell aids, as do some major department stores, such as Sears, which has a home care aids line of products. Individual health care insurance carriers should be consulted for their reimbursement for these items. Some organizations (e.g., churches, cancer associations, American Legions) provide financial assistance toward the purchase of these items. The local information and referral service can be called for more information.

Toxic Hazards in the Home

Radon gas

Studies by the Environmental Protection Agency indicate that as many as 10 percent of all American homes may have elevated levels of radon. Radon is a naturally occurring radioactive gas that seeps from bedrock and ground soil into

BOX 6-3	Modifications to Make the Home Safe and Functional

Handrails on stairways
Grab bars in shower/bathtub
Nonslip strips or finish on shower/bathtub floor
Replacement of steps with ramps
Telephones with large numbers
Smoke detectors
Lever rather than round faucet and door handles
Lighting in hallways, stairways
Hot water heater temperature control ≤ 100° F

homes and other buildings through foundation cracks, floor drains, joints, and pores in hollow-block concrete walls. Once radon enters a building, the radioactive particles can attach to dust and become airborne and eventually inhaled. Radon is not visible and has no odor. Regular exposure to radon can be deadly. Radon is the second leading cause of lung cancer, and smokers exposed to radon have a tenfold increase in their risk for developing lung cancer.

Radon detection kits can be purchased from hardware stores and used to measure the presence of radon. Radon levels can vary from one room to another and from one time of year to another, so more than one screening may need to be done.

The risks from radon can be reduced by providing good ventilation in the home (especially in the basement), sealing off radon entry routes, having radon gas suctioned from the soil, reducing time spent in areas of high radon concentration, and keeping crawl space vents open all the time. Of course, prohibiting smoking in the home not only reduces the risk of developing radon-caused lung cancer, but also has many other health benefits. State health departments usually have a radiation office that can provide information and guidance on detecting and correcting radon problems.

Electromagnetic fields

Some research has linked electromagnetic fields to cancer. The areas of concern not only implicate the electromagnetic fields generated by power lines, but also those emitted from ordinary domestic appliances. Some research has reported evidence that power lines and appliances are able to attract the radioactive products of radon, which are believed to be carcinogenic (Baltimore Sun, 1996). Additional research is needed before conclusions are drawn, but it may be prudent to avoid living in a home that is close to power lines and to limit exposure to electric blankets and other electrical appliances that have prolonged or close contact with the body.

A variety of symptoms can result from irritants and toxins in the home (Box 6-4). Some measures that can assist in reducing health hazards in the home are

BOX 6-4	Symptoms Associated with Unhealthy Conditions in the Home
Headache	Coughing
Dry or sore throat	Irritated, itchy, watery, red eyes
Fatigue	Nausea
Drowsiness	Skin rashes, itching
Insomnia	Joint pain
Dizziness	Confusion
Sneezing	Irritability
Sinus congestion	Behavioral changes
Difficulty breathing	

offered in Box 6-5, and a listing of resources for information on protecting the home is provided in Box 6-6.

Feng Shui

Finally, a variety of the sensory elements just discussed are combined in the environmental application arts. These go one step further than modifications for function and safety. The significance of environment on health and healing has long been appreciated by the Chinese, who have developed an art of the placement of items in the environment called feng shui (pronounced "fung shway"). Items are viewed as triggering joyful or energetic responses that can energize and facilitate the Ch'i, the vital energy flow. Feng shui concentrates on balancing yin (feminine, dark, cool, soft, wet, earth, moon) and yang (masculine, light, hot, hard, dry, sky, sun). All of the five elements (wood, fire, earth, metal, and water) need to be represented in the environment through furnishings and decorations.

The Human Environment's Influence on Health

Relationships can have a profound effect on health and healing. People who are pessimistic, critical, or unpleasant can be a source of stress and have a negative impact, whereas those who are optimistic, supportive, and fun can promote a sense of comfort and well-being that has many positive effects.

Whenever possible, it makes sense for clients to be involved with people who have a positive influence. This may entail developing and nurturing new relationships. In some circumstances, the terms of old relationships may need to be changed if they are more of a burden than a pleasure. Clients need to evaluate their relationships in terms of their therapeutic benefit; some questions for clients to consider in making this assessment include:

- Does the person make me feel cared about and important?
- Am I accepted in the relationship for who I am?
- Is this person honest with me and willing to offer constructive criticism?
- Will this individual help me to solve problems independently?
- Does this person encourage me to adopt and practice healthy behaviors?

BOX 6-5   General Measures to Reduce Health Hazards in the Home

- Whenever possible, open windows and operate fans to increase ventilation.
- Avoid cigarette smoking in the home.
- Test for radon; consult an expert to reduce radon if levels are elevated.
- Regularly check that gas appliances are properly operating.
- Vent furnaces, fireplaces, wood stoves, clothes dryers, and gas space heaters to the outdoors.
- Operate an exhaust fan when using a gas stove.
- Use dehumidifiers in damp areas of house; if closets are damp, keep an electric light lit inside the closets at all time to prevent mold.
- Use antimold tile cleaners in the bathroom.
- Change filters on heating and air conditioning systems according to manufacturer's recommendations.
- Avoid idling car inside a garage.
- Have asbestos removed by qualified professionals; do not handle it yourself.
- Keep dust levels down by frequent dusting with a damp cloth and eliminating dust catchers.
- Do not leave food on counters or garbage indoors overnight.
- Vacuum at least twice a week.
- Avoid consuming water (for drinking or cooking) from the hot water tap (heat makes lead in pipes more soluble).
- Consider installing a water purification system, preferably a reverse-osmosis unit.

- Remove peeling paint. Have it tested for lead and mercury, and if it is positive for these toxins, have the paint removed by a professional.
- Cover asbestos with plastic or duct tape, or have it removed by a professional.
- Avoid storing unneeded chemicals. When chemicals must be stored, ensure that they are in a well-ventilated area and out of the reach of children.
- Limit close exposure to electrical appliances (e.g., microwave ovens, VCR, electric blankets). Unplug appliances when not in use to prevent the existence of an electrical field.
- Control noise levels by replacing noisy appliances with quiet ones, installing acoustical tile ceilings, avoiding toys that make loud sounds. "White sound" or sleep sound generators can be purchased to camouflage or suppress noise.
- Avoid using aerosol products.
- Air dry-cleaned clothes outdoors for a day to reduce exposure to tetrachloroethylene (solvent used in dry cleaning that can have harmful effects).
- Leave windows open for two days in rooms where wall-to-wall carpeting has recently been installed.
- Do not use dishes or cookware that has been painted or glazed with lead paint. (Old dishes and pottery often have lead paint.)

BOX 6-6

Resources for Information About Protecting the Home

ALLERGENS
Allergy Testing Association
4727 Wilshire Boulevard #610
Los Angeles, CA 90010
(800) 522-8877
American Academy of Allergy and Immunology
611 E. Wells Street
Milwaukee, WI 53202
(800) 822-2762
www.aaaai.org/index.html
American College of Allergy and Immunology
800 E. Northwest Highway #1080
Palatine, IL 60067
(708) 359-2800
www.aaaai.org/index.html
Asthma and Allergy Foundation of America
1717 Massachusetts Avenue NW #305
Washington, DC 20036
(202) 265-0265
www.aafa.org
Mothers of Asthmatics
10875 Main Street #210
Fairfax, VA 22030
(703) 385-1103
www.podi.com/health/aanma
National Foundation for the Chemically Hypersensitive
PO Box 222
Ophelia, VA 22530
(517) 697-3989
www.social.com/health/nhic/data/hr2400/hr2442.html
National Institute of Allergy and Infectious Diseases
National Institutes of Health
Building 31, #7A32
Bethesda, MD 20892
(301) 496-5717
www.niaid.nih.gov
ASBESTOS
Asbestos Victims of America
PO Box 559
Capitola, CA 95010
(408) 476-3646
www.social.com/health/nhic/data/hr1800/hr1899.html
Environmental Protection Agency
TS-799
401 M Street SW
Washington, DC 20460

Environmental Protection Agency's Asbestos
Hotline: (202) 554-1404
www.epa.gov
Publications:
  Asbestos in the Home
  Guidance for Controlling Asbestos-Containing Materials in Buildings
  Managing Asbestos in Place: A Building Owner's Guide to Operations and Maintenance Programs for Asbestos-Containing Materials
White Lung Association
PO Box 1483
Baltimore, MD 21203
(410) 243-5864
www.social.com/health/nhic/data/hr2100/hr2116.html
ELECTROMAGNETIC FIELDS
Bonneville Power Administration
PO Box 12999
Portland, OR 97212
(800) 547-6048
www.bpa.gov
Publications:
  Electric and Biological Effects of Transmission Lines: A Review
  Electric and Magnetic Fields from 60-Hertz Electric Power: What Do We Know About Possible Health Risks
  Electric Power Lines: Questions and Answers on Research into Health Effects
INDOOR AIR QUALITY
U.S. Consumer Product Safety Commission
Washington, DC 20207
www.cpsc.gov
Publication: *An Update on Formaldehyde*
Consumer Federation of America
1424 16th Street NW
Washington, DC 20036
www.inresco.com/Bcorgs_cfa.html
Publication: *Formaldehyde: Everything You Wanted to Know But Were Afraid to Ask*
Environmental Protection Agency
401 M Street SW
Washington, DC 20460
www.epa.gov
Publications:
  Indoor Air Facts No. 5: Environmental Tobacco Smoke
  The Inside Story: A Guide to Indoor Air Quality

Public Information Center
US Environmental Protection Agency
PM-211B
401 M Street SW
Washington, DC 20460
www.epa.gov/earth100/records/a0115.html
Publication: *Residential Air-Cleaning Devices: A Summary of Available Information*

LEAD PAINT
For guidelines on lead removal:
Alliance to End Childhood Lead Poisoning
600 Pennsylvania Avenue SE
Suite 100
Washington, DC 20003
www.aeclp.org
Parents Against Lead
28 East Ostend Street
Baltimore, MD 21230
(410) 727-4226

NOISE
CertainTeed Corporation
PO Box 860
Valley Forge, PA 19482
www.certainteed.com
Publication: *Fire Resistance and Sound Control Guide*
Owens Corning
Insulation Operating Division
One Owens Corning Parkway
Toledo, OH 43659
www.owenscorning.com
Publication: *Noise Control Design in Residential Construction*
Manville Building Materials Corporation
Ken-Caryl Ranch
Denver, CO 80217
www.schuller.com
Publication: *Sound Control*
Mineral Insulation Manufacturers Association
1420 King Street
Alexandria, VA 22314
Publication: *Sound Control for Commercial and Residential Buildings*

PESTICIDES
Environmental Protection Agency
401 M Street SW
Washington, DC 20460
Environmental Protection Agency's Pesticide Hotline: (800) 858-7378
www.epa.gov
Publications:
   A Citizen's Guide to Pesticides
   Consumer's Guide to Safer Pesticide Use

RADON
Environmental Protection Agency
401 M Street SW
Washington, DC 20460
Environmental Protection Agency's Radon Hotline (800) SOS-RADO(N)
www.epa.gov
Publications:
   A Citizen's Guide to Radon; What It Is and What to Do About It.
   Application of Radon Reduction Methods
   Radon Reduction Methods: A Homeowner's Guide

WATER
Information on water testing laboratories:
American Association for Laboratory Accreditation
656 Quince Orchard Road
Gaithersburg, MD 20878
(301) 670-1377
www.a21a.org
Information on certified water purification system dealers:
Water Quality Association
4151 Naperville Road
Lisle, IL 60532
(708) 505-0160
www.wqa.org
Information on well water:
American Groundwater Trust
National Well Water Association
6375 Riverside Drive
Dublin, OH 43017
(800) 423-7748
www.h2o-ngwa.org
Environmental Protection Agency's Safe Drinking Water Hotline: (800) 426-4791

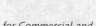

Relationships are a two-way street—in other words, one must be a good friend to promote a good friendship. Chronically ill individuals should try to develop interests and engage in conversations beyond their illnesses. This is not to imply that it is inappropriate to discuss health problems with significant others, but relationships with family and friends should not be limited to caregiving or "counseling" sessions. Although loved ones may be patient and accept illness-focused relationships, they may begin to view the relationship as a burden rather than a joy and perhaps avoid interactions. Likewise, chronically ill individuals need diversions from their illnesses and opportunities for relaxation and pleasure.

Related Diagnoses

The diagnoses pertinent to this chapter are those that either affect the client's perception of his or her health or that influence or alter health care behaviors.

Altered Health Maintenance

Description

Altered health maintenance refers to the inability to identify, seek, or engage in practices to maintain health. Factors that can contribute to this diagnosis include:
- impaired communication
- perceptual or cognitive impairment
- depression, anxiety
- impaired motor skills
- immobility
- worsening of chronic condition
- knowledge deficit
- religious, cultural beliefs
- ineffective family coping, family dysfunction
- threatened or actual loss of independence
- relocation
- unachieved developmental tasks
- insufficient financial resources, increased expenses
- substance abuse
- crisis

Client Goals
- to identify factor(s) responsible for altered health maintenance
- to describe at least one way to improve health maintenance
- to demonstrate at least one action to improve health maintenance

Interventions
- Discuss causative/contributing factors with client; guide client in identifying measures to improve health maintenance.
- Provide education to improve knowledge and skill.
- Assist client in fulfilling self-care needs (e.g., provide assistive device, arrange for personal care assistance, obtain financial aid).

- Ensure that client understands basic preventive health measures (e.g., principles of good nutrition, exercise program, self-examinations).
- Ensure that client possesses appropriate knowledge of chronic condition; provide education as necessary.
- Review signs and symptoms indicating complication or worsening of chronic condition, and resultant required actions.
- Help client identify and negotiate assistance of at least one support person or chronic care coach. Include this person in instructional activities.
- Teach client stress management and relaxation exercises as necessary.
- Assist family in developing effective communication patterns and coping strategies.
- Help client to recognize positive self-care practices. (Note: Clients with chronic illnesses may become discouraged that their conditions seem to be worsening despite their efforts; they will need assistance in recognizing that their actions do make a difference in that their conditions and general state of well-being may be superior to that which could have resulted without their actions.)
- Assist client in clarifying values and establishing goals.
- Refer client to appropriate resources (e.g., nutritionist, counselor, physical therapist, Medicaid office, Alcoholics Anonymous).

Risk for Infection

Description

A significant potential for pathogenic organisms to invade the individual constitutes a risk for infection. Chronically ill clients must develop more vigilant health maintenance strategies than healthy individuals if they want to avoid infections or recover from them. A variety of factors can cause chronically ill individuals to be vulnerable to infection, including:

- altered antigen-antibody reaction
- advanced age
- malnutrition
- immobility
- poor infection control practices
- invasive procedures
- effects of medications
- unhealthy environment
- altered cognition

Client Goals

- to verbalize and demonstrate practices to prevent infection
- to describe signs and symptoms of infection
- to be free from infection

Interventions

- Assess client's knowledge of infection prevention measures (e.g., handwashing, good hygienic practices, proper food handling and storage);

educate as needed.
- Promote good nutritional state.
- Encourage multivitamin supplements to promote a healthy nutritional state and improve immune response.
- Promote good, intact skin status.
- Advise client to avoid exposure to persons with suspected or known infections.
- Encourage client to obtain immunizations as appropriate.
- Help client to safely use the herb echinacea, which has been proven to be an effective immunity booster and antiinfective agent (Melchart et al., 1994).
- Guide client in use of relaxation exercises and imagery (Rider et al., 1990) directed at immunity boosting.
- Teach client signs and symptoms of infection and reporting process. (Note: Older clients can demonstrate altered signs of infection. For example, fever may be apparent at lower levels than what occurs with younger persons and pain may be absent or atypical. Altered cognition could be the first clue that an infection is present.)
- Encourage client to maintain clean, safe environment.
- Educate caregivers in infection prevention and control measures as needed.
- Aid in reducing risk of antibiotic resistance by using alternative to antibiotics when feasible (e.g., the natural antibiotic herb echinacea; homeopathic remedies).

Acquired Immune Deficiency Syndrome (AIDS)

Description

AIDS is a severe immune deficiency disease that results from the human immunodeficiency virus (HIV). As the virus attaches to and depletes the specialized white blood cells T4 or helper T cells, the immune response is hindered and the client is at risk for opportunistic infections.

To date, HIV is known to be transmitted through body secretions (e.g., blood, semen, vaginal secretions, breast milk, saliva, cerebrospinal fluid, tears, urine). High-risk groups for AIDS include homosexual males, IV drug users, babies born to infected mothers, and people who received blood transfusions prior to 1985.

The Centers for Disease Control and Prevention (CDC) defines AIDS as an illness characterized by one or more indicator diseases (specific cancers or opportunistic infections) and laboratory evidence of HIV infection (Box 6-7).

AIDS is a complex disease that not only affects multiple body systems, but also has a significant impact on psychosocial and spiritual health. Multiple diagnoses can be associated with this disease including: high risk for infection, ineffective breathing pattern, altered nutrition (less than body requirements), diarrhea, impaired skin integrity, altered thought processes, pain, activity intolerance, risk for injury, fatigue, spiritual distress, social isolation, body image disturbance, powerlessness, hopelessness and knowledge deficit.

BOX 6-7	Centers for Disease Control and Prevention Guidelines for Diagnosis of AIDS

Presence of one or more of the following indicator diseases *without laboratory evidence of HIV infection*:
- bronchitis, pneumonitis, or esophagitis of more than one month's duration
- candidiasis of esophagus, trachea, bronchi, lung
- extrapulmonary cryptococcosis
- cryptosporidiosis with diarrhea persisting more than 1 month
- cytomegalovirus (CMV) of an organ other than the liver, spleen, or lymph nodes in person older than one month of age
- herpes simplex virus ulcers persisting more than 1 month
- Kaposi's sarcoma in person under age 60
- lymphoid interstitial pneumonia, pulmonary lymphoid hyperplasia, or both (LIP/PLH complex) in person under age 13
- disseminated *Mycobacterium avium* or *M. kansasii* infection at a site other than or in addition to the lungs, skin, or cervical or hilar lymph nodes
- Pneumocystis carinii pneumonia (PCP)
- progressive multifocal leukoencephalopathy
- toxoplasmosis of the brain in person younger than one month of age

Presence of one or more of the above indicator diseases or one or more of the following indicator diseases with a positive test for HIV:
- disseminated coccidioidomycosis at a site other than or in addition to the lungs or cervical or hilar lymph nodes
- HIV encephalopathy
- disseminated histoplasmosis at a site other than the lungs
- isosporiasis with diarrhea persisting longer than 1 month
- Kaposi's sarcoma
- primary lymphoma of the brain
- other non-Hodgkin's lymphoma of B-cell or unknown immunologic phenotype
- disseminated mycobacterial disease caused by other than *M. tuberculosis* at a site other than or in addition to the lungs, skin, or cervical or hilar lymph nodes
- extrapulmonary disease caused by *M. tuberculosis*, involving at least one site
- recurrent Salmonella (nontyphoid) septicemia
- HIV wasting syndrome (emaciation)

Presumptive diagnosis of one or more of the following indicator diseases with positive test for HIV:
- candidiasis of the esophagus
- CMV retinitis with vision loss
- Kaposi's sarcoma
- LIP/PLH complex in a person under age 13
- disseminated mycobacterial disease (acid-fast bacilla with species not identified by culture) involving at least one site other than or in addition to the lungs, skin, or cervical or hilar lymph nodes
- PCP
- toxoplasmosis of the brain in a patient older than 1 month of age

Client Goals

- to be free from secondary infection
- to learn and practice infection control measures
- to verbalize signs and symptoms of infection and other complications
- to possess intact skin and oral mucous membrane
- to be free from pain/utilize effective pain control measures
- to breathe effectively
- to consume adequate nutrition (state specific requirements) and fluid
- to maintain body weight within ideal range
- to utilize protection to practice sex safely
- to verbalize feelings and needs
- to learn about and utilize community resources
- to utilize measures to boost immune function

Interventions

- Provide education about the disease and its care; review the following:
  - infection control practices
  - mouth care
  - skin care
  - medications (Box 6-8)
  - diet: importance of maintaining adequate nutritional intake to prevent weight loss and infection; benefit of eating small, frequent meals; high-calorie, high-protein foods
  - safe sexual practices
  - balance of activity and rest
- Assist client in locating community resources (e.g., Meals on Wheels, hospice, counseling).
- Encourage client to express feelings; refer for counseling as indicated.
- Teach progressive relaxation, meditation, and other stress management practices.
- Use massage and guided imagery to relax the client and promote a sense of well-being. (Note: massage for clients with AIDS may need to be modified to avoid rapid, deep massage that could overstimulate the adrenal system.)
- Refer client to counseling for addiction, if appropriate.
- Guide client in clarifying values and identifying a sense of purpose in life.
- Assist client in using alternative therapies wisely. (Note: One study reported that 40% of HIV-infected individuals used alternative therapies (Anderson et al., 1993); it is beneficial to ensure that clients are using safe therapies and not fads or high-risk therapies that are of little value.)
- If candidiasis is a problem, encourage nutritional interventions to control these yeast infections, such as reducing intake of simple carbohydrates and sugars, increasing complex carbohydrates, and adding garlic to the diet. Cultured dairy products (e.g., low-fat yogurt) and supplemental lactobacillus acidophilus can facilitate good bacteria growth while yeast is being controlled.

- Encourage good nutrition. Review with nutritionist or alternative specialist the value of supplements. (One study showed that HIV-infected mothers who were deficient in vitamin A were significantly more likely to transfer the virus to their babies than nondeficient mothers [Semba et al., 1994]).
- Help client to wisely use herbs that have an antiinfective action (e.g., echinacea, garlic, Chinese bitter melon, lentinan [extract of shitake mushroom], ginseng).
- Consult with acupuncturist regarding benefit of acupuncture in increasing immune function.
- Provide client with information on resources to find additional information and assistance, such as those listed in Box 6-9.

BOX 6-8   Examples of Medications Used for HIV-Related Infections

Co-trimoxazole (Septra, Bactrim): Drug of choice for treatment of Pneumocystis carinii pneumonia (PCP). Adverse effects include: pallor; fatigue, weakness; skin peeling, rash, redness; unusual bleeding, bruising; yellowing of eyes and skin; aching joints and muscles; anorexia, nausea, vomiting; photosensitivity.

Pentamidine (Lomidine, Pentam 300): May be used if client is allergic to sulfa drugs or if co-trimoxazole is ineffective. Can cause severe hypotension while being injected. Adverse effects include reduced WBC count, high risk for infections; unusual bleeding, bruising; drowsiness; flushed, dry skin; increased voiding, thirst; nausea, vomiting, metallic taste in mouth; fatigue, weakness; blurred vision; altered cognition, hallucinations: headache, dizziness.

Zidovudine (Retrovir): Can limit replication of HIV to slow progression of disease; used in HIV positive persons who do not have AIDS. Adverse effects include chills, fever, pallor, sore throat, unusual bleeding or bruising; fatigue, weakness; altered taste perception, anorexia, nausea, vomiting, diarrhea; insomnia, restlessness, agitation; rash. (Most adverse effects subside within several weeks of therapy.) Long-term use can cause anemia and granulocytopenia; dosage may be decreased if granulocyte count decreases and increased when count rises.

BOX 6-9

Resources for Information About Assistance with AIDS

AIDS Alternative Health Project
3223 N. Sheffield Avenue
Chicago, IL 60657
(312) 327-6437

AIDS Health Project
Box 0884
San Francisco, CA 94143
(415) 476-6430

Cure Now
PO Box 29386
Los Angeles, CA 90026
(213) 660-7563

Gay Men's Health Crisis
PO Box 274
129 West 20th Street
New York, NY 10011
(212) 807-6655
www.gmhc.org

HEAL
16 East 16th Street
New York, NY 10003
(212) 674-HOPE
www.aidsnyc.org/heal/index.htm

Health Education Resource Organization (HERO)
101 West Read Street
Suite 825
Baltimore, MD 21201
(410) 685-1180
www.carr.lib.md.us/comminfo/H/F000023.htm

Mothers of AIDS Patients (MAP)
PO Box 3132
San Diego, CA 92013
(619) 234-3432

National AIDS Hotline
Centers for Disease Control (CDC)
(800) 342-AIDS
www.cac.gov/nchstp/od/hotline.htm

National AIDS Network
2033 M Street NW
Suite 800
Washington, DC 20036
(202) 293-2437

National Association of People with AIDS (NAPA)
1413 K Street NW
Suite 7
Washington, DC 20005
(202) 898-0414
www.thecure.org

Pneumonia

Description

Pneumonia is a severe inflammation of the lungs that can involve part of the lung (lobular or segmental), the entire lung (lobar), or the alveoli adjacent to the bronchi (bronchopneumonia).

The very young and the elderly are more highly susceptible to developing pneumonia. Other high-risk groups include persons with chronic respiratory conditions, debilitated individuals, and immune-compromised persons, including those with AIDS and substance abusers. Clients who chronically use antibiotics may be susceptible to the devastating effects of pneumonia due to pathogens becoming resistant to common antibiotics.

The pattern of onset varies, with pneumococcal and Klebsiella pneumonias having a rapid onset accompanied by shaking and chills, and staphylococcal pneumonias developing slowly and subtly. General signs include the following: fever; rapid, shallow respirations; elevated pulse; productive cough; restricted chest movement; chest pain; cyanosis; nausea, vomiting; anorexia, weight loss; altered mental status; abnormal breath sounds; dull percussion sounds over affected area; elevated WBCs; and radiologic evidence of consolidation.

Age-related changes can alter the clinical presentation of symptoms in older adults. For example, lower normal body temperature in some older adults can cause fever to be manifested at temperatures that may not cause alarm in younger persons, and altered pain sensations can cause a significant infection to be present without chest pain. Often, confusion and weight loss are apparent before other clinical signs.

Client Goals

- to recover from pneumonia
- to regain or maintain patent airway
- to obtain adequate rest and sleep
- to be free from pain and anxiety
- to be free from secondary complications of pneumonia
- to learn and demonstrate measures to prevent pneumonia

Interventions

- Refer for and assist with diagnostic tests to confirm diagnosis and evaluate ongoing status.
- Administer and/or teach client to administer prescribed medications (e.g., antibiotics, analgesics, antipyretics, expectorants, cough suppressants).
- Observe and teach client to recognize signs of complications.
- Encourage adequate hydration, nutritional status, for instance:
  - encourage intake of fresh garlic, cayenne peppers, and chili peppers, which can be effective in preventing and treating pneumonia.
  - avoid dairy and processed foods.
  - promote good intake of vitamins A and C, beta-carotene, and zinc.
- Assist client in loosening and removing secretions through the use of:
  - the juice of fruit and yellow and green vegetables.
  - the herbs lobelia and saguinaria.
  - chest massage, especially using a tapping action.
- Help client to wisely use herbs that have an antiinfective action (e.g., echinacea, hydrastis, uva ursi).
- Instruct client in deep breathing exercises to promote good ventilation and movement of secretions; encourage yoga exercises.
- Teach client infection control practices.
- Assist client in controlling pain and anxiety; strategies might include guided imagery, progressive relaxation, touch therapy, and/or music.
- Use aromatherapy with essential oils of eucalyptus, camphor, lavender, lemon, or teatree.
- Ensure client has received pneumococcal and influenza vaccinations unless contraindicated. (At one time it was believed that one pneumo-

coccal vaccine would last a lifetime, but the current recommendation is for revaccination every six years for those who are chronically ill.)
- Instruct client in measures to prevent and identify signs of pneumonia.

Risk for Injury

Description

Risk for injury refers to the potential for accidental injury or trauma because of perceptual, cognitive or physiologic alteration. A variety of factors can contribute to the risk for injury, including:
- altered cognition or level of consciousness
- immobility
- impaired sensory function
- fatigue
- debilitated state
- dependency on others for caregiving and protection
- poor coordination
- gait disturbance
- incontinence
- knowledge deficit regarding safe practices
- unsafe behaviors (e.g., smoking in bed, driving while experiencing effects of drugs)
- advanced age (e.g., slower response and reaction time, sensory changes)
- physiological and psychological immaturity to protect self
- malnutrition
- unsafe use of medications, adverse effects of medications
- use of special equipment (e.g., oxygen, lift, wheelchair, IVs)
- environmental hazards (e.g., malfunctioning appliances, clutter, leaks)
- unfamiliar environment
- incapable or careless caregiver

Client Goals
- to be free from injury
- to learn and use measures to prevent injury
- to improve status in order to protect against injury

Interventions
- Assess risk factors for injury; discuss with client.
- Assist client in reducing risk for injury, e.g.:
  - teach safe self-care practices
  - improve general health status
  - ensure use of eyeglasses, hearing aids
  - orient to new surroundings
- Evaluate home safety. Recommend improvements to environment to promote safety; refer for assistance as needed.

- Assist caregivers of cognitively impaired client to safeguard environment.
- Educate caregivers as needed.
- Ensure that alternative therapies are used safely (e.g., treatments obtained from certified or competent therapists, not ingesting herbal preparation intended for topical use, heeding precautions, advising therapists of medical conditions prior to engaging in treatments).

Falls

Description

Many of the effects of chronic illnesses can increase the risk for falls; some of these effects include postural hypotension, altered cognition, weakness, dizziness, poor vision, altered mobility, paralysis, edema, and pain. Antihypertensives, antipsychotics, sedatives, and other medications that may be used by clients can produce side effects that contribute to falls. The inability to maintain a safe home can create risks that promote falls. Equipment intended to be assistive (such as wheelchairs, canes, and walkers) can be a source of falls. Also, the unsafe practices (e.g., leaving clutter on the floor or failing to clean a spill) or lack of a timely response by caregivers can facilitate falls. Once a client has fallen, the risk of future falls increases. Some clients may become sufficiently anxious after they've experienced a fall that they unnecessarily impose restrictions on themselves to avoid future falls.

Client Goals

- to be free from falls
- to identify and reduce risk factors for falls
- to learn and use appropriate measures when a fall occurs

Interventions

- Assess client's risk for falls; plan strategies to minimize specific risks (e.g., if client has postural hypotension, teach how to change positions slowly; if vision is poor, encourage client to wear glasses at all times and have rooms well lighted).
- Evaluate environment for factors contributing to falls and assist client in reducing these risks; ensure that environment is safe, e.g.:
  - no loose carpeting
  - good lighting
  - nonslippery floor and tub surfaces
  - handrails in stairways
- Advise client to wear safe shoes and clothing.
- Instruct client in ways to fall safely when a fall is unavoidable.
- Advise client that when a fall occurs ensure that no injury is present before moving. (Be aware that fractures may not be apparent immediately following the fall; signs may be evident after client resumes activity.)
- For clients who are alone and at high risk for falling, recommend use of an emergency alarm system that can be worn on their person to use in the event that they fall and need help.

- Teach caregivers proper lifting and transfer techniques and other measures to reduce risk for falls.
- Monitor clinical status for effects of the disease, medications, and treatments that could promote falls; assist client in correcting problem as appropriate.

Risk for Poisoning

Description

Risk for poisoning refers to the accentuated risk of accidental exposure or ingestion of drugs or dangerous products in doses sufficient to cause harm.

Client Goals

- to be free from poisoning
- to be free from harmful effects of drugs
- to identify and reduce risks for poisoning

Interventions

- Identify risks for poisoning, e.g.:
  - altered cognitive or emotional state
  - poor vision
  - polypharmacy
  - large amount of drugs in home
  - misuse of herbal remedies or other nutritional products
  - environmental hazards (lead paint, contaminated drinking supply)

Plan interventions to reduce specific risks.

- Ensure that medications are used appropriately (Box 6-10):
  - Recommend use of alternative therapies rather than drugs when appropriate (e.g., massages rather than tranquilizers, echinacea rather than antibiotics, ginger rather than an antiemetic drug, progressive relaxation rather than an antihypertensive drug); consult with physician as to appropriateness of alternative therapy.
  - Ensure that drugs are prescribed in appropriate doses, remembering that older adults may require smaller doses than other age groups.
  - Review drugs for drug-drug and drug-food interactions; consult with pharmacist as needed.
  - Evaluate effects of drugs to ensure that they continue to be of therapeutic value and are producing greater benefit than harm.
  - Instruct client in proper administration, recognition of adverse effects, and interactions.
- Ensure that herbal remedies are used correctly (refer to Box 5-20 for specific precautions).
- Refer client for screening for toxicity from lead, mercury, and other toxins as needed.

BOX 6-10   Considerations for Maximizing Benefits from Medications

Medications are widely used in the treatment of chronic diseases. It is not uncommon to find that a client is consuming multiple drugs daily, on a long-term basis. The chronic use of medications can create unique problems. For instance:

- as new medications are added to the set of drugs already used, there can be a greater risk for interactions, particularly if the health care practitioner does not review the complete medication history prior to prescribing a drug, or if the client begins using an over-the-counter drug without having the potential for interactions reviewed;
- as the client ages or the status of the disease changes, drug dosages may become inappropriate.

Further, health care providers may not be 100% conscientious in overseeing drug therapy. For instance, the Physician Insurers Association of America in an analysis of malpractice claims discovered most errors, in frequency of occurrence, to be (Crane, 1993):

27.2% incorrect dose

24.9% inappropriate drug for condition

20.6% failure to monitor for side effects

18.1% poor communication by physician

13.2% failure to monitor drug levels

13.2% lack of knowledge about drug

13.0% failure to use most appropriate drug

12.7% inappropriate length of treatment

12.5% failure to monitor drug's effectiveness

12.2% inadequate medication history

 9.9% inadequate notes in chart

 9.7% failure to notice allergy toward drug

In order to maximize the benefits and reduce the risks associated with medications, measures should be taken to:

Ensure that drugs are used only as necessary and not when nonpharmacologic measures can substitute. Many alternative therapies can assist clients to manage symptoms and maintain health without the risks associated with drugs. For instance, progressive relaxation can help to keep blood pressure under control; biofeedback, touch therapy, and acupuncture can control pain; echinacea and other herbs can boost immunity to fight infections; and meditation, massage, and guided imagery can relieve stress.

Determine if dosages are appropriate. Most people with chronic illnesses are of advanced age; drug absorption, metabolism, detoxification, and excretion can be altered due to resulting age-related changes. Dosages that are appropriate for a middle-aged individual can be excessive for an older person, thus they may need to be adjusted. Consideration also must be given to adjusting the dosage of any drug that has been used by the client for several years to accommodate for aging-related changes.

(continued)

Prevent drug-drug and drug-food interactions. Many of the drugs commonly used for chronic conditions can interact with each other. Due to the scope and complexity of these interactions, computer cross-checks for interactions or consultation with a pharmacist can be beneficial. Clients should be advised to use the services of a single pharmacy that can maintain a drug profile and perform interaction checks.

Create an informed consumer. Clients should be helped in gaining knowledge regarding the purpose, proper administration, precautions, side effects, interactions, adverse reactions to report, and special storage requirements for every drug used. Clients should be encouraged to keep a record of all drugs (prescription and nonprescription) used for their own reference and to review this record with their health care providers (Figure 6-1).

Encourage the use of the body's internal healing system to maximize the benefits of the drug. Beliefs and expectations regarding a drug's benefit can influence the body's reaction to the drug, demonstrated by the placebo effect. Clients should understand the therapeutic intent of the drugs they take and have confidence that these effects will be achieved. Guided imagery can assist in enhancing the outcomes of medications by helping clients to develop an image of the actions of the drug on the body and the intended response.

Noncompliance

Description

The personal choice to reject or deviate from advice given by health care professionals is considered noncompliance. Many factors can cause clients to fail to comply with recommended health practices, including:

- altered cognition or mood
- physical limitation, pain
- knowledge deficit
- poor motivation
- limited finances
- insufficient support systems
- family dysfunction
- nonassertiveness
- conflict between recommended health practices and values or belief system
- lack of confidence in therapy or therapist

Client Goals

- to verbalize understanding of benefits of complying with therapy and risks in not doing so
- to identify obstacles to compliance and measures to minimize them
- to demonstrate compliance with care plan, self-care practices

Interventions

- Assist client in identifying obstacles to compliance and developing strategies to reduce or eliminate them, such as:

- improving knowledge of self-care techniques
- eliciting help of a chronic care coach, caregiver
- obtaining financial aid
- negotiating compromised care plan with therapist, physician
- learning assertiveness skills
- obtaining assistive devices
- controlling physical symptoms
- Encourage client to express feelings and concerns. Advocate on client's behalf as needed.
- Utilize guided imagery to help client visualize steps in achieving goals and outcomes.
- Offer positive reinforcement for desirable health care practices.
- Help client evaluate effectiveness and safety of alternative therapies. If necessary, consult with specialist in field (e.g., acupuncturist, homeopathic practitioner, herbalist), research (Internet, library searches); contact National Institute of Health's Office of Alternative Medicine (800-531-1794).
- Monitor health status to ensure that client does not develop complications.
- Recognize that adherence to the care plan can vary over time; therefore, ongoing assessment for noncompliance and prompt intervention are essential.

Medication	Dosage	Route	Administration time(s)	Purpose	Possible side effects	Unusual symptoms to report	Special precautions

FIGURE 6-1

Client's Drug Record.

References

Anderson W, et al.: Patient use and assessment of conventional and alternative therapies for HIV infection and AIDS, *AIDS* 7:561-66, 1993.

Associated Press: British physicists explore link of cancer, electromagnetic fields, *Baltimore Sun*, February 14, 1996, p 14A.

Crane M: The medication errors that get doctors sued, *Medical Economics*, November 22, 1993, pp. 36-41.

Garland FC: Occupational sunlight exposure and melanoma in the US Navy, *Archives of Environmental Health* 45:261-267, 1990.

Knasko SC: Ambient odor's effect on creativity, mood, and perceived health, *Chemical Senses* 17(1):27-35, 1993.

Kobrick JL and Fine BJ: Climate and human performance. In Osborne DJ, Gruneberg MM, eds: *The physical environment at work*, New York, 1983, John Wiley and Sons.

Ornstein R and Sobel D: *The healing brain*, New York, 1987, Simon and Schuster.

Melchart D, et al.: Immunomodulation with echinacea: a systematic review of controlled clinical trials, *Phytomedicine* 1:245-54, 1994.

Miller JF: *Coping with chronic illness: overcoming powerlessness*, Philadelphia, 1992, F.A. Davis.

Rider MS, et al.: Effect of immune system imagery on secretory IgA, *Biofeedback and Self-Regulation* 15(4):317-33, 1990.

Rose JE and Behm FM: Inhalation of vapor from black pepper extract reduces smoking withdrawal symptoms, *Drug and Alcohol Dependence* 34:225-29, 1994.

Semba RD, et al.: Maternal vitamin A deficiency and mother-to-child transmission of HIV-1, *Lancet* 343:1593-97, 1994.

Stanhope M: Economics of health care delivery. In Stanhope M and Lancaster J, eds: *Community health nursing: process and practice for promoting health*, St Louis, 1988, Mosby.

Stevenson C: The psychophysiological effects of aromatherapy massage following cardiac surgery, *Complementary Therapies in Medicine* 2(1):27-35, 1994.

Wilkinson S: Aromatherapy and massage in palliative care, *International Journal of Palliative Nursing* 1(1):21-30, 1995.

Recommended Readings

Amber RB: *Color therapy*, Santa Fe, 1983, Aurora Press.

Buckingham SL: *Practitioner's guide to neuropsychiatry of HIV/AIDS*, New York, 1998, Guilford Publishing Co.

Callen M: *Surviving AIDS*, New York, 1990, Harper Collins.

Campbell D: *Music and miracles*, Wheaton, IL, 1992, Quest Books.

Campbell D: *Music: physician for times to come*, Wheaton, IL, 1991, Quest Books.

Frandzel S: The sound of healing: the role of music, *Alternative and Complementary Therapies* 2(4):225-29, 1996.

Kohl M: Chemical sensitivity: the environmental illness controversy, *Alternative and Complementary Therapies* 2(1):42-45, 1996.

Lauritson J: *The AIDS war*, New York, 1993, Asklepios.

Liberman J: *Light: medicine of the future*, Santa Fe, 1993, Bear and Co. Publishing.

Lynn L: Alternative living with HIV: the Chinese medicine HIV treatment center, *Alternative and Complementary Therapies* 2(1):35-41, 1996.

Merritt S: *Mind, music, and imagery*, New York, 1990, Plume Press.

Muir M: Antibiotic resistance: the collapse of the miracle cure, *Alternative and Complementary Therapies* 2(3):140-144, 1996.

Murray M and Pizzorno J: *Encyclopedia of natural medicine*, Rocklin, CA, 1991, Prima Publishing.

Ott J: *Health and light*, Old Greenwich, CT, 1988, The Devin-Adair Co.

Root-Bernstein R: *Rethinking AIDS*, New York, 1993, The Free Press.

Spintge R: *Music medicine*, St Louis, 1992, MMB Music.

Stashower ME, et al.: Chaparral and liver toxicity, *Journal of the American Medical Association* 274(11):871-73, 1995.

Tomatis A: *The conscious ear*, Tarrytown, NY, 1991, Staton Hill Books.

Whipple B and Scura KW: The overlooked epidemic: HIV in older adults, *American Journal of Nursing* 96(2):22-29, 1996.

Nutrition and

Metabolic

*D*iet plays a central role in health and healing. Poor nutrition can be the source of chronic health problems, such as obesity and anemia. By the same token, careful attention to nutrients can help to keep a chronic condition under control, as is exemplified with dietary management of diabetes mellitus and diverticulosis.

Over the years attitudes and practices toward nutrition have changed. For instance, the consumption of red meat has declined, while grains, fruits, and vegetables have become the foundation of the healthy diet (Fig. 7-1). Vegetarian diets, once viewed as the practice of fringe populations, are now promoted as a healthy choice for the mainstream. The daily multivitamin has been replaced by a carefully selected group of supplements. The issue of toxins in the food chain have heightened concern over not only what we eat, but what we need to avoid.

Adherence to a special diet is required for some chronic conditions. Even without the need for a modified diet, persons with chronic conditions are challenged to use nutrition as a means to boost immunity, enhance energy, and optimize general function and well-being.

Assessment Considerations

A variety of subjective and objective data are used to assess nutritional status. These include:

- **Food intake and habits.** Clients can be asked to describe their eating patterns and preferences. A 24-hour record of intake on a typical day can provide insight into the types of foods consumed and schedule of eating. Specific questions can be asked regarding the consumption of alcohol and caffeine, snacking patterns, and special practices. The use of vitamins, minerals, and herbs should be noted. Religious restrictions should be reviewed, as well as the impact of finances on the ability to consume a healthy diet.
- **Clinical indicators.** The general appearance of the client can give clues to nutritional status. In addition to body size, the physical status of body organs and function can offer insights into nutritional status (Box 7-1). If the client demonstrates evidence of weakness, paralysis, or other signs that the independent preparation and consumption of food could be a problem, a determination needs to be made of assistance required by and available to the client. Further assessment indicators include the client's appraisal of appetite, digestion, and elimination patterns, as well as symptoms such as nausea, indigestion, and cramping.
- **Anthropometric assessment.** Height, weight, triceps skinfold measurement, and arm circumference yield insights into nutritional status. Changes in weight should be reviewed.
- **Biochemical assessment.** Laboratory evaluation of various body fluids and tissues can aid in identifying nutritional problems.

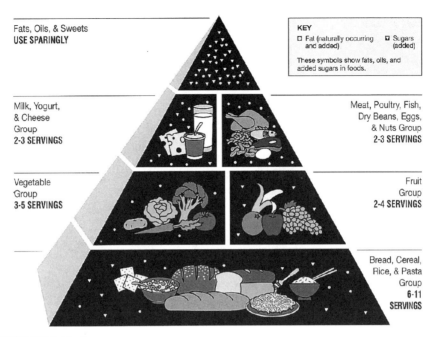

Fats, Oils, & Sweets
USE SPARINGLY

KEY
☐ Fat (naturally occurring   ☑ Sugars
   and added)   (added)
These symbols show fats, oils, and
added sugars in foods.

Milk, Yogurt,
& Cheese
Group
2-3 SERVINGS

Meat, Poultry, Fish,
Dry Beans, Eggs,
& Nuts Group
2-3 SERVINGS

Vegetable
Group
3-5 SERVINGS

Fruit
Group
2-4 SERVINGS

Bread, Cereal,
Rice, & Pasta
Group
6-11
SERVINGS

FIGURE 7-1

The Food Guide Pyramid. From U.S. Department of Agriculture: USDA's food guide pyramid, USDA Human Nutrition Information Pub No. 249, Washington, DC, 1992.

BOX 7-1	Signs Suggestive of Malnutrition

Skin: dry, rough, rash, flaky, swollen, excessively light or dark, petechiae, thin appearance

Hair: lack of shine, dull, dry, brittle, thin, falling out, color change

Face: depigmentation, dark areas under eyes, skin flaking, swelling, scaling around nostrils

Eyes: pale, dry, dull, redness of conjunctiva, bloodshot appearance

Lips: swelling, dryness, fissures

Tongue: swelling, bright red, smooth, sore, hypertrophic or atrophic papillae

Teeth: lost, loose, discolored, caries

Gums: receding, bleeding, soft, painful

Glands: enlarged thyroid or parotid

Nails: ridged, brittle, soft, spoon-shaped

Muscles: wasted appearance, weakness, tenderness

Pulse: tachycardia, abnormal rhythm

Blood pressure: elevated, excessively low

Mental status: confusion, irritability, depression

Physical status: fatigue, lethargy, headache, delayed healing, frequent infections, bruising, unplanned weight loss > 5% in one month, > 10% in 6 months

Determining Nutritional Needs

Age, height, activity level, and health status are among the factors considered in determining nutritional needs and a recommended daily allowance (RDA). Consultation with a nutritionist is beneficial in determining the ideal diet that meets a client's unique needs.

The issue of nutritional supplements is a controversial one. Increasingly, evidence emerges supporting the therapeutic value of supplements. The RDAs that have been in use are considered by many nutritional experts and alternative practitioners to be too low to meet the challenges of life today (e.g., stressful lifestyles, exposure to pollutants). Often, there are wide ranges offered by various therapists as to desirable RDA. Clinicians must keep this in mind and advise clients to use supplements carefully, reminding them that some supplements taken in high doses can produce serious adverse effects; one can get too much of a good thing! Box 7-2 offers a discussion of basic nutrients required for healthy living.

BOX 7-2	Nutrients for Healthy Living

RDA refers to the recommended dietary allowances as established by the Food and Nutrition Board of the National Research Council, National Academy of Sciences

EDA refers to the estimated dietary allowances for nutrients that do not have established RDA

Protein

Function: Large complex molecules made of amino acids, each of which has a specific function. General functions include building, repairing and maintaining body tissue, detoxifying harmful substances, producing antibodies, regulating acid-base balance

Sources: Complete proteins (provide all amino acids in proper amounts needed by body): meat and dairy products. Incomplete proteins (must be combined in certain ways or with a complete protein to provide correct balance of amino acids): nuts, grains, legumes

RDA: 70 gm, adult man; 60 gm, adult woman

Carbohydrates

Function: Provide energy for body

Sources: Simple carbohydrates: table sugars, fruits. Complex carbohydrates: starches (e.g., potatoes, rice, cereals)

RDA: No specific recommendation, although a high intake of complex carbohydrates and a low intake of simple carbohydrates are advisable

Fats

Function: Provide concentrated energy, help synthesize essential compounds in body, aid in control of body temperature

Sources: Whole-milk products, meats, eggs, nuts, peanut butter, olives, avocados, vegetable oils

RDA: No specific recommendation

Fat-Soluble Vitamins

Vitamin A (Retinol)

Function: Acts as antioxidant; promotes nonspecific resistance to infection, aids in production of lysozymes in tears, saliva and sweat that help fight bacteria; stimulates cell-mediated and humoral immunity, promotes good vision and healthy tissue and hair. Beta-carotene metabolizes into vitamin A in the body and is a stronger antioxidant than vitamin A

Sources: Milk, butter, liver, green and yellow vegetables

RDA: 5000 IU, men; 4000, women (Doses in excess of 10,000 IU per day during pregnancy have been shown to significantly increase the risk of birth defects); at least 15 mg of beta-carotene daily is recommended

Vitamin D

Function: Promotes strong bones and teeth, calcium-phosphorus metabolism; aids the immune system to some extent

Sources: Sunlight, egg yolk, organ meats, fish

RDA: 200 IU, 400 IU for pregnant women and for children

Vitamin E

Function: Institutes antioxidant properties that aid in the prevention of free radicals; enhances antibody production, maintains circulatory system; stronger immune-boosting effect when taken with selenium

Sources: Dark green vegetables, eggs, liver, wheat germ, vegetable oil, oatmeal, peanuts, tomatoes

RDA: 12 IU, 15 IU for pregnant and nursing women (although 100 IU recommended for cardiovascular and immune-boosting effect)

Vitamin F (Unsaturated fatty acids)

Function: Promotes healthy skin, blood coagulation, cholesterol, glandular activity

Sources: Sunflower seeds, vegetable oils

RDA: No specific recommendation

Vitamin K (Menadione)

Function: Blood clotting

Sources: Green leafy vegetables, yogurt, molasses

RDA: 80 mcg men; 65 mcg women

Water-Soluble Vitamins

Vitamin B_1 (Thiamine)

Function: Promotes resistance to infection, primary immunoglobulin response, digestion, cardiovascular function, energy production

Sources: Peas, lima beans, asparagus, corn, potatoes, blackstrap molasses, brown rice, meat, nuts, poultry, wheat germ

RDA: 1.5 mg

Vitamin B_2 (Riboflavin)

Function: Along with other B-complex vitamins, helps to maintain mucosal barriers that protect against infection; aids in production of antibodies and red blood cells, skin repair

Sources: Brewer's yeast, broccoli, spinach, asparagus, Brussels sprouts, peas, corn, blackstrap molasses, nuts, organ meats, whole grains

RDA: 1.7 mg   (continued)

Vitamin B$_6$ (Pyridoxine)

Function: Promotes health of mucous membranes and blood vessels; involved in antibody formation, red blood cell formation; affects immune function more than other B vitamins

Sources: Bananas, avocados, carrots, kale, spinach, sweet potatoes, apples, wheat germ, grains

RDA: 2-4 mg

Vitamin B$_{12}$ (Cobalamin)

Function: Aids development of red blood cells; maintains nervous system; believed to exert regulatory influence on T helper and suppressor cells

Sources: Cheese, fish, milk, milk products, organ meats, eggs

RDA: 2 mcg, 2.2 mcg for pregnant women

Niacin (Niacinamide, B$_3$)

Function: Converts food to energy; promotes healthy skin, nervous system, cell metabolism

Sources: Cereals, yeast, lean meat, liver, eggs

RDA: 19 mg men, 15 mg women, 17 mg pregnant women

Biotin (Vitamin H)

Function: Contributes to metabolism of protein, carbohydrates, and fats; promotes health of skin and circulatory system

Sources: Egg yolk, green leafy vegetables, milk, organ meats

EDA: 200 mcg

Vitamin C (Ascorbic Acid)

Function: Acts as antioxidant; promotes wound healing, healthy gums; believed to promote phagocytic function, boosting immunity (Linus Pauling claimed vitamin C was important in preventing common cold and influenza)

Sources: Citrus fruits, berries, green peppers, broccoli, Brussel sprouts, spinach

RDA: 60 mg, 70 mg pregnant women (many experts recommend 200 mg)

Folic Acid (Folacin, Folate, Vitamin B$_9$)

Function: Aids in production of red blood cells; enhances immune system, normal growth

Sources: green leafy vegetables, milk and other dairy products, organ meats, oysters, salmon, Brewer's yeast, dates, tuna, whole grains

RDA: 200 mcg, 400 mcg women of childbearing age

Pantothenic Acid

Function: Enhances immune system, promotes antibody formation; helps convert proteins, carbohydrates and fats into energy

Sources: Brewer's yeast, legumes, organ meats, salmon, wheat germ, whole grains, mushrooms

RDA: 5-10 mg

Choline (Lecithin)

Function: Regulates liver and gallbladder, cell membrane structure, nerve transmission

Sources: Yeast, eggs, fish, lecithin, wheat germ, organ meats, soy

RDA: No specific recommendation

Inositol

Function: Promotes metabolism of fat and cholesterol, nerve function

Sources: Molasses, yeast, lecithin, fruits, meat, milk, nuts

RDA: No specific recommendation

Para-aminobenzoic Acid (PABA)

Function: Contributes to pigmentation of skin, maintains hair color and health of blood vessel wall

Sources: Molasses, eggs, liver, milk, rice, yeast, wheat germ, bran

RDA: No specific recommendation

Vitamin P (Bioflavonoids)

Function: Supports maintenance of blood vessel wall

Sources: Skin and pulp of fruits

RDA: No specific recommendation

Minerals

Calcium

Function: Promotes growth and maintenance of teeth and bones, muscle contraction, nerve transmission

Sources: Milk, cheese, green vegetables

RDA: 800 mg, 1200 mg pregnant women and young adults

Chromium

Function: Assists carbohydrate metabolism, energy production, glucose utilization

Sources: Yeast, whole grains, vegetable oils

EDA: 200 mcg

Copper

Function: Aids in hemoglobin production, enzyme activity, protection from infection

Sources: Nuts, seeds, organ meats, raisins, molasses, seafood

EDA: 2 mg

Iodine

Function: Contributes to production of thyroid hormone, regulation of metabolism

Sources: Seafood, kelp, iodized salt

RDA: 150 mcg

Iron

Function: Transports oxygen to tissues, supports enzyme activity, immune function

Sources: Spinach, lima beans, peas, Brussel sprouts, broccoli, strawberries, asparagus, blackstrap molasses, eggs, fish, poultry, wheat germ, shredded wheat

RDA: 10 mg postmenopausal women and men, 15 mg premenopausal women, 30 mg pregnant women

Magnesium

Function: Supports enzyme activity, regulation of acid-base balance, glucose metabolism, nerve function, protein production; enhances immune system function

Sources: Honey, bran, green vegetables, nuts, seafood, spinach, kelp

RDA: 350 mg, men; 280 mg, women

(continued)

Manganese
Function: Aids in enzyme activity in reproduction, growth, fat metabolism; enhances immune system function
Sources: Whole grains, eggs, nuts, green vegetables
EDA: 2.5–5 mg

Phosphorus
Function: Contributes to formation of bones and teeth, muscle contraction, kidney function, nerve and muscle activity
Sources: Eggs, fish, meat, poultry, grains, cheese
RDA: 800 mg, 1200 mg young adults and pregnant women

Potassium
Function: Maintains fluid-electrolyte balance, pH balance of blood, nerve and muscle function
Sources: Dates, raisins, figs, peaches, sunflower seeds
EDA: 99 mg

Selenium
Function: Acts as antioxidant (with vitamin E), protects cell membrane, promotes humoral immunity, potentiates activity of phagocytes
Sources: Butter, wheat germ, whole grains, seafood, eggs, brown rice, apple cider, vinegar, garlic
RDA: 70 mcg (some experts recommend 200 mcg) Note: Excess doses (i.e., >400 mcg) are toxic.

Zinc
Function: Stimulates T cell immunity (but decreases phagocytic immunity), wound healing, development and growth of reproductive organs, production of male hormone
Sources: Brewer's yeast, liver, seafood, soybeans, spinach, sunflower seeds, mushrooms
RDA: 15 mg

Vegetarian Diets

As commented earlier, there was a time when vegetarian diets were viewed as being for people with specific religious beliefs or nonconforming attitudes. Today, increasing numbers of Americans are selecting vegetarian diets as an informed effort to improve their health status. Vegetarians tend to consume less total and saturated fat and cholesterol, and greater amounts of fiber and antioxidants than nonvegetarians, and have lower rates of cancer, heart disease, diabetes, obesity, hypertension, gallstones, and kidney stones (Messina and Messina, 1996).

There are several types of vegetarian diets (Table 7-1) that can be followed, a point clinicians must remember when assessing dietary patterns. Information regarding vegetarian diets can be obtained through dieticians and the organizations listed in Box 7-3.

TABLE 7-1
Types of Vegetarian Diets

Type	Foods Included	Foods Avoided
Lacto-ovo	Grains, legumes, nuts, seeds, vegetables, fruits, dairy products, eggs	Meat, poultry, fish
Vegan	Grains, legumes, nuts, seeds, vegetables, fruits	Meat, poultry, fish, dairy products, eggs, foods that have had animal products added or involve animal processing (e.g., white sugar, beer)
Macrobiotic	Grains, legumes, nuts, seeds, vegetables (particularly sea vegetables), soy products, some followers may include seafood	Meat, poultry, fish, dairy products, eggs, tropical fruits, vegetables of nightshade family, processed sweeteners
Fruitarian	Fruits, vegetables that are botanically fruits (tomatoes, eggplant, zucchini, avocado)	Meat, poultry, fish, dairy products, grains, legumes, most vegetables
Raw Foods	Fruits, vegetables, nuts, seeds, sprouted grains and beans in raw form, some followers may include raw dairy products	Meat, poultry, fish, cooked plant foods
Natural Hygiene	Raw vegetables and fruits, whole grains, legumes, nuts, seeds, sprouted grains	Meat (although this varies), dairy products, eggs

BOX 7-3
Resources for Information About Vegetarianism

American Vegan Society
501 Old Harding Highway
Malaga, NJ 08328
(609) 694-2887
www.social.com/health/nhic/data/hr0100/hr01
14.html
North American Vegetarian Society
PO Box 72
Dolgeville, NY 13329
(518) 568-7970
www.cyberveg.org/navs

Vegetarian Education Network (VE Net)
PO Box 3347
West Chester, PA 19381
Vegetarian Nutrition Dietetic Practice Group
c/o American Dietetic Association
216 West Jackson Boulevard
Suite 800
Chicago, IL 60606
www.eatright.org
Vegetarian Resource Group
PO Box 1463
Baltimore, MD 21203
(410) 366-8343
www.vrg.org

Food Allergies

Many individuals possess chronic symptoms that could be associated with food allergies. A food allergy is an abnormal response, a hypersensitivity, to a food. For the person with a food allergy, when the food is digested, it triggers the production of specific immunoglobulin E (IgE). The IgE is released and attaches to the surface of mast cells. The next time the food is consumed, it interacts with the IgE on the surface of the mast cells and stimulates the release of histamine, which causes symptoms of food allergy (Box 7-4).

In adults, the most common foods that cause allergic reactions include shellfish, crayfish, lobster, crab, peanuts, walnuts, fish, and eggs. In children, the most common causes of food allergy are eggs, milk, and peanuts.

Sometimes, diagnosis is simple in that the reaction clearly is linked to the intake of a specific food. However, sometimes the history alone cannot isolate the responsible food, and diagnostic testing is warranted; these tests can include a scratch skin test (contraindicated in persons with extensive eczema and severe allergic reactions) and blood tests (e.g., RAST, ELISA).

Avoiding the food that is responsible for the reaction is the treatment used for food allergy. This appears simple on the surface, but in some situations, the food can be missed because it is a small ingredient in another product. For instance, someone with an egg allergy may avoid eating an egg dish but not consider that the dressing they put on their salad or a soup they are eating has been made with eggs. Advise clients to check the labels of the foods they eat.

Nutrition and The Healing Process

Although the general principles of healthy eating have been widely publicized, it is helpful to reinforce them for clients in an effort to promote health. Issues helpful to reinforce include the following:

- avoiding an overweight condition by balancing intake with energy expenditure
- increasing fiber intake
- reducing daily fat consumption to less than 30% of caloric intake, reducing saturated fats
- increasing consumption of whole grains, vegetables and fruits and reducing animal foods

BOX 7-4	Symptoms of Food Allergy	
Vomiting		Sneezing
Diarrhea		Runny nose
Abdominal pain		Dyspnea
Urticaria		Asthma
Swelling		Anaphylaxis

- substituting natural complex carbohydrates for refined, processed sugars
- consuming caffeine and sodium in moderation

In addition to promoting a healthy state, some nutrients are believed to have a role in the treatment of specific diseases. Some of these are discussed below.

Cancer

- High levels of beta-carotene have been shown to be protective against squamous cell carcinoma of the lung (Mendes et al., 1986).
- High dietary intake of folate protects against colorectal cancer (Giovannucci et al., 1993).
- Some studies have found persons with cancer to have lower levels of selenium than healthy individuals, suggesting the importance of this nutrient (Combs, 1989).
- Oral and throat cancer rates were lower in persons who regularly took vitamin E supplements than in persons who did not (Grudley et al., 1992).

Cardiovascular Disease

- Studies have shown that beta-carotene is useful in the prevention and treatment of cardiovascular disease. One study revealed that myocardial infarction victims had lower levels of beta-carotene than a control group (Kardinaal et al., 1993).
- Persons with intermittent claudication experienced an improvement in their conditions when they used inositol nicotinate (O'Hara et al., 1988).
- A group of hypertensive men who took chromium for several months experienced a rise in HDL cholesterol (Roeback et al., 1991).
- Persons who had undergone coronary angioplasty who used fish oil had a reduced rate of arterial blockage as compared to persons who did not use fish oil (Gapinski et al., 1993). Fish oil also has been shown to maintain normal coagulation and reduce blood pressure in hypertensive individuals (Morris et al., 1993).
- Persons with atrial fibrillation who were given magnesium recovered more quickly than those persons who did not receive the mineral (Brodsky et al., 1994).
- Persons who received magnesium after a myocardial infarction lived longer than persons not receiving magnesium (Woods and Fletcher, 1994).
- Several studies have shown that people who took at least 100 IUs of vitamin E daily had lower rates of coronary artery disease than those who did not use the supplement (Rimm et al., 1993).

Respiratory Disease

- Smokers who had a high consumption of fish had less COPD as compared to smokers without high consumption (Shahar et al., 1994).
- Fish oil helped persons with cystic fibrosis experience an improvement in lung function (Lawrence and Sorrell, 1993).

Musculoskeletal Disease

- The use of fish oil by persons with rheumatoid arthritis resulted in a reduction in morning stiffness and pain, and an improvement in grip strength (Cleland et al., 1988).

Gastrointestinal Disease

- Persons with ulcerative colitis who took fish oil gained weight and had improvement in intestinal tissue (Stenson et al., 1992).

Neurologic Disease

- A group of individuals with multiple sclerosis who ate a low-fat diet and were followed for over 30 years demonstrated less deterioration, higher levels of function, and lower death rates than persons with multiple sclerosis who didn't reduce fat intake (Swank and Dugan, 1990).
- A prospective study of a group of nurses showed those taking vitamin C supplements had a decreased incidence of cataracts (Hankinson et al., 1992).

Clinicians should be aware of special diets that have received wide popularity in recent years (Box 7-5). The risks and benefits of these diets should be reviewed with the client's physician and nutritionist to determine the appropriateness for the client.

As time progresses, knowledge will increase regarding the therapeutic role of nutrients. Clinicians and chronically ill individuals need to be alert to new research findings.

Boosting Immunity

The promotion of immunologic health is important to persons with chronic illnesses because many of these conditions compromise immune functioning (Box 7-6). An important goal in chronic care is to boost immune functioning, and there are several steps clients can take to achieve this goal:

Diet

Diet can influence immune functioning. Some of the foods that have a positive effect on immunity include: milk, yogurt, nonfat cottage cheese, eggs, fresh fish, fruits, vegetables, grains, nuts, garlic, onion, sprouts, pure honey, and unsulfured molasses.

BOX 7-5   Popular Diets

Atkins Diet

Purposes: weight reduction and maintenance; cardiac health

Features:

- low carbohydrates
- pure proteins (meat, fish, fowl, shellfish)
- pure fats (butter, olive oil, mayonnaise)
- combinations of proteins and fats (mainstay of diet)
- use of nutritional supplements

Dr. Dean Ornish's Life Choice Diet

Purposes: weight reduction; cardiac health; reversing cardiac disease

Features:

- less than 10% diet from fat
- high complex carbohydrates
- high fiber
- vegetarian
- eat beans, legumes, fruits, grains, vegetables until hunger satisfied
- eat nonfat dairy products and other nonfat or very low-fat products in moderation
- avoid meats, oils, avocados, olives, nuts, seeds, sugar, simple sugar derivatives, high-fat or low-fat dairy products, alcohol, any commercially available product with more than two grams of fat per serving

Pritikin Diet

Purposes: weight reduction; blood pressure reduction; cholesterol reduction; cardiac health

Features:

- low total fat, cholesterol, sodium
- rich in unrefined carbohydrates, vitamins, minerals, dietary fiber
- moderate in protein
- whole grains, vegetables, fruits, legumes, chestnuts, nonfat dairy, juices, herbal teas, soybean products, fish preferred over fowl, fowl preferred over red meat
- excludes animal fats, tropical oils, hydrogenated oils, fatty meats, organ meats, processed meats, whole dairy products, coconuts, macadamia nuts, salt products, egg yolks, fried foods, saccharin, caffeinated beverages

Sears' Zone-Favorable Diet

Purpose: achieve and maintain the zone (a state in which the body and mind work at their best)

Features:

- ingestion of a beneficial ratio of protein to carbohydrate with each food intake
- caloric consumption consisting of 30% protein, 30% fat, and 40% carbohydrates

(continued)

- determination of individual protein requirement based on lean body mass and activity level
- low-fat protein
- "favorable" carbohydrates, emphasizes those with low glycemic indexes (i.e., those that enter bloodstream slowly)
- "favorable" fats, emphasizes monounsaturated
- do not allow more than five hours to pass without eating meal or snack to control entry rates of protein and carbohydrate into bloodstream, thereby controlling resulting hormonal response
- use of supplements: antioxidants (vitamins C and E, beta carotene) and enzymatic cofactors (vitamins B_3 and B_6, zinc, magnesium)

See Recommended Reading list for information on texts describing these diets in detail.

BOX 7-6   How the Immune System Works

The *white blood cells (WBCs)* serve as the main defenses of the immune system. These cells circulate to the tissues of the body, identify foreign invaders that threaten the body's health, and destroy these invaders. The specific types of white blood cells are:

B cells: These cells get their name for being bone marrow-derived. They produce antibodies that neutralize or destroy antigens. (An antigen is a substance that induces sensitivity when it comes in contact with tissue and causes antibodies to be formed. A specific antibody reacts with the antigen and creates immunity to the antigen.)

T cells: The name of these cells comes from *thymus-derived*. T-cells consist of T helper cells that induce B cells to respond to an antigen and T suppressor cells that stop certain activity of immunologic response. The T helper and T suppressor cells are in a delicate balance; immune malfunction results when this balance is disrupted. Examples of diseases that result when there is an abnormal ratio of helper to suppressor cells include systemic lupus erythematosus, AIDS, multiple sclerosis, and chronic active hepatitis.

NK cells: These natural killer cells function without B cell involvement by killing foreign invaders on direct contact. They do so by producing cytotoxin, a cell poison.
    B and T cells in the thymus and bone marrow are unspecialized and produce antibodies in response to antigens that they identify.

Macrophages: These are large white blood cells produced in the bone marrow that are responsible for phagocytosis. Phagocytosis is a process in which antigens are consumed, much like "Pac Man" gobbles an opponent.
The *lymphatic system* consists of all the organs of the immune system. The organs are divided into primary organs (the thymus and bone marrow) and secondary organs (lymph nodes, spleen, tonsils, and appendix).

Thymus gland: This gland, located beneath the breastbone, is made of tiny lobules. It reaches maximum size in early childhood, then begins to shrink. T-cells mature in the outer cortex of the lobe and migrate to an area inside the lobe, called the medulla, where they are stored for later use.

Bone marrow: Marrow is the soft material in the hollow interior of the long bones of the arms and legs. Red blood cells and macrophages are produced in the marrow, and B and T cells undergo development here.

Lymph nodes: These small pea-shaped organs are located throughout the body and are connected by a network of vessels that receive drainage. Areas within the lymph nodes trap and filter antigens from the lymphatic fluid.

Spleen: This spongy, bloody organ is located on the left side of the abdominal cavity below the ribs. The spleen helps to produce antibodies, maintain cellular immunity, and recirculate white blood cells. Blood circulates B cells, T cells, antigens, macrophages and antigen-reactive cells to the spleen.

Tonsils: These are groups of lymphoid tissues located in several different areas of the throat. They contain B and T cells.

Other minor organs: The appendix, Peyer's patches, and intestinal nodes are the sites of B cell maturation and antibody production for the intestinal region.

The way in which these structures of the immune system work to produce highly specialized functions is indeed amazing. Antigens and antibodies are protein-containing agents. Antibodies recognize the distinct shape and chemical structure of various antigens and attack the antigens as foreign material that is threatening the body. The five types of antibodies known by their abbreviations: IgG, IgA, IgM, IgD, and IgE. (Ig stands for immunoglobulins.)

Once the body has been exposed to an antigen, the immune system stores the information about the antigen in its memory system. This is the reason we do not become as ill with future exposures to an antigen as we did on the first exposure.

Vaccination is a process in which a weakened or dead strain of an antigen is injected into the body. The immune system stores information about the antigen in its memory and fights future exposure to the antigen.

The brain has an important role in regulating immunity. Neurotransmitters are chemical messengers that stimulate the nervous system. Three neurotransmitters that influence immunity are acetylcholine, serotonin, and catecholamines (epinephrine and dopamine). Acetylcholine stimulates a nucleic acid that activates B and T cell response. Receptors for acetylcholine are in the thymus. Serotonin is an immunosuppressant in that it has an inverse relationship with antibody production, meaning that the greater the serotonin the lower the antibody production. Dopamine stimulates immune function. It is believed that B cells may be increased by low dopamine levels. In fact, people with Parkinson's disease, who characteristically have dopamine deficiencies, have reduced T cells and T cell response.

Amino acids, the building blocks of protein, are necessary to increase levels of neurotransmitters, and can be affected by diet. Amino acid supplements can ensure an adequate intake to enhance neurotransmitter levels. (Reducing the dietary intake of protein improves the efficacy of amino acid supplements.)

Many health advocates believe that the RDAs are not adequate for the daily stresses and environmental insults to which people are exposed today and that higher minimum levels must be ingested to ensure good immune functioning. Some of the specific vitamins and minerals that affect the immune system are included in Box 7-2.

Psychological Factors

Studies have identified psychological traits that are commonly seen among individuals with strong immune systems; these include the following (Dreher, 1996):

- awareness of positive and negative mind-body signals, such as anger, pain, pleasure
- willingness to be open and confide in others
- commitment to one's work
- control over one's life
- acceptance of stress as a challenge rather than a threat
- assertiveness
- ability to trust and offer unconditional love
- altruism
- development and exercise of multiple facets of personality

By understanding the relationship of these traits to their ability to maintain health and facilitate healing, individuals can attempt to change patterns and behaviors that will nurture these characteristics.

Immune-Boosting Herbs

Echinacea is highly regarded as an effective immune system stimulant. It has long been used by Native Americans for its wound-healing and antiinflammatory effects, and often is referred to as a natural antibiotic. Research has shown that when taken internally, echinacea increases the number and activity of white blood cells, including a promotion of phagocytosis (Melchart et al., 1994).

Garlic is known for its antibiotic, antifungal, and antiviral properties (in addition to the many other benefits it offers). In addition to garlic cloves that can be eaten in the diet, a variety of garlic preparations are on the market, some of which are odor-free.

Ginseng is another herb with a wide range of therapeutic uses, including stimulation of immune system activity.

Goldenseal is a widely used American herb that stimulates the immune response. Its antimicrobial properties are due to berberine and other alkaloids that it contains. Because it can stimulate contractions, it should not be used during pregnancy.

Stress Management

Because the thymus, spleen, and lymph nodes are intimately involved in the stress response, stress affects immune function.

Some stress-related diseases are accompanied by an elevation in the level of cortisol in the blood. Cortisol is a powerful immunosuppressant that breaks down lymphoid tissue, decreases the level of T helper cells, increases T suppressor cells, inhibits the production of natural killer cells, and reduces virus-fighting interferon. Some diseases associated with high cortisol levels include arthritis, depression, cancer, hypertension, and diabetes. The chronic use of vitamin C, salicylates (aspirin), dilantin, and cimetidine lower cortisol levels.

Effective stress management is important to enhancing the function of the immune system. (See Chapter 15 for further discussion on stress).

Exercise

Immunity is enhanced through any type of moderate, regular activity. Vigorous exercise is known to increase endorphins that produce a sense of well-being.

Other Therapies

Meditation, yoga, and guided imagery can be used to stimulate immune functioning. (For more information on these therapies, see Chapter 5.)

Care in Using Antibiotics

Antibiotics are commonly prescribed to fight infections, but along with their benefits are some risks to the immune system. Overuse of antibiotics can disrupt the body's balance and enable other infections to easily develop. (Women who have developed yeast infections after taking an antibiotic are well aware of this side effect.) Also, excess use of antibiotics can lead to the pathogens becoming resistant to the drugs. To promote more benefit than risks from antibiotics and to ensure that they do not result in suppressing the function of the immune system, be sure to use antibiotics only when absolutely necessary and as infrequently as possible.

Related Diagnoses

Altered Nutrition: Less Than Body Requirements

Description

This diagnosis refers to an insufficient quality and quantity of nutrient intake to meet body's needs.

Client Goals

- to consume at least _____ calories daily
- to gain ____ pounds within _____ (time period)
- to maintain weight between _____ and _____ pounds
- to possess serum levels that fall within a normal range
- to describe prescribed diet
- to be free from clinical signs of malnutrition

Interventions

- Assist client in identifying factors that contribute to nutritional alteration and correcting them (e.g., improving oral health, obtaining help with meal preparation, accepting instructions on diet).
- Consult with dietician regarding special dietary needs, supplements.
- If appropriate, develop eating contract with client that describes agreed-on daily food consumption.
- Stimulate appetite by:
  - promoting oral hygiene
  - providing a pleasant environment for meals
  - controlling pain and other symptoms
  - suggesting wine prior to meals (unless contraindicated)
  - assisting with stress reduction
- Provide assistive devices and feeding assistance as needed.
- Advise client or caregiver to maintain food intake record; review and intervene as needed.
- Obtain client's weight at regular intervals; review laboratory values.
- Teach client to use imagery to visualize improved nutritional status and affirmations (e.g., "I will gain five pounds"; "I can enjoy eating more vegetables").
- Ensure that pain, nausea, and other symptoms are controlled. Advise client that ginger is effective in controlling nausea and vomiting (Bone et al., 1990; Fischer-Rasmussen et al., 1990).
- Consult with appropriate therapists regarding psychotherapy, behavioral modification, etc.
- Provide positive reinforcement and feedback.

Anorexia

Description

Anorexia is a loss of appetite or disinterest in food. This condition often accompanies cancer, COPD, depression, and other chronic diseases. Appetite can also be reduced by medications used to treat chronic diseases, such as antipsychotic and antianxiety drugs. Inactivity and social isolation can contribute to anorexia, as can the grief associated with the losses confronted by chronically ill clients.

In addition to the obvious signs of disinterest in food and weight loss, anorexic clients can display fatigue, weakness, and altered cognition.

Client Goals

- to consume minimum daily requirements of nutrients
- to gain _____ pounds within _____ (time period)

Interventions

- Assess factors that contribute to poor appetite and assist client in reducing them.
- Elicit help of family and chronic care coach to assist in preparing favorite foods for client.
- Assist in providing good oral hygiene before meals.
- Coordinate with physician and other therapists as appropriate in recommending use of nutritional supplements.
- Support therapies used to improve underlying problem.
- Refer to organizations for education and support (see Box 7-7).

BOX 7-7

Resources for Information About Anorexia

American Anorexia/Bulimia Association
425 East 61st Street
New York, NY 10021
(212) 891-8686
www.social.com/health/nhic/data/hr0100/hr01
23.html

National Anorexic Aid Society
445 East Granville Road
Worthington, OH 43085
(614) 436-1112

National Association of Anorexia Nervosa and Associated Disorders
PO Box 7
Highland Park, IL 60035
(708) 831-3438
www.medpatients.com/Health%20Resources/
NAANAD.htm

RESOURCES

Anemia

Description

Anemic individuals have reduced red blood cells, hemoglobins, or hematocrits. Several types of anemia include the following:

iron deficiency the most common form, in which there is insufficient dietary intake of iron, impaired iron absorption, or excessive blood loss

pernicious caused by impaired absorption of vitamin B_{12} or folic acid, or stomach cancer

aplastic resulting from radiation, chemicals, or certain drugs

Client Goals

- to correct underlying cause of anemia as possible
- to maintain red blood cell count, hemoglobin and hematocrit levels within normal range
- to be free from complications associated with anemia

Interventions

- Assist client in having underlying cause identified and corrected.
- For iron deficiency anemia, teach client dietary habits that will promote improvement, including consumption of iron-rich foods, use of vitamin C (ascorbic acid promotes iron absorption).
- Teach client proper administration and effects of medications.
- Be aware that folic acid can compromise the effectiveness of methotrexate, colchicine, trimethoprim, phenytoin, and other drugs (Butterworth and Tamura, 1989). Advise client to have pharmacist review drugs for potential interactions when folic acid is prescribed.
- Suggest ways that energy can be conserved while counts are low.
- Teach client signs of complications that should be reported.
- Refer to organizations for support and education (see Box 7-8).

BOX 7-8

Resources for Information About Anemia

Aplastic Anemia Foundation of America
PO Box 22689
Baltimore, MD 21203
(800) 747-2820
www.teleport.com/nonprofit/aafa

Cooley's Anemia Foundation
129-09 26th Avenue #203
Flushing, NY 11354
(800) 522-7222
www.thalassemia.org

Cirrhosis

Description

This progressive disease involves irreversible damage to liver cells that can ultimately cause liver failure and death. Most often, cirrhosis is an outgrowth of chronic alcoholism, although hepatitis and biliary obstruction can be responsible for this condition also.

Client Goals

- to prevent additional liver damage by adhering to treatment plan
- to maintain body chemistry within normal range
- to be free from complications associated with cirrhosis (e.g., impaired skin integrity, altered level of consciousness, impaired respiration, portal hypertension, infections)
- to obtain treatment for alcoholism (if applicable)

Interventions

- Teach client about liver function and impact of cirrhosis.
- Teach and reinforce diet, e.g., high-protein, high-calorie, low-fat, sodium-restricted. (If serum ammonia is elevated, a low-protein diet may be prescribed to prevent uremia.) To avoid stressors on the liver, it is

helpful for the client to avoid highly processed foods and additives. Beet, carrot, and wheat grass juice could be helpful.

- Encourage client to eat several small meals daily rather than three large ones to avoid bloating; recommend protein supplements between meals unless contraindicated.
- Advise client to take safe doses of vitamins A, B complex, D and K to compensate for liver's inability to store them, and vitamin B_{12}, folic acid, and thiamin to correct anemia. (Excess doses of vitamin A and niacin should be avoided because they can result in liver toxicity. Cod liver oil should be avoided.)
- If nausea is present, suggest the use of ginger (e.g., about ten drops of tincture of ginger in a small amount of liquid); use antiemetic medication if ginger is ineffective.
- Teach client how to administer drugs safely and what adverse reactions to report.
- Advise client to monitor weight and report weekly weight gain that exceeds five pounds or that increases a few pounds daily; this can indicate fluid retention.
- Advise client to avoid alcohol to prevent further destruction of liver cells. If alcoholism is a problem, assist client in seeking treatment (see Chapter 15).
- Discuss with client and health care provider use of silymarin, a component of the herb milk thistle with other active ingredients. (Milk thistle offers protection of the liver.) Studies have shown that persons with cirrhosis who took silymarin had lower death rates than those who received a placebo (Ferenci et al., 1989).
- Caution client about the use of herbs containing pyrrolizidine alkaloids, which can cause liver problems; these herbs include comfrey, borage, coltsfoot, chaparral and germander (Gordon et al., 1995).
- Advise client to plan several rest periods during the day to conserve energy and decrease metabolic demands.
- Monitor intake and output; observe for ascites and other signs of edema.
- Promote good skin care as pruritus can be a problem.
- Monitor laboratory values.
- Observe and teach client and caregivers to observe for signs of impending hepatic coma, including nausea, vomiting, low-grade fever, diarrhea, and abdominal discomfort.
- Observe and teach client and caregivers to observe for signs of hepatic encephalopathy, including euphoria, fatigue, irritability, restlessness, poor judgment, confusion.
- Recommend aromatherapy using essential oils of juniper, rosemary, or rose.
- Refer to organizations for education and support (see Box 7-9).

BOX 7-9
Resources for Information About Cirrhosis

American Liver Foundation
1425 Pompton Avenue
Cedar Grove, NJ 07009
(800) 223-0179
sadieo.ucsf.edu/alf/alffinal/homepagealf.html

American Share Foundation (transplants)
15314 Gault Street #314
Van Nuys, CA 91406
(818) 994-6848
www.asf.org

Altered Nutrition: More Than Body Requirements

Description

This is a state in which the body's intake exceeds metabolic demand.

Client Goals

- to demonstrate positive dietary practices
- to lose _____ pounds within _____ (time frame)
- to maintain weight between _____ and _____ pounds
- to participate in a regular exercise program

Interventions

- Consult with nutritionist to determine client's caloric needs and restrictions. Encourage whole-grain, high-complex carbohydrate, high-fiber, and low-fat diet that incorporates client's unique dietary needs.
- Recommend use of nutritional supplements that have benefit for weight loss and weight management including chromium, beta-carotene, biotin, and vitamins A, B_3, B_6, C, and E (Morris, 1992).
- Develop a contract with client to meet dietary goals.
- Assist client in identifying unhealthy eating patterns that contribute to problem.
- Help client identify factors that contribute to problem (e.g., depression, anxiety) and refer for counseling as needed.
- Counsel family on changes in their behaviors that can be supportive of client's efforts (e.g., altered cooking style, taking walks after dinner, limiting snacks, omitting high-calorie foods from social activities).
- Help client develop an exercise program.
- Refer to weight loss groups, support groups, therapist as needed.
- Refer for hypnosis, if appropriate. Several studies have demonstrated hypnosis to be effective in weight loss (Barabasz and Spiegel, 1989).
- Guide client in safe use of herbs: *ephedra sineca (ma-huang)* for enhancing metabolic rate, cayenne for stimulating metabolism, *coryanthe johimbe* for burning fat, plantain for decreasing fat absorption and creating feeling of fullness, kelp to boost thyroid gland activity, and fennel seed for promoting digestion. (Ephedra used for weight reduction can be effective but

should be used under medical supervision; it should be avoided by persons with hypertension, heart disease, thyroid disease, diabetes, and benign prostatic hypertrophy, pregnancy, and persons using antidepressants.)
- Assist client in use of guided imagery to visualize burning of fat cells, and in constructing image of self as thinner.
- Refer obese clients to local support groups (see Box 7-10).

BOX 7-10

Resources for Information About Altered Nutrition

American Society of Bariatric Physicians
5600 S. Quebec Street
Suite 160-D
Englewood, CO 80111
(303) 779-4833
www.social.com/health/nhic/data/hr1400/hr14
99.html

National Association to Advance Fat Acceptance (NAAFA)
PO Box 188620
Sacramento, CA 95818
(916) 558-6880
naafa.org

Overeaters Anonymous
World Services Office
PO Box 92870
Los Angeles, CA 90009
(213) 936-4206
www.hiwaay.net/recovery

Diabetes Mellitus

Description

Diabetes mellitus is a chronic metabolic disease in which there is an abnormally high blood glucose level. This condition can arise in a variety of manners, giving rise to the two major classifications of diabetes:

Type I (Insulin dependent): primarily juvenile form but can begin later in life if pancreas malfunctions due to injury or disease; body is unable to produce insulin; accounts for 10% of cases

Type II (Noninsulin-dependent): production of insulin ineffective or insufficient to meet body's demands; primarily affects people over age 40

Client Goals

- to verbalize knowledge of disease process, prescribed diet, medications, activity considerations, weight management, foot care, glucose monitoring, complications, resources
- to ingest prescribed diet that meets metabolic needs
- to maintain weight within _____ to _____ pounds
- to administer prescribed medications correctly (Fig.7-2)
- to be free from complications associated with the disease
- to recognize signs of complications (e.g., hyperglycemia, hypoglycemia (Box 7-11), peripheral vascular disease, hypertension, retinopathy, neuropathy, infection)

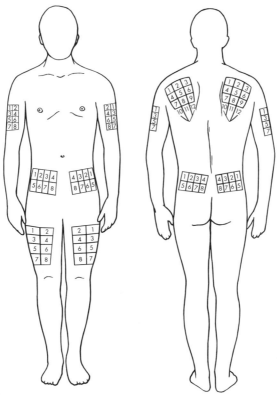

FIGURE 7-2

Subcutaneous Injection Sites. From Potter P, Perry A: *Fundamentals of Nursing*, ed 4, St. Louis, 1997, Mosby.

BOX 7-11	Signs of Hyperglycemia and Hypoglycemia

Hyperglycemia	Hypoglycemia
Thirst	Confusion
Sweet, fruity-smelling breath	Trembling
Dry mouth	Weakness
Anorexia	Hunger
Nausea, vomiting	Irritability
Excess voiding	Tachycardia
Abdominal pain	Perspiration
Disorientation	Tingling fingers, mouth
Labored breathing	Headache
Dry, flushed skin	Slurred speech
Drowsiness	Unsteady gait
Coma	Seizure

Interventions

- Assess client's knowledge of disease; develop and implement teaching plan based on assessed needs; collaborate with nutritionist as appropriate. Ensure that client is knowledgeable concerning:
  - disease process
  - diet, weight management
  - glucose monitoring
  - physical activity considerations
  - antidiabetic medications
  - foot care
  - signs of complications
  - resources
- Educate caregiver, coach, and significant others as necessary.
- Encourage physical activity, which has been shown to lower blood glucose. (Note: studies have demonstrated that the incidence of diabetes is significantly lower in persons who regularly exercised than in those who did not [Manson et al., 1992]). Instruct in yoga, tai chi, and other forms of exercise that can promote circulation.
- Instruct client in use of progressive relaxation and biofeedback-assisted relaxation, which have been shown to promote peripheral circulation (Rice and Schindler, 1992).
- Consult with nutritionist regarding benefits of soya diet for client. Soya has been shown to be beneficial in raising insulin levels, smoothing glucose tolerance curves, promoting cholesterol synthesis, improving glomerular filtration, lowering blood pressure, and providing good nutrition with low caloric content (Holt et al., 1996).
- Review herbal supplements that client uses for those that have proven hypoglycemic properties; these include bilberry, goat's rue, fenugreek, bitter melon, dandelion, onion, garlic, mulberry leaves, olive leaves, and ginseng (Ivorra et al., 1989; Kroll 1996). Advise client to consult with practitioner if these herbs will be used on a regular basis or if they are being discontinued after long-term use as blood glucose levels can be affected. (Reinforce that herbal therapies complement but do not substitute for conventional treatment of diabetes.)
- Help client to wisely use herbs that can have a positive impact on cardiovascular function, e.g., ginkgo biloba, hawthorn berry.
- Regularly evaluate for presence of complications, e.g., poor peripheral circulation, infection, delirium. Teach client and caregivers signs to note and report.
- If the client has pain associated with diabetic neuropathy, consider use of capsaicin cream (derivative of chili pepper), which has been shown to be effective in reducing the intensity of pain (Capsaicin Study Group, 1991).
- As appropriate, suggest client discuss new treatments with physician, including implantable probes and pumps, pancreas transplants, pancreas

islet cell grafts, glycemic index, and treatment with cyclosporine (immunosuppressant that helps to prevent islet beta-cell destruction).
- Refer client to sources of additional information and support (see Box 7-12).

BOX 7-12
Resources for Information About Diabetes

American Diabetes Association
1660 Duke Street
Alexandria, VA 22314
(800) 232-3472
www.diabetes.org
Diabetes Education Center
4959 Excelsior Boulevard
Minneapolis, MN 55416
(612) 927-3393
www.lilly.com/diabetes/diabetes_education.html

Juvenile Diabetes Foundation International
432 Park Avenue South
New York, NY 10016
(800) 223-1138
www.jdfcure.com
National Diabetes Information Clearinghouse
National Institutes of Health
9000 Rockville Pike
Box NDIC
Bethesda, MD 20892
(301) 468-2162
www.niddk.nih.gov/Brochures/NDIC.htm

Hiatal Hernia

Description

A protrusion of a portion of the stomach through the esophageal hiatus of the diaphragm is a hiatal hernia. There are two types:

sliding hernia: most common; part of the stomach rolls up through the diaphragm causing displacement of organs and esophageal spasms when client is recumbent or with certain activities

rolling (paraesophageal) hernia: stomach rises alongside the esophagus while esophagogastric junction stays in place

Contributing factors include obesity, age-related degenerative changes, and conditions that increase abdominal pressure.

Client Goals

- to be free from discomfort related to hiatal hernia
- to consume prescribed diet to prevent/relieve reflux and indigestion
- to avoid activities that increase intra-abdominal pressure

Interventions

- Consult with nutritionist and physician to develop diet plan appropriate for client; instruct in diet.
- Advise client to eat five or six small meals rather than three large ones.
- Assist client in identifying foods that increase symptoms (e.g., spicy foods, fried foods, caffeine, carbonated drinks, peppers).
- Teach and support weight reduction diet if indicated.

- Teach client to identify and avoid activities that increase symptoms such as eating before bedtime, heavy lifting, bending forward, wearing tight girdles or bras, straining to have bowel movement).
- Advise client to use antacids safely. Teach client that antacids can interact with other drugs (e.g., chlorpromazine, digoxin, iron preparations, isoniazid, oral anticoagulants, penicillins, phenytoin, phenylbutazone, salicylates, sulfonamides, tetracyclines, and vitamins A and C). Advise client to monitor bowel habits as aluminum hydroxide and calcium carbonate can cause constipation; magnesium carbonate can cause severe diarrhea.
- Instruct client in deep breathing exercises to strengthen diaphragm muscles and promote good respirations.
- Advise client to practice yoga and other stress reduction practices.
- If client smokes, assist with smoking cessation.
- Recommend that client sleep in position that maintains head above level of stomach.
- To reduce gastric irritation and symptoms, recommend that several times during the day the client drink a cup of an infusion of equal parts comfrey root, marshmallow root, and meadowsweet.
- To reduce nausea, suggest that the client use ginger; if this is ineffective, consult with physician regarding antiemetic.
- If dietary and activity changes and medication fail to relieve symptoms, consult with physician regarding possibility of surgery.

Fluid Volume Deficit

Description

A fluid volume deficit is a reduction in vascular, cellular, and intracellular fluid. Chronic conditions can contribute to dehydration by:
- reducing the ability to request, obtain, and consume fluids (e.g., dementia, aphasia, paralysis, swallowing impairment, pain)
- increasing fluid loss (diarrhea, draining wound, vomiting)
- requiring treatments that promote excessive loss (e.g., diuretics, drainage tubes)

Client Goals

- to possess fluid and electrolyte levels within normal range
- to ingest at least 1500 ml of fluids daily (unless contraindicated)
- to be free from complications associated with dehydration

Interventions

- Identify clients at high risk for dehydration and caution about risk. (Clients at high risk include those with altered cognition, depression, immobility, anorexia, vomiting, fatigue, drainage tubes; those being tube fed; those taking diuretics, laxatives, sedatives, tranquilizers).
- Suggest at-risk client follow regular plan to ensure adequate consumption of fluid; educate caregiver as indicated.

- Reinforce importance of increasing fluid consumption during times of warm weather, exercise, and fever.
- Teach client and caregiver signs of dehydration and measures to correct.
- Assist with correction of fluid volume deficit as necessary.

Altered Fluid Volume: Excess

Description

Fluid volume excess is a state of vascular, cellular, or extracellular fluid overload. A variety of chronic conditions can cause increased fluid retention and edema, including congestive heart failure, cirrhosis, and nephrosis. Excess sodium intake, steroid therapy, hormonal disturbances, and rapid infusion of intravenous fluids can contribute to this diagnosis, also.

Client Goals

- to possess a balanced fluid intake and output
- to be free from signs of circulatory overload, edema
- to be free from complications associated with fluid volume excess

Interventions

- Teach high-risk client signs of fluid retention; encourage client to weigh daily, observe for signs of edema.
- Encourage activity and frequent position changes.
- Monitor skin status; implement strategies to prevent skin breakdown.
- Consult with dietician regarding dietary modifications. Teach client to use seasonings other than salt and to check food labels for sodium content.
- Advise client to avoid clothing and shoes that may fit improperly when edema is present.
- Recommend that client avoid prolonged sitting or standing and crossing legs.
- Offer and recommend therapeutic massage to aid in reducing edema.
- Advise client to avoid long-term use of the herb licorice which has been shown to promote edema (Farese et al., 1991).

Congestive Heart Failure

Description

Congestive heart failure is a condition in which the heart is unable to pump sufficient blood to meet the metabolic needs of the tissues. The inability of the heart to circulate blood causes excess fluid to accumulate in the body's tissues. Congestive heart failure can result from congenital, rheumatic, or coronary heart disease; hypertension; mitral stenosis; acute myocardial infarction; or fluid overload.

Client Goals

- to possess fluid and electrolyte balance
- to be able to participate in light to moderate activities without dyspnea, pain, or dysrhythmias

Interventions

- Assist client in identifying and controlling factors that contribute to congestive heart failure.
- Teach and reinforce prescribed treatment.
- Encourage client to follow good diet to promote healthy heart function and prevent further disease.
- Consult with health care provider regarding use of coenzyme Q10 (CoQ10). A randomized, double-blind, controlled trial of individuals with congestive heart failure demonstrated that people receiving CoQ10 experienced fewer complications and hospitalizations than the control group (Morisco et al., 1993).
- Advise client to schedule rest periods after activities.
- Monitor skin status; teach client and caregiver measures to prevent impairment of skin integrity.
- Teach client and caregivers signs of congestive heart failure and related complications (e.g., altered mental status, irregular and/or elevated pulse, dyspnea, decreased activity tolerance, decreased blood pressure, cough, nocturia, distended neck veins, peripheral edema, ascites, abdominal discomfort, weight gain.

Altered Oral Mucous Membrane

Description

A disruption in the integrity of the mucosal lining of the oral cavity is altered oral mucous membrane. Cancer, anemia, periodontal disease, malnutrition, and some infections can threaten the status of the oral mucosa, as can years of smoking and the use of certain medications (e.g., anticholinergics, antibiotics, and chemotherapeutic agents). Irritation and burns from food or drink can threaten the oral mucosa; this can occur easily when clients have reduced sensations or altered cognition.

Client Goals

- to possess healthy, intact gums, teeth, lips, and tongue
- to demonstrate good oral hygiene practices
- to be free from complications associated with impaired oral mucous membrane (e.g., malnutrition, pain, infection)

Interventions

- Instruct client in good oral hygiene practices. Provide assistive devices as necessary.

- Inspect client's mouth on a regular basis.
- If mouth ulcers are present, recommend use of vitamin E oil, which can facilitate faster healing (Wadleigh et al., 1992).

Impaired Skin Integrity

Description

A disruption to the healthy, normal status of the skin is a state of impaired skin integrity. This can be a potential state, in which the skin is at risk for breakdown, or an actual state, in which an alteration to the skin's status exists. Some chronic conditions increase the risk of impaired skin integrity; these include diabetes mellitus, emaciation, peripheral vascular disease, obesity, paralysis, incontinence, and immobility.

Client Goals

- to possess intact skin
- to restore skin integrity

Interventions

- Identify client at high risk for impaired skin integrity and teach client and caregivers ways to maintain intact skin. Strategies should include the following practices:
  - keeping skin clean and dry
  - changing positions frequently enough to prevent pressure
  - avoiding shearing forces
  - using moisturizer to prevent dryness
  - avoiding harsh soaps
  - preventing excessive exposure to sunlight
  - obtaining treatment of skin conditions
- Encourage good nutrition.
- Evaluate for environmental sensitivities that could promote skin disorders.
- Consult with homeopathic practitioner regarding remedies to treat skin conditions.
- Use massage therapeutically. Avoid massage to bony prominences.
- Recommend the use of essential oils topically for their specific therapeutic benefits:
  - thyme oil: antiseptic
  - neroli oil: rejuvenating
  - oils of rosemary and carrot seed: cell regeneration
  - oils of cinnamon, garlic, lavender, lemon, sage and thyme: relief of stings and bites
- Recommend the therapeutic use of herbs topically:
  - aloe vera as an effective emollient
  - chamomile baths and irrigations for relief of inflamed areas

- goldenseal for eczema, ringworm
- nettle for eczema
- peppermint for pruritus, urticaria
- St. John's wort to facilitate wound healing
- witch hazel as an astringent

Pressure Ulcer

Description

As the title implies, a pressure ulcer is an area of necrosis (Box 7-13) caused by pressure to an area that results in tissue hypoxia. Risk factors include immobility, malnutrition, emaciation, shearing forces, incontinence, heavy perspiration, conditions that impair circulation, and medications or diseases that decrease mobility or sensations.

Client Goals

- to be free from pressure ulcers
- to heal an existing pressure ulcer; to decrease from stage ____ to stage ____
- to be free from complications related to pressure ulcer

Interventions

- Assess the amount of time the client can remain in a position without showing signs of pressure and develop individualized turning schedule accordingly. To determine repositioning schedule required, examine the client's pressure points after one-half hour in the same position. If redness is present, develop a q 1/2 hour turning schedule; if there are not signs of pressure, allow the client to remain in the same position and check after one hour. Continue adding one-half hour increments until pressure is observed, to a maximum of two hours in one position.

BOX 7-13   Stages of Pressure Ulcers

Stage 1
Persistent area of skin redness without break in skin; it does not disappear when pressure is relieved.

Stage 2
Partial-thickness loss of skin layers that presents clinically as an abrasion, blister, or shallow crater, no necrotic area.

Stage 3
Full thickness loss of skin exposing subcutaneous tissues; presents as deep crater with or without undermining adjacent tissue.

Stage 4
Full thickness loss of skin and subcutaneous tissue that exposes muscle and/or bone.

- Assist client in obtaining alternating pressure mattress and other pressure-relieving devices.
- Implement prescribed treatment plan; monitor progress.
- Consult with nutritionist regarding diet; teach and reinforce to client. Promote protein intake unless contraindicated.
- Ensure good intake of zinc, beta-carotene, and vitamins A, B-complex, C, and D to promote healing. Also, recommend the therapeutic use of herbs: garlic, comfrey, echinacea, goldenseal, and slippery elm.
- Use massage and touch therapy to promote circulation; avoid massage of bony prominences.
- Use aloe vera as an emollient.
- Guide client in use of imagery to visualize healing of ulcer and improved circulation to area.
- Consult with homeopathic practitioner regarding remedies (e.g., *Calendula*, *Hypericum*, *Chamomilla*, *Phosphorus*, *Hamamelis*, *Silicea*, and *Belladonna*).
- Consult with health care provider regarding pressure ulcer treatment with pulse electromagnetic energy treatment. Research is supporting the healing benefits of electromagnetic therapy; one randomized, double-blind study of pressure ulcer treatment showed that 84% of ulcers receiving electromagnetic energy treatments healed versus 40% of those in the untreated group (Salzberg et al., 1995).

Psoriasis

Description

Psoriasis is a chronic hereditary disorder characterized by an accelerated turnover (mitotic activity) of the skin. Elevated, erythematous scaling plaques appear on the skin. This is a common condition that can be exacerbated by stress, anxiety, food allergies, illness, surgery, trauma, infection, a change in climate, and certain drugs (e.g., beta-blockers).

Client Goals

- to state nature of condition, management, and factors to control in order to minimize recurrence
- to be free from complications related to psoriasis (e.g., infection, pain, social isolation)

Interventions

- Teach client and caregivers facts about disease, care, and factors that could contribute to exacerbations.
- Assist client, as needed, with prescribed treatment, which could include:
  - wet dressings
  - application of antimitotic products (e.g., anthralin)
  - topical steroids with occlusive wraps
  - phototherapy with ultraviolet B (UV-B)

- PUVA therapy (Psoralen with long-wave ultraviolet light)
    - coal tar preparations (topical, bath, or in combination with ultraviolet light)
- Assist client in identifying factors that precipitate attacks and ways to avoid or minimize them.
- Advise client to avoid harsh soaps and detergents and extremes in temperature, and to expose affected areas to sunlight in moderation.
- Encourage good intake of unsaturated fatty acids, folic acid, lecithin, zinc, and vitamins A, B-complex, B_6, and C with bioflavoids.
- Teach progressive relaxation, deep breathing exercises, and other stress reduction strategies.
- Reinforce that psoriasis is a noninfectious, noncontagious disease.
- Suggest use of fish oil supplements. Although the results have been divided, some studies have demonstrated improvement in psoriasis with the use of fish oil (Lassus et al., 1990). Because of the lack of adverse effects associated with fish oil, its use to determine effectiveness for the individual client should carry minimal, if any, risk.
- Guide client in the use of imagery to visualize healing of lesions and promote relaxation.
- Suggest baths in sea salt (approximately one pound of sea salt in a tub of body temperature bath water) unless contraindicated.
- Encourage client to discuss emotional impact of disease. Promote socialization and normal lifestyle.
- Use bergamot and lavender in aromatherapy.
- Consult with homeopathic practitioner regarding use of *Psorinum*, *Sulfur*, *Graphites*, *Arsenicum album*, and *Cuprum metallicum*.
- Refer for additional information and support (see Box 7-14).

BOX 7-14
Resources for Information About Psoriasis

National Psoriasis Foundation
6600 SW 92nd Avenue
Suite 300
Portland, OR 97223
(800) 248-0886
www.psoriasis.org

References

Barabasz M, Spiegel D: Hypnotizability and weight loss in obese subjects, *International Journal of Eating Disorders* 8(3):335-41, 1989.

Bone ME, et al.: Ginger root: a new antiemetic. The effect of ginger root on postoperative nausea and vomiting after major gynecological surgery, *Anesthesia* 45:669-71, 1990.

Brodsky MA, et al.: Magnesium therapy in new-onset atrial fibrillation, *American Journal of Cardiology* 73:1227-29, 1994.

Butterworth CE and Tamura T: Folic acid safety and toxicity: a brief review, *American Journal of Clinical Nutrition* 50:353-58, 1989.

Capsaicin Study Group: Treatment of painful diabetic neuropathy with topical capsaicin, *Archives of Internal Medicine* 151:2225-29, 1991.

Cleland LG, et al.: Clinical and biochemical effects of dietary fish oil supplements in rheumatoid arthritis, *Journal of Rheumatology* 15:1471-75, 1988.

Combs GF: Selenium. In Moon TE, Micozzi MS, eds: *Nutrition and cancer prevention: investigating the role of micronutrients*, New York, 1989, Marcel Dekker.

Dreher H: *The immune power personality: 7 traits you can develop to stay healthy*, New York, 1996, Penguin.

Farese RV, et al.: Licorice-induced hypermineralocorticoidism, *New England Journal of Medicine* 325(17):1223-27, 1991.

Ferenci P, et al.: Randomized controlled trial of silymarin treatment in patients with cirrhosis of the liver, *Journal of Hepatology* 9:105-113, 1989.

Fischer-Rasmussen W, et al.: Ginger treatment of hyperemesis gravidarum, *European Journal of Obstetrics & Gynecology and Reproductive Biology* 38:19-24, 1990.

Gapinski P, et al.: Preventing restenosis with fish oils following coronary angioplasty, *Archives of Internal Medicine* 153:1595-1601, 1993.

Giovannucci E, et al.: Folate, methionine, and alcohol intake and risk of colorectal adenoma, *Journal of the National Cancer Institute* 85(11):875-84, 1993.

Gordon DW, et al.: Chaparral ingestion: the broadening spectrum of liver injury caused by herbal medications, *Journal of the American Medical Association* 27(96):489-90, 1995.

Grudley G, et al.: Vitamin supplement use and reduced risk of oral and pharyngeal cancer, *American Journal of Epidemiology* 135:1083-92, 1992.

Hankinson SE, et al.: Nutrient intake and cataract extraction in women, *British Medical Journal* 305:335-39, 1992.

Holt S, Muntyan I, Likver L: Soya-based diets for diabetes mellitus, *Alternative and Complementary Therapies* 2(2):79-82, March-April 1996.

Ivorra MD, Paya M, and Villar A: A review of natural products and plants as potential anti-diabetic drugs, *Journal of Ethnopharmacology* 27(3):243-275, December 1989.

Kardinaal AFM, et al.: Antioxidants in adipose tissue and risk of myocardial infarction: the Euramic study, *Lancet* 342:1379-84, 1993.

Kroll D: Treating diabetes with herbs: gentler and less costly, *Alternative and Complementary Therapies* 2(2):75-78, March-April 1996.

Lassus A, et al.: Effects of dietary supplementation with polyunsaturated ethyl ester lipids (Angiosan) in patients with psoriasis and psoriatic arthritis, *Journal of International Medical Research* 18:68-73, 1990.

Lawrence R and Sorrell T: Eicasopentaenoic acid in cystic fibrosis; evidence of a pathogenic role for leukotriene B4, *Lancet* 342:465-69, 1993.

Manson JE, et al.: A prospective study of exercise and incidence of diabetes among US male physicians, *Journal of the American Medical Association* 268:63-67, 1992.

Melchart D, et al.: Immunomodulation with echinacea: a systematic review of controlled clinical trials, *Phytomedicine* 1:245-54, 1994.

Mendes MS, Comstock GW and Vuilleumier JP: Serum beta-carotene, vitamins A and E, selenium, and the risk of lung cancer, *New England Journal of Medicine* 315:1250-54, 1986.

Messina M and Messina V: *The dietician's guide to vegetarian diets: Issues and applications*, Gaithersburg, MD, 1996, Aspen Publications.

Morisco C, Trimarco B, Condrelli M: Effect of coenzyme CoQ10 therapy in patients with congestive heart failure: a long-term multi-center randomized study, *Clinical Investigator* 71:S134-S136, 1993.

Morris BW: The trace element chromium: a role in glucose homeostasis, *American Journal of Clinical Nutrition* 55(5):989-991, 1992.

Morris MC, Sacks F, Rosner B: Does fish oil lower blood pressure? *Circulation* 88:523-33, 1993.

O'Hara JO, Jolly PN, Nicol CG: The therapeutic efficacy of inositol nicotinate in intermittent claudication: a controlled trial, *British Journal of Clinical Practice* 42:377-83, 1988.

Rice BI and Schindler JV: Effect of thermal biofeedback-assisted relaxation training on blood circulation in the lower extremities of a population with diabetes, *Diabetes Care* 15(7):853-858, July 1992.

Rimm EB, et al.: Vitamin E consumption and the risk of coronary heart disease in men, *New England Journal of Medicine* 328:1450-56, 1993.

Roeback JR, et al.: Effects of chromium supplementation on serum high-density lipoprotein cholesterol levels in men taking beta-blockers, *Annals of Internal Medicine* 115:917-24, 1991.

Salzberg CA, et al.: The effects of non-thermal pulsed electromagnetic energy on wound healing of pressure ulcers in spinal cord-injured patients: a randomized, double-blind study, *Ostomy/Wound Management* 41(3):42-48, 1995.

Shahar E, et al.: Dietary n-3 polyunsaturated fatty acids and smoking-related chronic obstructive pulmonary disease, *New England Journal of Medicine* 33:228-33, 1994.

Stenson WF, et al.: Dietary supplementation with fish oil in ulcerative colitis, *Annals of Internal Medicine* 116:609-14, 1992.

Swank RL and Dugan BB: Effect of low saturated fat diet in early and late cases of multiple sclerosis, *Lancet* 336:37-39, 1990.

Wadleigh RG, et al.: Vitamin E in the treatment of chemotherapy-induced mucositis, *American Journal of Medicine* 92:481-84, 1992.

Woods KL and Fletcher S: Long-term outcome after intravenous magnesium sulfate in suspected acute myocardial infarction, *Lancet* 343:816-19, 1994.

Recommended Readings

Atkins RC: *Dr. Atkins' new diet revolution*, New York, 1992, M. Evans and Co., Inc.

Ayello EA: Keeping pressure ulcers in check, *Nursing 96* 26(10):62-63, 1996.

Balch J and Balch P: *Prescription for nutritional healing*, ed 2, Garden City Park, NY, 1997, Avery Publishing.

Chaitow L: *Body/mind purification program*, New York, 1990, Simon and Schuster.

Cirone N and Schwartz N: Diabetes in the elderly, *Nursing 96* 26(3):34-47, 1996.

Dross JA: Caring for the patient with insulin-dependent diabetes mellitus, *Nursing 96* 26(8):46-47, 1996.

Elson H: *Staying healthy with nutrition*, Berkeley, CA, 1992, Celestial Arts.

Fishman TD, Freedline DPM, Kahn D: Putting the best foot forward, *Nursing 96* 26(1):58-60, 1996.

Garner DM and Garfinkle PE: *Handbook of treatment for eating disorders*, ed 2, New York, 1997, Guilford Publishing Co.

Haas E: *Staying healthy with nutrition*, Berkeley, CA, 1992, Celestial Arts Publishing.

Holt S: The Dietary Supplement and Health Education Act: far-reaching consequences for consumers and manufacturers, *Alternative and Complementary Therapies* 2(4):259-63, 1996.

Jonnalagadda SS, et al.: Effects of individual fatty acids on chronic diseases, *Nutrition Today* 31(3):90-107, 1996.

Lieberman S and Bruning N: *The real vitamin and mineral book*, Garden City Park, NY, 1990, Avery Publishing Group.

Marcus AO: Diabetes mellitus: nephropathy and hypertension, *Clinical Diabetes* 14(4):91-95, 1996.

Murray M: *The complete book of juicing*, Rocklin, CA, 1992, Prima Publishing.

Ni M and McNease C: *Tao of nutrition*, Santa Monica, CA, 1993, Seven Star Communications.

Ornish D: *Eat more, weigh less*, New York, 1993, Harper Collins Publishers.

Perkin S: *Gastrointestinal health*, New York, 1992, Harper Perennial.

Philpott WH: *Victory over diabetes*, New Canaan, CT, 1992, Keats Publishing, Inc.

Pierdinock J: Using homemade salves to soothe the skin, *Country Journal* 23(4):62-65, 1996.

Pritikin R: *The new Pritikin program*, New York, 1990, Simon and Schuster.

Roth E and Streicher S: *Good cholesterol, bad cholesterol*, Rocklin, CA, 1993, Prima Publishers.

Rood RP: Patient and physician responsibility in the treatment of chronic illness: the case of diabetes, *American Behavioral Scientist* 39(6):729-52, 1996.

Rubin R: *Psyching out diabetes: a positive approach to your negative emotions*, Los Angeles, 1992, Lowell House.

Salloum TK: *Fasting signs and symptoms: a clinical guide*, East Palestine, OH, 1992, Buckeye Naturopathic Press.

Sears B: *Enter the zone*, New York, 1995, HarperCollins.

Shelton HM: *Fasting can save your life*, Tampa, FL, 1991, American Natural Hygiene Society, Inc.

Simone CB: *Cancer and nutrition*, Garden City Park, NY, 1994, Avery Publishing Group.

Simopoulos AP: Genetic variation, nutrition, and chronic diseases, *Nutrition Today* 30(5):194-207, 1995.

Trickett S: *Irritable bowel syndrome and diverticulosis*, London, 1992, Thorson's/HarperCollins.

Werbach MA: *Nutritional influences on illness*, ed 2, Tarzana, CA, 1992, Third Lane Press.

Wright JV: *Dr. Wright's guide to healing with nutrition*, New Canaan, CT, 1990, Keats Publishing.

The essential function of removing wastes from the body normally is conducted without considerable planning or thought. Typically, it isn't until we are faced with an alteration in this process that we appreciate the significant degree to which eliminatory processes affect our general health and well-being. For instance, diarrhea can make us uncomfortable, deplete our energy, cause anxiety over the possibility of involuntary expulsion of wastes, and prevent us from engaging in work and social activities.

Many chronic diseases carry a risk of altered urinary or bowel elimination, necessitating active assessment and care planning for the prevention or reduction of elimination problems. When elimination problems are present, consideration must be given to the multiple variables contributing to these problems and the impact on all aspects of the individual's health and quality of life.

Assessment Considerations

Certain chronic conditions can give clues to potential or actual elimination problems. The type and pattern of food and fluid intake should be reviewed, along with the client's complaints or concerns regarding elimination. The physical and mental ability of the client to recognize and understand signals to eliminate and appropriately toilet are important in identifying functional incontinence problems. In addition, there are specific considerations for urinary and bowel elimination.

Urinary Elimination

Question the client as to the frequency and times of voiding and the volume of urine eliminated with each voiding. Review symptoms related to altered urinary elimination (e.g., pain, hesitancy, incontinence, sense of pressure in bladder area, dribbling, blood-tinged urine). If the client is incontinent, review the factors outlined in Box 8-1.

If retention-related symptoms are described, examine the abdomen for the presence of a distended bladder.

Obtain a urine sample and note color (Table 8-1) and odor. As indicated, have urine tested for specific gravity, pH, protein, and culture and sensitivity.

Bowel Elimination

Question the client as to the regular pattern of bowel elimination, recent changes in bowel function, and symptoms. Discuss factors that the client uses to promote bowel elimination.

Inspect the abdomen for skin color, contour and activity. Auscultate bowel sounds; percuss to determine presence of fluid, gas, and masses; palpate for tenderness and masses. Inspect the perianal region for hemorrhoids, lesions, rectal prolapse, tumors, fissures, inflammation, and other problems. If indicated, perform a rectal examination for masses, impactions, and, for males, enlarged prostate gland.

BOX 8-1	Factors to Consider in Assessing the Client with Urinary Incontinence

Onset: date first noticed, pattern when started (partial or complete incontinence), related factors (e.g., began new medication, had an infection)

Pattern: frequency of voiding, amount, times (instruct client to maintain 24-hour record if necessary)

Related factors: activities or symptoms that accompany or precipitate

Symptoms: presence of urgency, burning, vaginal itching, sense of pressure in bladder area, dribbling, pain, fever, dehydration

Functional status: awareness of sensation to void, ability to control, toileting independence, mental status

Bowel elimination pattern (fecal impaction can be cause of urinary incontinence)

Diseases, health conditions: e.g., urinary tract infection, diabetes, dementia, congestive heart failure

Environmental factors: accessibility of bathroom, ability to reach commode/urinal

Medications that can affect continence: diuretics, sedatives, antipsychotics, antidepressants, antiparkinson, antihistamines, alpha stimulants

Urinalysis, urine culture

Post-void residual (amount of urine remaining in bladder after voiding, determined via catheterization)

Bladder stress test (loss of urine after vigorous coughing or laughing)

Urodynamic testing: e.g., cystoscopy, cystometry, uroflowmetry

TABLE 8-1

Examples of Conditions That Can Discolor Urine

Urine color	Possible cause
Red, rust	Blood in urine, infection, bladder tumor
Yellow-brown, green-brown	Jaundice, obstructive bile duct
Orange	Bile in urine, ingestion of pyridium
Smoky, cloudy	Hematuria, presence of prostatic fluid or semen

Related Diagnoses

Altered Urinary Elimination: Incontinence

Description

The inability to voluntarily control the release of urine is urinary incontinence. There are various types of incontinence including:

Stress: leakage of urine resulting from sudden increase in intra-abdominal pressure (e.g., during laughing, coughing, sneezing, lifting heavy object); associated with weak pelvic muscles or damaged urinary sphincter

Urge: sudden urge to void accompanied by involuntary passage of urine; can be due to irritation or spasms of bladder wall secondary to urinary tract infection, prostatic hypertrophy, diverticulosis

Reflex: involuntary loss of urine when a specific volume is reached; related to uninhibited bladder contractions or spasms

Overflow: excess accumulation of urine in bladder that causes overflow; associated with bladder neck obstructions, medications, neurogenic bladder

Functional: inability to toilet in time; related to immobility, dementia, inability to undress, inaccessible bathroom, toileting dependency

Total: constant loss of urine without awareness of bladder filling or incontinence

Client Goals

- to partially/totally restore bladder function
- to maintain or regain positive self-concept and dignity
- to be free from complications related to incontinence (e.g., falls, skin breakdown, social isolation)

Interventions

- Assist with identification and correction (as possible) of underlying cause:
  - record intake and output
  - describe diagnostic tests
- Consult with physician/urologist regarding the potential for continence (based on the diagnosed cause). Discuss usefulness of medications, pessary, surgery, intermittent self-catheterization, and other approaches; support treatment plan and provide education to client as needed.
- Help client and caregivers in providing easily accessible toilet facilities:
  - relocate client's bedroom to room nearest bathroom
  - provide bedside commode, bedpan, urinal
- For stress incontinence, teach pelvic muscle exercises to strengthen pelvic floor (Box 8-2). Advise the client that these exercises must be done regularly to achieve benefit and that improvement may not be noted for several months. Advise caregivers or coach to provide encouragement and reinforcement.
- For client who experiences once-a-day or fewer episodes of incontinence, who can recognize urge to void and is aware when incontinence has occurred, teach *prompted voiding.* This consists of a caregiver checking the client every two hours and prompting (asked if they feel the need to void). The client toilets if the need to void is sensed.
- For client with good cognitive function and the ability to regain bladder control, use *bladder retraining* (Box 8-3).
- For the client with altered cognition who is not a good candidate for bladder retraining or prompted voiding, use *habit training,* in which the client is toileted before voiding occurs. (This differs from bladder retraining in that the client does not control voiding but toilets before voiding occurs.) Instruct the caregiver to remind or toilet the client one-half hour

---

BOX 8-2   **Teaching Plan for Pelvic Strengthening (Kegel) Exercises**

Instruct the client to:
- *Locate the pubococcygeal muscle.* This can be done by:
  - voluntarily stopping and starting the flow of urine during voiding.
  - squeezing the rectal muscles as though you are trying to prevent flatus from being expelled or holding a pencil between the buttocks.

If the above measures are not effective in helping the client identify the correct muscle, insert a gloved finger into the rectum and ask the client to tighten the muscles around the finger.
- *Perform the muscle-strengthening exercise.* To do this:
  - tighten the muscle in similar fashion as used to locate it;
  - hold the muscle tight for the count of 10;
  - relax the muscle;
  - repeat 15-20 times;
  - do the exercise in the morning, afternoon, and night (minimally).
- *Stay with it!* The exercises must be done correctly and regularly for several months in order for improvement to be noted.

BOX 8-3   **Bladder Retraining Program**

- Encourage good fluid intake during the day.
- If diuretics are prescribed, administer them early in the day.
- Record client's voiding pattern and related factors (relationship of voiding to activity, fluid ingestion) for several days. Review and determine amount of time client can hold urine.
- Advise client to toilet approximately 30 minutes before expected voiding time.
- Encourage voiding by running water, placing client's hands in warm water, pouring warm water over vulva or penis, rocking back and forth, massaging over bladder area.
- Measure amount voided.
- Maintain record of results.
- Praise client for continence.
- If client is incontinent between scheduled times, discuss reasons and alter schedule accordingly.

before anticipated time of voiding (based on record of client's voiding pattern over several days). Encourage the caregiver to document results for one week (i.e., note on flow chart if client was wet or dry at time checked for toileting). Evaluate after one week; if the client is wet more than one-half of the time, more frequent toileting should be done.

- Suggest use of biofeedback, which has been shown to improve urinary and fecal incontinence (Urinary Incontinence Guideline Panel, 1992); refer to appropriate therapist.
- Recommend adult briefs and condom catheters as appropriate. Remind client and caregivers that good cleansing of the skin is necessary when changing these containment devices because although skin may be dry, salts from the urine can dry on the skin and cause irritation.
- Emphasize importance of cleaning urine spills from floor immediately to prevent falls.
- Recommend environmental modifications to accommodate effects of incontinence, e.g.:
  - removing rugs from floor
  - using a mattress with a washable surface or washable cover to protect mattress
  - using pads or covers on upholstered furniture
  - cleaning furniture and floor surfaces with disinfectant
  - airing room, using room deodorizers
- Advise caregivers to manage incontinent episodes in matter-of-fact style and avoid discussing incontinent episodes in presence of others to preserve dignity of client.
- Encourage client to express feelings.
- Refer client and caregivers to resources for information and support (see Box 8-4).

BOX 8-4

Resources for Information About Incontinence

Continence Restored, Inc.
785 Park Avenue
New York, NY 10021
(212) 879-3131

Help for Incontinent People
Box 544
Union, SC 29389
(803) 585-8789

Kimberly Clark Corporation
2001 Marathon Avenue
Neenah, WI 54946
(414) 721-2000
www.kimberly-clark.com

Procter and Gamble
Procter and Gamble Plaza
Cincinnati, OH 45202
(800) 428-8363
www.pg.com

Simon Foundation for Incontinence
PO Box 835
Wilmette, IL 60091
(800) 23-SIMON
www.laborie.com/simon.html

Benign Prostatic Hypertrophy

Description

Benign prostatic hypertrophy is an enlargement of the prostate gland due to a non-cancerous growth. The risk of prostatic hypertrophy increases with each decade of life. Bladder outlet obstruction, urinary retention, and bladder distension can result.

Client Goals

- to eliminate urine effectively
- to be free from urinary retention
- to be free from urinary tract infection
- to have a balanced fluid intake and output

Interventions

- Assist with and educate client about diagnostic tests.
- Educate client about disease and its management. Review and clarify misconceptions concerning relationship of prostate problems to sexual function.
- Assist client with treatment, e.g.:
  - administration of urinary antiseptics if infection is present, drugs to reduce hyperplasia
  - prostatic massage to relieve congestion
  - preparation for surgery (transurethral resection, open prostatectomy)
- Encourage good fluid intake.
- Advise client and/or caregivers to monitor intake and output.
- Encourage regular physical activity.
- Advise client and/or caregivers to observe for and report signs of urinary tract infection and prostatitis, e.g., fever, chills, dysuria, flank pain, pain between legs.
- Encourage client to express concerns; encourage wife/partner to ask questions and express concerns.
- Discuss wise use of zinc, vitamins C and E, and the herb saw palmetto, which has been shown to reduce the size of the prostate, improve urinary flow and reduce nocturia (Champault et al., 1984; Walker 1991).
- Consult with homeopathic practitioner for remedies to treat prostatic enlargement, and acupuncturist regarding use of acupuncture.
- Guide client in use of imagery to visualize reduction in size of gland and unobstructed flow of urine.
- When prostatitis is present, use lavender, cypress, or thyme in aromatherapy.
- Consult with physician regarding use of contrasting temperature sitz baths (three minutes warm, thirty seconds cold), which have been shown to increase blood flow to the gland and improve function (Boyle and Saine, 1991). Be sure to advise client in safety precautions, e.g., measuring water temperature.
- Encourage client to receive prostate examination at least annually.
- Refer client to sources of additional information and support (see Box 8-5).

BOX 8-5
Resources for Information About Benign Prostatic Hypertrophy

Prostate Information
(800) 543-9632
Prostate Cancer Resource Network
PO Box 966
Fort Richey, FL 34656
(813) 847-1619
www.hmri.com
Women's Suffrage for Prostate Cancer Awareness and Support
743 Caribou Court
Sunnyvale, CA 94087
(888) 776-2262
info@pcawomen.org

Center for Prostate Disease Research
Department of Surgery
Uniformed Services University of Health Sciences
4301 Jones Bridge Road
Bethesda, MD 20814
(301) 295-9826
//surgery.usuhs.mil/CPDR.HTML

RESOURCES

Chronic Renal Failure

Description

Chronic renal failure is a progressive, irreversible loss of nephron function that results in the kidneys losing their ability to filter wastes from the body and maintain homeostasis. It can be caused by a variety of conditions including: congenital or developmental disorders, glomerulonephritis, neoplasms, tubular disorders, and systemic diseases (e.g., diabetes mellitus, hyperparathyroidism, scleroderma, gout). Chronic renal failure is divided into three stages:

- Reduced renal reserve: kidneys function at 40% to 75% normal capacity; usually asymptomatic with homeostasis maintained
- Renal insufficiency: kidneys function at 20% to 40% of normal capacity; increased BUN and serum creatinine, polyuria, nocturia, anemia, azotemia, decreased ability to maintain homeostasis
- End-stage renal disease (ESRD): kidneys function at less than 15% of normal capacity; significantly elevated BUN and creatinine, anemia, hyperphosphatemia, hypocalcemia, hyperuricemia, hyperkalemia, metabolic acidosis, oliguria, fluid overload, uremic syndrome; requires renal replacement therapy (dialysis, kidney transplant)

Compliance with the treatment plan can slow the progression of the disease and reduce the risk of complications.

Client Goals

- to correctly describe the disease, its self-care requirements, and complications
- to comply with prescribed diet
- to possess sufficient energy and comfort to engage in activities of daily living
- to use prescribed medications correctly

- to be free from infection, fluid retention, and other complications related to chronic renal failure

Interventions

- Teach client and caregivers/coach about disease and related care (Box 8-6).
- Assist with medication administration; medications could include:
  - antihypertensives
  - diuretics
  - calcium carbonate or calcium acetate to decrease hyperphosphatemia
  - calcium, vitamin D to facilitate calcium absorption
  - histamine H_2 receptor antagonists to reduce gastric irritation and ulceration
  - epoietin alfa (EPO) for anemia
- Recommend B complex vitamins, folic acid, and vitamins B_6 and C to compensate for dietary restrictions and replace loss of water-soluble vitamins during dialysis. Suggest use of fish oil, which has been shown to have positive effect on renal function, including lower rate of rejection of transplanted kidneys (Van der Heide et al., 1993).
- Reinforce strict adherence to dietary and fluid restrictions. Recommended diet often includes high calories and reduced protein, sodium, phosphorus, and potassium. Advise client to avoid salt substitutes due to their high potassium content.
- Encourage good oral hygiene to reduce irritation and bad taste associated with decreased salivary flow and ammonia from urea breakdown.
- Encourage frequent showers with mild soap if pruritus is present.
- Help client to plan rest periods between activities to conserve energy.
- Guide client in use of imagery to visualize good renal flow.

BOX 8-6   Topics to Include in Teaching Plan for the Client with Chronic Renal Failure

- Nature of disease
- Diet (e.g., strict adherence to restrictions of protein, sodium, phosphate) and changing dietary needs as disease progresses; fluid restriction
- Medications; cautious use of drugs that potentially can be nephrotoxic
- Responsibilities related to specific treatments (e.g., hemodialysis, peritoneal dialysis) or surgery
- Importance of exercise to promote muscle strength and prevent bone demineralization
- Scheduling rest periods to prevent fatigue
- Skin care
- Signs and symptoms to report (e.g., edema, weakness, fever, cough)
- Resources

BOX 8-7

Resources for Information About Renal Failure

American Association of Kidney Patients
100 South Ashley Drive
Suite 280
Tampa, FL 33602
(800) 749-2257
American Kidney Foundation
6110 Executive Boulevard
Suite 1010
Rockville, MD 20852
(800) 638-8299
cybermart.com/aakpaz/aakp.html

National Kidney Foundation
2 Park Avenue
New York, NY 10003
(212) 889-2210
www.kidney.org

- Suggest aromatherapy using hyssop or juniper.
- Encourage client to express feelings. Chronic renal disease can necessitate lifestyle changes with which client could need support.
- Refer to resources for additional information and support (see Box 8-7).

Constipation

Description

Constipation is an infrequent elimination of feces; the feces is of a hard, dry consistency and difficult or painful to expel. Many chronic conditions can cause constipation, including cirrhosis, diabetic neuropathy, multiple sclerosis, spinal cord injury, Crohn's disease, diverticulitis, and hemorrhoids. Antacids, analgesics, antihypertensives, anticholinergics, and antipsychotics are among the drugs that can reduce bowel elimination. A diet low in fiber and fluid, inactivity, advanced age, stress, depression, calcium supplements, and failure to allot time for toileting are factors contributing to this problem, also.

There is a difference in opinion between conventional and alternative practitioners regarding bowel elimination requirements. Most conventional practitioners would not label a person as constipated because he or she failed to have a daily bowel movement; however, many alternative practitioners believe at least one bowel movement daily is essential for health.

Client Goals

- to identify and, if possible, correct underlying cause of constipation
- to eliminate feces on a regular basis
- to be free from risks associated with constipation

Interventions

- Assist client in identifying factors that cause or contribute to constipation and developing a plan to correct factors (e.g., dietary modification, increasing appetite, changing medication, treating depression). Support prescribed treatments.

- Review client's history of preventing and correcting constipation; be alert to laxative misuse that aggravates problem.
- Encourage diet to facilitate regular elimination:
  - high fiber (inclusion of bran in diet)
  - high fluid intake (particularly if bran is used, to prevent blockage)
  - reduction in highly processed foods
  - two glasses of juice daily (e.g., carrot and apple, carrot and spinach, celery, beet)
- Advise client to chew foods slowly and thoroughly.
- Suggest the use of vitamin C supplements several times a day until stool softening is noted. (Ensure that client does not exceed 5000 mg per day.)
- Recommend herbs with laxative effects: aloe, dandelion root, *Cascara sagrada*, senna, rhubarb.
- Ensure that client allocates adequate time for toileting. Older clients may find that they have incomplete emptying of the bowel at one sitting and may need to complete their bowel movement 30 to 45 minutes after their first movement.
- Advise bedbound client to use commode rather than bedpan for bowel movements. The use of the bedpan while in bed forces the extension of the legs, abdominal hyperextension, and defecation without muscular help, causing unnecessary strain.
- Assist client in developing an exercise program to increase activity. To strengthen pelvic floor and abdominal muscles instruct client to do leg lifts (straight or bent legs), bent-knee sit-ups, and alternating contraction and relaxation of perineal muscles while seated.
- Consult with acupuncturist regarding treatments to restore peristalsis.
- Massage in circular motion around abdomen with essential oil of rose, marjoram, fennel, or rosemary.
- Discourage client who has cardiac disorder from straining or using enemas as this can stimulate the vagus nerve and inhibit heart function.
- If laxatives must be used, teach client to use them safely.
- Consult with homeopathic practitioner regarding use of *Alumina, Bryonia, Graphites, Natrum muriaticum, Nux vomica, Silicea.*
- Teach client to use progressive relaxation and other stress reduction measures if appropriate.

Diverticular Disease

Description

Diverticulosis is a condition in which multiple pouches form along the intestinal wall. Chronic constipation, obesity, a low-residue diet, and genetic predisposition are contributing factors to the development of this problem. When undigested food particles and small seeds (e.g., from berries) accumulate in these pouches, irritation and inflammation can occur; this inflammation of the diverticula is diverticulitis.

Client Goals

- to eliminate feces from the bowels regularly and without strain or discomfort
- to prevent and/or treat episodes of diverticulits

Interventions

- Assist client in identifying and reducing/eliminating contributing factors and adapting measures to control diverticular disease, e.g.:
  - high-fiber, low-residue diet
  - avoiding foods known to aggravate condition
  - preventing intraabdominal pressure (avoiding straining during bowel movements, heavy lifting, constricting clothing)
  - identifying possible food allergies and removing sensitive foods from diet
  - reducing weight
  - maintaining regular pattern of bowel elimination
- Assist client in relieving pain, e.g., use of guided imagery, biofeedback, safe use of analgesics.
- Consult with homeopathic practitioner regarding use of *Colocynthis*, *Bryonia*, and *Belladonna*.
- If antibiotics are ordered, ensure that client and/or caregivers administer them correctly and safely.

Hemorrhoids

Description

A hemorrhoid is a varicose vein in the anal region. Internal hemorrhoids occur above the anorectal line, whereas external hemorrhoids arise below and are visible on inspection. Chronic constipation, obesity, straining while having a bowel movement, long periods of sitting or standing, and heavy lifting are among the factors contributing to this condition.

Client Goals

- to be free from discomfort
- to prevent complications associated with hemorrhoids (e.g., infection, bleeding)

Interventions

- Assist client in establishing regular pattern of bowel elimination (refer to nursing interventions under "Constipation")
- Recommend a high-fiber intake. Insoluble fiber in foods such as whole-grain breads, wheat bran, fresh fruits, and vegetables absorb water to produce softer stool and may be more beneficial than soluble fiber (e.g., oat bran), which does not absorb water.
- Encourage a good fluid intake.
- Suggest use of sitz baths to relieve pain. Teach client and caregivers safety

measures associated with this procedure (e.g., ensuring water temperature of 100° to 105°F, observing for dizziness caused by blood being pulled to lower extremity).

- Advise client to use witch hazel compresses after bowel movements for comfort.
- For thrombosed external hemorrhoid, an ice pack can be applied to relieve pain and reduce the clot. This should be applied only for a few minutes at a time usually for a period of no more than a few hours.
- Encourage client to do Kegel-type exercises (alternating relaxation and contraction of perineal muscles) to facilitate circulation in anorectal area.
- Consult with physician regarding other treatments if self-care measures are not effective; such measures could include banding, excision, injection therapy, infrared coagulation, cryosurgery, and laser therapy.

Diarrhea

Description

The frequent passage of loose, unformed stools is known as diarrhea. This condition can be associated with diverticular disease, lactose intolerance, cancer, vitamin deficiencies, large doses of vitamin C, some artificial sweeteners, malabsorption, stress, infections, and drug reactions (e.g., antibiotics, laxatives).

Client Goals

- to prevent/correct diarrhea
- to establish pattern of regular bowel elimination
- to be free from complications associated with diarrhea (e.g., dehydration, impaired skin integrity)

Interventions

- Assist client in identifying and correcting underlying cause. Review medications used by client for those that can cause diarrhea (e.g., antibiotics, magnesium-based antacids, anticancer drugs, ascorbic acid, cardiac glycosides, cimetidine, gold salts, muscle relaxants, nonsteroid antiinflammatory drugs, potassium preparations, and vitamin E). Keep in mind that chronic diarrhea can be associated with food allergies; an elimination diet to identify sensitive foods may be needed.
- Advise client and caregivers to use good infection control practices.
- Ensure that client drinks adequate fluids; monitor intake and output.
- Teach client and caregivers to properly cleanse rectal area and to apply petroleum gel to prevent excoriation.
- Suggest use of natural substances for controlling diarrhea such as rice water or barley water (made by boiling rice or barley and straining the water for drinking), potatoes, tomatoes, apples (including the peel, which contains pectin) and carrots; the herb goldenseal is helpful.
- Teach stress reduction measures if stress is contributing factor.
- Consult with homeopathic practitioner regarding use of remedies:

Chamomilla, Colchicum, Sulphur, Arsenicum album, Nux vomica, Argentum nitricum, Ipecacuanha, Apis mellifica, Veratrum album, Mercurius sulphuricus, Calcarea carbonica, and *Natrum sulphuricum.*

- Use aromatherapy; essential oils with antispasmodic effects include eucalyptus, cypress, and chamomile.

Bowel Incontinence

Description

The inability to control the elimination of feces is bowel incontinence. Fecal impaction is a common cause of bowel incontinence, as is diarrhea. This condition can arise from some diseases, such as carcinoma of the rectum, and dementia. Rectal prolapse and the inability to toilet independently also can contribute to the problem.

Client Goals

- to regain bowel control
- to demonstrate regular pattern of bowel elimination
- to be free from complications associated with bowel incontinence (e.g., impaired skin integrity, social isolation, falls)

Interventions

- Assist client in identifying and correcting underlying cause.
- Recommend at least 2000 ml of fluid and high-fiber diet (unless contraindicated) to facilitate formed stool.
- Teach client and caregivers proper hygienic practices and infection control measures.
- Establish bowel retraining program (Box 8-8).
- Suggest use of biofeedback which has been shown to improve urinary and fecal incontinence (Urinary Incontinence Guideline Panel, 1992); refer to appropriate therapist.
- Guide client in use of imagery to assist in retraining efforts.
- Assist with use of adult briefs or other containment device.
- Encourage client to maintain or re-establish normal lifestyle.
- Ensure that caregivers treat client with dignity.

BOX 8-8   Bowel Retraining

- Maintain record of bowel elimination pattern and related factors (relationship to meals, drugs, activities) for one week; review to identify time when bowel elimination can be anticipated.
- Identify stimuli for bowel movement (e.g., activity, warm drink).
- Establish time for toileting based on record; advise or assist client to toilet approximately 20 minutes prior to that time.
- Insert a glycerin suppository approximately 30 minutes prior to scheduled time. (Mechanical stimulation may not be necessary after a routine is established.)
- Encourage client to use commode rather than bedpan. Place a footstool under feet to raise knees above level of hips.
- Instruct client to take several deep breaths, tighten abdomen, press hands on abdomen, and bear down. Rocking the trunk back and forth can be helpful.
- Advise client not to remain on the toilet for more than 10 minutes after anticipated time of elimination.
- Record results.
- Offer positive reinforcement for successes.

References

Boyle W and Saine A: *Lectures in naturopathic hydrotherapy*, East Palestine, OH, 1991, Buckeye Naturopathic Press.

Champault G, Patel JC, and Bonnard AM: A double-blind trial of an extract of the plant *Serenoa repens* in benign prostatic hyperplasia, *British Journal of Clinical Pharmacology* 18:461-2, 1984.

Urinary Incontinence Guideline Panel: Urinary incontinence in adults: clinical practice guideline, AHCPR Pub. No. 92-0038. Rockville, MD, Agency for Health Care Policy Research, Public Health Service, U.S. Dept. of Health and Human Services, March 1992.

Van der Heide JJH, et al.: Effect of dietary fish oil on renal function and rejection in cyclosporine-treated recipients of renal transplants, *New England Journal of Medicine* 329:769-73, 1993.

Walker M: *Serenoa repens* extract (saw palmetto) relief for benign prostatic hypertrophy, *Townsend Letter for Doctors*, February/March 1991.

Recommended Readings

Fantl JA, et al.: Managing acute and chronic urinary incontinence, clinical practice guideline, *Quick Reference Guide for Clinicians*, No. 2, 1996 Update.

U.S. Dept. of Health and Human Services, Public Health Service, Agency for Health Care Policy and Research: AHCPR Pub. No. 96-0686, Rockville, MD, March 1996.

Holt S, Likver L, and Muntyan I: The vegetarian way to a healthy urinary tract, *Alternative and Complementary Therapies* 2(3):168-172, 1996.

Kelly M: Clinical snapshot: chronic renal failure, *American Journal of Nursing* 96(1):36-37, 1996.

Klag MJ: Blood pressure and end-stage renal disease in men, *Journal of the American Medical Association* 275(20):1526, 1996.

Passmore AP, et al.: Chronic constipation in long stay elderly patients: a comparison of lactulose and a senna-fibre combination, *British Medical Journal* 307(6731):769-72, 1993.

Steefel L: Irritable bowel syndrome: complementary therapies for a mind-body illness, *Alternative and Complementary Therapies* 2(2):71-74, 1996.

Activity and Exercise

*A*ctivity is an essential component of a healthy state. Activity enables us to exercise the body, fulfill self-care requirements, enjoy satisfying interests, be engaged with society, and achieve feelings of normalcy and well-being.

Chronic illnesses can have a profound effect on activity. Independent movement can be threatened and the seemingly simple task of going from one place to another can be a tremendous challenge. There can be interference in the ability to fulfill the activities of daily living (ADLs) and the instrumental activities of daily living (IADLs). Restrictions in activity can cause chronically ill individuals to be treated differently and have limitations imposed upon them; this, in turn, can significantly affect psychological, social, and financial well-being. Roles and responsibilities may be inadequately fulfilled.

Some of the ways in which exercise can be achieved were discussed in Chapter 4. Basically, these programs aim toward increasing flexibility, strength, and endurance. Exercise programs are tailored to meet individual needs and capabilities.

Assessment Considerations

Be it the dizziness associated with hypertension, the inability to remember how to climb stairs due to the effects of a dementia, or the loss of the use of a limb, there are many ways that a chronic condition can affect the pattern of activity and exercise; therefore an assessment of this functional pattern is critical.

A determination of the client's level of independence in the ADLs (Table 9-1) and IADLs (Table 9-2) gives a basic overview of functional capacity. Scores from assessment tools are important, not only to understanding current level of function, but also to identifying changes over time. For example, a change indicating the need for more in-depth evaluation would be a client's IADL score hitting 15 in February and 10 in the following June. A review of the client's typical day can yield insight into the pattern of activity and exercise. Specific areas to discuss include frequency and type of exercise, leisure activities, and household management responsibilities. When deficits are discovered, questions should be asked concerning when the deficits were first noted, strategies the client uses to compensate for them, and impact on the client's life.

Strength and energy level should be evaluated. Specific questions concerning fatigue, weakness, pain, and vertigo can assist in identifying problems. Along with these, vital signs should be assessed, both in a resting state and following both physical and mental activity. During this assessment, consideration should be given to mental activity and exercise. Mental stimulation and challenges promote physical health and a sense of well-being.

The client's diagnoses are important to review in determining the impact of the chronic condition on activity and exercise. Table 9-3 lists examples of ways in which common chronic diseases can affect activity. For instance, questions should be asked concerning the use of assistive devices and mobility aids. It is important

TABLE 9-1

Standards of Activities of Daily Living

	Level I independent	Level II requires mechanical assistance	Level III requires human assistance	Level IV totally dependent
Feeding	Able to eat without assistance	Needs special eating utensils	Needs food served and cut, packages opened, reminders to eat	Needs to be fed
Bathing	Able to get in and out of tub or shower and bathe all body parts	Needs grab bars, tub seats, adjusted faucet handles	Needs to be supported or lifted into tub or shower, back or other body part bathed	Needs complete bathing assistance
Dressing	Able to pick out appropriate garments and dress completely	Needs clothing and shoes modified with snaps or Velcro	Needs assistance with some garments and/or reminders of order in which to dress	Needs to be fully dressed
Continence	Able to completely control bowel and bladder elimination	Needs enemas, catheters	Periodically incontinent of urine or feces, needs to be reminded to toilet	Totally unable to control bowel or bladder elimination, catheterized
Toileting	Able to use toilet or bedpan and use proper related hygiene techniques	Needs bedside commode, bedpan, urinal	Needs assistance using commode or bedpan, wiping and cleansing after toileting	Unable to use toilet independently or clean self after elimination
Mobility	Able to walk and transfer from bed to chair	Needs cane, walker, crutch, wheelchair, brace, trapeze	Can walk, transfer, or use mobility aid with assistance	Totally unable to transfer, ambulate, or propel wheelchair

From Eliopoulos C: *Manual of gerontologic nursing,* St. Louis, 1995, Mosby.

TABLE 9-2

Instrumental Activities of Daily Living

Action	Score	Action	Score
A. ABILITY TO USE TELEPHONE		E. LAUNDRY	
1. Operates telephone on own initiative—looks up and dials numbers, etc.	1	1. Does personal laundry completely	1
2. Dials a few well-known numbers	1	2. Launders small items-rinses socks, stockings, etc.	1
3. Answers telephone but does not dial	1	3. All laundry must be done by others	0
4. Does not use telephone at all	0	F. MODE OF TRANSPORTATION	
B. SHOPPING		1. Travels independently on public transportation or drives own care	1
1. Takes care of all shopping needs independently	1	2. Arranges own travel via taxi but does not otherwise use public transportation	1
2. Shops independently for small purchases	0	3. Travels on public transportation when assisted or accompanied by another	1
3. Needs to be accompanied on any shopping trip	0	4. Travel limited to taxi or automobile with assistance of another	0
4. Completely unable to shop	0	5. Does not travel at all	0
C. FOOD PREPARATION		G. RESPONSIBILITY FOR OWN MEDICATIONS	
1. Plans, prepares, and serves adequate meals independently	1	1. Is responsible for taking medication in correct dosages at correct times	1
2. Prepares adequate meals if supplied with ingredients	0	2. Takes responsibility if medication is prepared in advance in separate dosages	0
3. Heats and serves prepared meals or prepares meals but does not maintain adequate diet	0	3. Is not capable of dispensing own medication	0
4. Needs to have meals prepared and served	0	H. ABILITY TO HANDLE FINANCES	
D. HOUSEKEEPING		1. Manages financial matters independently (budgets, writes checks, pays rent, bills, goes to bank), collects and keeps track of income	1
1. Maintains house alone or with occasional assistance (e.g., "heavy work-domestic help")	1	2. Manages day-to-day purchases but needs help with banking, major purchases, etc.	1
2. Performs light daily tasks such as dish washing, bed making	1	3. Incapable of handling money	0
3. Performs light daily tasks but cannot maintain acceptable level of cleanliness	1		
4. Needs help with all home maintenance tasks	1		
5. Does not participate in any housekeeping tasks	0		

From Lawton MP, Brody E: Assessment of older people: self-maintaining and instrumental activities of daily living, *Gerontologist* 9:181, 1969.

TABLE 9-3

Effects of Chronic Disease on Activity-Exercise Pattern

Chronic disease	Related symptoms that can affect activity and/or exercise
AIDS	Fatigue
Alzheimer's disease	Confusion, fatigue, pacing, wandering
Arthritis	Pain, restricted mobility
Asthma	Wheezing, dyspnea
Cancer	Pain, fatigue
Cirrhosis	Fatigue, dyspnea, edema, muscle atrophy
Chronic obstructive pulmonary disease	Shortness of breath, fatigue
Chronic renal failure	Fatigue, diminished exercise tolerance, weakness, dyspnea
Congestive heart failure	Shortness of breath, edema, fatigue
Coronary artery disease	Angina, muscle cramps, shortness of breath, fatigue, palpitations
Depression	Lethargy, fatigue, disinterest
Diabetes mellitus	Hypoglycemia, fatigue
Hypertension	Dizziness, fatigue secondary to antihypertensives
Multiple sclerosis	Tremors, spasms, hearing and visual disturbances
Parkinson's disease	Gait disturbance, tremors, dysarthria

to determine whether canes, wheelchairs, and other aids are properly sized and correctly used.

In addition to the actual activity limitations imposed by chronic conditions, a determination of the potential impact of these conditions on activity is beneficial so that risks can be identified and plans developed to prevent problems.

Related Diagnoses

Activity Intolerance

Description

Activity intolerance is a state in which the client experiences an inability to endure an increase in activity due to physiological or psychological factors.

Client Goals

- to increase activity to maximum level possible, while maintaining a healthy balance between activity and rest
- to verbalize decreased fatigue, weakness
- to express satisfaction with activity level
- to be free from complications related to activity intolerance

Interventions

- Assist client in identifying factors responsible for activity intolerance and planning specific interventions (e.g., obtaining counseling for depression, treating physical disorder, managing pain, improving dietary intake). Consult with occupational and physical therapists as needed.

- Teach client energy-saving techniques. Assist client in scheduling rest between activities and learning to balance activity and rest.
- Assist and/or teach caregivers to assist client with activities, exercise, and care as needed.
- Monitor vital signs before and after activities.
- Recommend ways to combine physical activity with a leisure or social function.
- Suggest client engage in yoga, tai chi, and other forms of activity.
- Review diet and ensure adequate nutrition.
- Advise client to boost energy with the use of vitamin supplements and the herbs ginseng and cayenne. To assist in protecting the body from the effects of stress from activity, suggest the use of the herbs valerian and ginseng.
- Recommend use of essential oils of black spruce and peppermint to promote energy, and citronella, mandarin and lavender for relaxation.
- Teach and encourage use of stress management and progressive relaxation techniques.
- Assist client in obtaining devices to improve independence and mobility, such as cane, wheelchair, long-handled utensils.

Chronic Fatigue Syndrome

Description

The Centers for Disease Control officially recognized chronic fatigue syndrome as a disease in 1988; prior to that time, many health care professionals dismissed the condition as an imaginary one. As the name implies, extreme, long-term (usually six months or more), unrelieved, and unexplained fatigue characterizes chronic fatigue syndrome. Other symptoms include muscle and joint pain, headache, memory disturbances, poor concentration, gastrointestinal disturbances, low grade fever, recurring infections, increased sensitivities/allergies, dizziness, depression, and, in some cases, confusion, hypersensitivity to heat and cold, night sweats, and irregular heartbeat. Symptoms can fluctuate from day to day.

Client Goals

- to increase activity tolerance
- to demonstrate independence in ADLs and IADLs
- to be free from complications associated with chronic fatigue syndrome

Interventions

- Support prescribed treatment plan (e.g., administration of antibiotics, dietary supplements).
- Ensure that other potential causes of fatigue are ruled out (Box 9-1).
- Encourage diet high in protein and complex carbohydrates, and low in simple carbohydrates and fats. Encourage good fluid intake.

- Suggest use of herbs to boost immune function and to help treat infections, such as echinacea, ginseng, goldenseal, and licorice.
- Recommend multivitamin and mineral supplement; some alternative practitioners recommend use of wheatgrass juice.
- If depression is present, refer for treatment; support treatment plan.
- Refer to acupuncturist for treatments to boost immunity.
- Guide client in use of imagery to boost immunity and energy.
- Refer to resources for additional information and support (see Box 9-2).

BOX 9-1	Possible Causes of Fatigue Other Than Chronic Fatigue Syndrome

Nutritional deficiencies	Diabetes mellitus
Stress	Cardiac disease
Sleep disturbance (e.g., sleep apnea)	Hypothyroidism
Obesity	Infection
Anemia	Adrenal insufficiency
Allergy	Medications (e.g., antipsychotics,
Depression	sedatives, antihistamines, anal-
Hypoglycemia	gesics, antihypertensives)

BOX 9-2

Resources for Information About Chronic Fatigue Syndrome

CFIDS Association, Inc.
PO Box 220398
Charlotte, NC 28222
(800) 442-3437
http://www.cfids.org/
CFIDS Buyer's Club
1187 Coast Village Road
#1-280
Santa Barbara, CA 93108
(800) 366-6056

CFS Survival Association
PO Box 1889
Davis, CA 95617
(916) 756-9242
National Chronic Fatigue Syndrome and Fibromyalgia Association
3521 Broadway
Suite 222
Kansas City, MO 64111
(816) 931-4777

Ineffective Airway Clearance

Description

An impairment in the passage of air through the respiratory tract due to the presence of an obstruction or the ineffective removal of secretions is ineffective airway clearance. When secretions slowly build up, this condition can lead not only to complete obstruction or infection but to fatigue and activity intolerance.

Client Goals

- to maintain or regain patent airway
- to effectively remove secretions from airway
- to be free from infections related to ineffective airway clearance
- to maximize ability to participate in physical activities

Interventions

- Assist client with diagnosis and treatment of underlying cause.
- Teach client and caregivers correct procedures for treatments:
  - intermittent positive-pressure breathing
  - oxygen therapy
  - suctioning
  - postural drainage
  - administration of medications (e.g., antibiotics, steroids, cough preparations, bronchodilators, antipyretics)
- Teach deep breathing exercises and encourage client to do them every 2 hours while awake.
- Encourage client to consume at least 1500 ml daily unless contraindicated.
- Recommend use of humidifier; if this is unavailable, suggest pan of water be placed on top of radiator or other heat source (review safety precautions).
- Encourage frequent oral hygiene.
- Monitor vital signs and sputum production.
- Reinforce infection control practices.
- Teach client and caregivers/coach signs of respiratory infection (e.g., increased cough or sputum production, tightness in chest, dyspnea, fever, sputum of yellow, green or gray color.
- Review status of influenza and pneumonia vaccination; arrange for immunization if warranted.

Asthma

Description

Asthma is a chronic respiratory disorder in which there is a sudden narrowing of the airway and dyspnea as a reaction to allergens, pollutants, stress, or infection. It is common among all age groups, but is a leading cause of disease and disability in children between ages two and seventeen years. For many children, fear may encourage a restriction of physical activities that is often unwarranted. Because many of the medications used to treat asthma potentially have serious effects (e.g., steroids), natural methods to prevent and manage asthma attacks can have significant long-term benefits for the client.

Client Goals

- to identify and control factors that cause attacks
- to state measures to prevent and treat asthma

- to describe appropriate steps in seeking help for acute attacks
- to demonstrate correct use of inhaler
- to maximize ability to engage in physical activities

Interventions

- Assist in diagnostic evaluation to determine cause of attacks.
- Teach client and caregivers/coach about disease and its management including:
  - description of disease and its effects
  - signs of attack
  - precipitating factors
  - preventive measures, e.g., smoking cessation, control of triggers (Box 9-3), prevention of infection, reducing irritants in home environment)
  - treatment of attack
  - proper use of medication, including inhaler
  - breathing exercises
  - relaxation techniques
  - lifestyle adjustments: diet, activity
- Ensure that inhaler is properly used; discourage overuse.
- Determine whether client breathes through the mouth rather than the nose. (Many asthmatics are mouth breathers, which can promote easier entry of unfiltered dust, organisms and cold air into lungs.) Assist client with breathing retraining to facilitate breathing through the nose.
- Suggest that client eliminate substances that could promote allergic reactions, such as tobacco, alcohol, caffeine, sugar, and foods containing preservatives. Refer to smoking cessation program if appropriate.

BOX 9-3   Potential Asthma Triggers

- Cold air, hot air, sudden changes in temperature
- High humidity
- Tobacco smoke
- Dust
- Vapors, fumes
- Mold spores
- Pollens
- Dander from animals
- Feather or hair-stuffed pillows or toys
- Upholstered furniture
- Draperies
- Insects (e.g., roaches)
- Fluorocarbon spray products
- Perfumes and scented products
- Dirty air conditioner and heating system filters
- Smog
- Automobile exhaust
- Medications
- Stress
- Overexertion
- Respiratory illnesses (e.g., colds, flu)

- Discuss supplementation of diet with niacinamide, magnesium (shown to significantly improve airflow rates in asthmatics not sufficiently helped by inhalers [Skobeloff et al., 1989]), calcium glycerophosphate, beta carotene, selenium, manganese and vitamins C, B_6, and B_{12} (Anibarro et al., 1992).
- Discuss the safe use of herbs that are helpful for asthma; these include ephedra, ginkgo biloba, thyme, mullein, marshmallow, capsaicin, onions, green tea, garlic, licorice, and slippery elm.
- Encourage client to include juices in diet: carrot and spinach, carrot and celery, grapefruit, lemon juice and water.
- Suggest that client consult with homeopathic practitioner regarding use of remedies such as *Antimonium tartaricom* and *Nux vomica*. Homeopathic immunotherapy has been shown to be effective in the treatment of asthma (Reilly et al., 1994).
- Teach client use of progressive relaxation and biofeedback.
- Guide client in the use of imagery to promote relaxation and to visualize widening of the airway. Research has supported a reduction in medication use and improvement in quality of life for persons with asthma who used imagery (Epstein et al., 1997).
- Use aromatherapy with essential oils of bergamot, camphor, eucalyptus, lavender, hyssop, or marjoram.
- Refer client to hypnotherapist. (Hypnotherapy has been shown to reduce asthma attacks.)
- Advise client to learn and practice yoga. Studies have shown that yoga training significantly increased pulmonary function, decreased respiratory symptoms, and reduced the need for asthma medications (Jain et al., 1991).
- Refer client to resources for additional information and support (see Box 9-4).

BOX 9-4

Resources for Information About Asthma

American Lung Association
1740 Broadway
New York, NY 10019
(212) 315-8700
www.lungusa.org/

Asthma and Allergy Foundation of America
1125 15th Street NW
Suite 502
Washington, DC 20005
(800) 7-ASTHMA
www.aafa.org/

Asthma Hotline
(800) 222-LUNG

National Institute of Allergy and Infectious Diseases
9000 Rockville Pike
Building 31, Room 7A-03
Bethesda, MD 20205
(301) 496-4000
www.niaid.nih.gov/

Risk for Aspiration

Description

The entry of secretions, food or other foreign matter into the tracheobronchial tree is aspiration. Many chronic conditions can predispose the client to this risk, including cerebrovascular accident, Parkinson's disease, multiple sclerosis, vocal cord paralysis, reduced level of consciousness, and dementia; medications that depress reflexes or dry oral cavity and artificial nutritional devices (e.g., NG tube) increase the risk for aspiration also.

Client Goals

- to swallow foods appropriately without aspiration
- to be free from complications related to aspiration

Interventions

- Assist client in identifying and reducing risk factors.
- Ensure that secretions have been cleared from mouth and pharynx prior to feeding.
- Advise client and caregivers to promote feeding safety by having client:
  - sit at 90° angle during ingestion of food and fluids and for approximately 45 minutes thereafter
  - flex head forward during swallowing (chin tuck)
  - keep head in midline
  - place food on uninvolved side (if paralysis present)
  - ingest 1/2 to 3/4 teaspoon at a time
  - hold breath and then swallow
  - swallow a second time
  - massage upward on laryngeal area to facilitate swallowing
- Instruct client to cut food into small pieces, chew thoroughly, and eat slowly.
- Teach client to use thermogustatory stimulation to facilitate swallowing; to do this, alternate small amount of lemon-flavored Italian ice with food while eating.
- Recommend frequent small-portioned feedings rather than three large meals.
- If client has decreased sensations in mouth or throat, encourage pureed or soft foods rather than liquids whenever feasible (e.g., gelatin, custard, sherbet).
- If client has nausea, suggest use of ginger.
- If aspiration is a frequent problem, ensure that suction equipment is available; teach caregivers how to suction and use Heimlich maneuver.
- Assess lung sounds, respiratory status frequently.

Impaired Gas Exchange

Description

A decreased passage of oxygen or carbon dioxide between the alveoli and vascular system is referred to as impaired gas exchange. Chronic obstructive pulmonary disease, chronic bronchitis, and pneumonia are among the conditions that can be responsible for this diagnosis.

Client Goals

- to have arterial blood gases within a normal range
- to be free from complications associated with impaired gas exchange

Interventions

- Support plan to monitor blood gases.
- Support and teach treatment plan, e.g., administration of bronchodilators or expectorants, postural drainage.
- Encourage at least 2000 ml fluids daily unless contraindicated.
- If prescribed, ensure that oxygen is used correctly and safely.
- Instruct client and caregivers to keep head of bed elevated 30° unless contraindicated.
- Teach client diaphragmatic, deep breathing exercises (Fig. 9-1).
- Assess lung sounds, respiratory status.
- Review impact of respiratory problem on sexual function. Offer suggestions, such as positions to conserve energy, resting before sexual activity.
- Use biofeedback and guided imagery to promote good lung expansion.

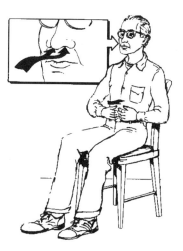

FIGURE 9-1

Diaphragmatic, deep breathing exercises. Inhaling air should cause client's hands to move out with the expanding abdomen. As client exhales, the abdomen and hands will move again. From Hoeman S:*Rehabilitative/restorative care in the community*, St. Louis, 1990, Mosby.

- Advise client and caregivers/coach to recognize and report signs and symptoms of impaired gas exchange, e.g., cyanosis, dyspnea, orthopnea, change in respiratory rate, retracted breathing, cough, increase in amount or viscosity of sputum, edema, reduced output.
- Suggest use of yoga to promote respiratory function.
- Encourage client to express concerns.

Chronic Obstructive Pulmonary Disease (COPD)

Description

Chronic bronchitis is a form of COPD characterized by repeated inflammation of the bronchi with production of large amounts of mucus that obstruct the airways (Fig. 9-2). The irritation from cigarette smoke (including second-hand smoke) can contribute to this problem, as can infections of the respiratory tract.

Another type of COPD is emphysema, which is characterized by a distension and reduced number of alveoli. This disorder is frequently associated with a resul-

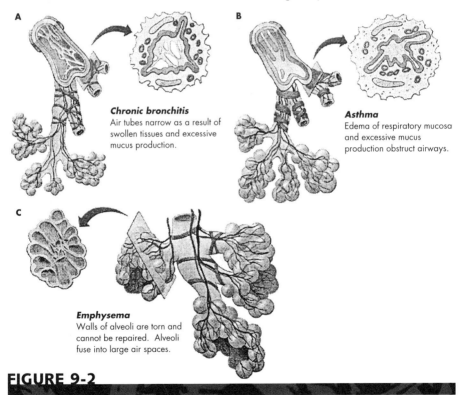

Chronic bronchitis
Air tubes narrow as a result of swollen tissues and excessive mucus production.

Asthma
Edema of respiratory mucosa and excessive mucus production obstruct airways.

Emphysema
Walls of alveoli are torn and cannot be repaired. Alveoli fuse into large air spaces.

FIGURE 9-2

Disorders of the airways in patients with chronic bronchitis, asthma, and emphysema. A, Chronic bronchitis. Excessive amounts of mucus accumulate in the airways obstructing airflow and impairing ciliary function. B, Asthma. Bronchial smooth muscle constricts in response to irritants, resulting in airflow obstruction and wheezing. C, Emphysema. Proteolytic enzymes destroy lung tissue resulting in enlarged air sacs and impaired gas exchange. From Thibodeau A, Patton K: *Anatomy and physiology,* ed 3, 1996, Mosby.

tant exhaustion and high activity intolerance. Cigarette smoking is the major risk factor for emphysema, along with infections, chronic irritation from pollutants, and other causes.

Client Goals

- to learn and utilize measures to promote effective respirations and gas exchange
- to maintain patent airway
- to adapt to necessary lifestyle changes (e.g., smoking cessation, improved nutrition)
- to be free from complications associated with COPD (e.g., infection, peptic ulcer, adverse drug reactions)
- to find strategies for both using and conserving energy efficiently
- to describe strategies to maximize ADL and IADL involvement and independence

Interventions

- Instruct client and caregivers/coach in realities of disease and its management.
- Assist client in identifying and reducing/eliminating contributing factors, e.g.:
  - smoking cessation
  - avoidance of second-hand smoke
  - avoidance of air pollutants
- Support and instruct client and caregivers/coach in prescribed treatments, including:
  - medications (e.g., bronchodilators, antibiotics)
  - IPPB treatments
  - oxygen
  - chest physiotherapy (postural drainage, percussion, coughing)
- Determine impact of disease on ADL and IADL independence. Assist client in developing measures to promote independence (e.g., scheduling rest between activities, using a cart to carry groceries).
- Encourage good diet with adequate caloric intake to compensate for extra calories expended during breathing. Suggest:
  - frequent oral hygiene
  - eating small meals several times throughout the day rather than three large ones
  - performing chest physiotherapy approximately one hour before meals
  - resting before meals
  - consuming nutritious snacks
  - utilizing Meals on Wheels if meal preparation is a problem
- Recommend use of fish oil, which has been shown to reduce the risk of COPD in smokers and is believed to have a beneficial effect on the lungs (Shahar et al., 1994).

- Encourage consumption of hot, spicy foods (chili peppers, onion, garlic, horseradish) which can assist in opening airways, and raw juices (e.g., carrot, spinach, celery).
- Discourage large amounts of dairy products, starches, sugars, and eggs in diet; these foods can increase mucus production.
- Recommend vitamins A, B_{12}, C, and E, zinc, selenium, lethicin, and bioflavonoids as supplements.
- Teach and advise client and caregivers to report signs of peptic ulcer, a complication associated with COPD.
- Instruct client in the safe use of herbs: Echinacea, horehound, goldenseal, garlic and ginseng; also herbal teas that can provide relief:
  - coltsfoot tea to assist with expectoration and decrease the amount of mucus produced
  - mixture of coltsfoot, mullein, and licorice to soothe coughing
  - blend of poke root, licorice, echinacea, grindelia and lobelia for bronchitis relief
- Advise client to consume at least 2000 ml of fluids daily unless contraindicated. Promote fluid intake in other forms, such as gelatins, sherbets, soups.
- Review measures that client should follow to avoid respiratory infection, such as:
  - avoidance of crowds and contact with people who have colds or other respiratory infections
  - adherence to good infection control measures
  - influenza and pneumonia vaccinations
- Review general measures to boost immunity (see Chapter 7).
- Teach client to use guided imagery, biofeedback, meditation, and yoga to improve respirations and control symptoms.
- Offer and teach caregivers to massage client to promote respiratory function.
- Use aromatherapy with essential oils of:
  - blend of clove, cinnamon, melissa, and lavender for bronchitis
  - eucalyptus, lavender, or pine for emphysema or bronchitis
- Consult with homeopathic practitioner regarding use of *Aconite, Bryonia, Phosphorus, Ferrous phosphoricum*, and *Calcarea sulphurica* for bronchitis, and *Aspidosperma* and *Carbo vegetabilis* for emphysema.
- Refer client to resources for additional information and support (see Box 9-5).

BOX 9-5

Resources for Information About Chronic Obstructive Pulmonary Disease

American Lung Association
1740 Broadway
New York, NY 10019
(800) 586-4872
www.lungusa.org/

Nicotine Anonymous
PO Box 1585
New York, NY 10113
(800) 977-4325

Altered Tissue Perfusion

Description

Altered tissue perfusion results from a decrease in nutrition and oxygenation at the cellular level secondary to a reduced capillary blood supply. Clients at high risk for this diagnosis are those with arteriosclerotic heart disease, hypertension, congestive heart failure, pulmonary edema, aneurysms, varicosities, diabetes, and anemia.

Client Goals

- to be free from signs of altered tissue perfusion
- to learn and adapt to practices/activities to improve circulation
- to be free from complications related to altered tissue perfusion

Interventions

- Assist client in identifying and reducing or eliminating contributing factors (e.g., preventing angina attacks, smoking cessation, keeping extremities warm, reducing weight, not wearing constricting clothing).
- Support and teach client and caregivers/coach prescribed treatment plan:
  - medications (e.g., anticoagulants, antihypertensives, vasodilators)
  - antiembolism stockings
  - range-of-motion, Buerger-Allen exercises
  - diet restrictions (e.g., low calorie, low cholesterol, low fat, low sodium, no alcohol)
  - monitoring vital signs
- Promote good skin care, including foot care, and frequent position changes.
- Advise client to avoid the following:
  - extremes in temperature
  - prolonged standing, sitting
  - crossing legs
  - constipation
  - inactivity
  - cigarette smoking
  - rapid changes in position
- Teach and encourage client to use progressive relaxation, meditation, biofeedback, and yoga for stress reduction and promotion of circulation.
- Assist client in developing appropriate exercise program. Consult with physical therapist as needed.
- If poor peripheral circulation is present, encourage client to do any or all of the following, as applicable:
  - walk unless symptoms are experienced
  - protect feet from injury
  - wash feet and dry thoroughly, apply lotion to prevent dryness
  - keep toenails cut straight across

- avoid stockings with dyes that bleed
- wear appropriate-fitting shoes, avoid going barefoot
- obtain podiatry care for foot disorders
- massage feet daily unless contraindicated (Box 9-6)
- promptly recognize abnormalities that should be reported (e.g., numbness, ulcers, discoloration, unusual coldness or warmth, swelling)

Angina Pectoris

Description

Angina pectoris is a clinical syndrome characterized by pain in the chest and radiating to the shoulder and left arm caused by ischemia of the heart muscle. Although the most common cause is atherosclerosis, risk factors include diabetes mellitus, hypertension, aortic regurgitation or insufficiency, and severe anemia. Exercise becomes limited because it can be a precipitating factor.

Client Goals

- to identify and control precipitating factors
- to be free from complications associated with angina pectoris

Interventions

- Assist client in identifying precipitating factors that trigger attack and in developing measures to adjust for, reduce or eliminate them; these factors include:
  - physical exertion
  - emotional stress
  - cold weather
  - cigarette smoking or smoke
  - large, heavy meal
  - sexual activity

BOX 9-6   Foot Massage

Unless thrombosis or another contraindication exists, foot massages should be promoted as a means to promote relaxation and circulation. Instruct the caregiver to:
- soak the feet (water temperature should not exceed 105°F) and dry thoroughly
- inspect for breaks, discolorations and other problems
- apply lotion to the hands
- cradle the client's foot in both hands for a few seconds
- using the thumb, make circular motions over the sole
- roll knuckles over the sole
- gently rotate and pull each toe
- knead the heel and ankle
- massage the heel firmly
- allow the client a few minutes of relaxation before rising

- Reinforce importance of preventing attacks rather than merely correcting them after they are present. Repeated anginal attacks can leave fibrotic scars that increase risk of serious myocardial disease.
- Instruct client and caregivers/coach in proper use of medications (e.g., nitrates, beta-adrenergic blocking agents, calcium channel blockers) and recognition of adverse effects.
- Teach client use of progressive relaxation, meditation, yoga, and biofeedback to reduce stress.
- Discuss use of L-carnitine supplement, which has been shown to increase maximum exercise workload, reduce attacks, and reduce mortality (Davini et al., 1992), and CoQ10, which has been beneficial in increasing exercise tolerance in persons with chronic angina (Kamikawa et al., 1985).
- Consult with acupuncturist regarding benefit of treatment for client. Some studies have shown acupuncture to cause a reduction in the number and severity of angina attacks (Richter et al., 1991).

Hypertension

Description

Hypertension is an above normal blood pressure (Table 9-4). Over 60 million Americans suffer from this chronic condition with a higher incidence in black Americans than in white Americans. Hypertension can be:

Essential or primary: accounts for most cases; no known cause.

Secondary: related to underlying disease or condition, such as renal arterial or parenchymal disease, endocrine disorders, coarctation of aorta, head trauma, cranial tumor, and pregnancy

The asymptomatic nature of hypertension can cause clients to be lax in their adherence to the treatment plan, thereby necessitating ongoing reinforcement.

TABLE 9-4

Classification of Hypertension

The Joint National Committee on the Detection, Evaluation, and Treatment of High Blood Pressure classifies hypertension according to the following guidelines:

Systolic	Diastolic	Classification	Recommended Action
< 140	< 90	Normal	Routine screening
140-159	< 90	Borderline systolic hypertension	Re-evaluate in 2 months
≥ 160	< 90	Systolic hypertension	Re-evaluate in 2 months
	85-89	High-normal diastolic	Re-evaluate in 2 months
	90-104	Mild hypertension	Re-evaluate in 2 months
	105-114	Moderate hypertension	Refer for evaluation < 2 weeks
	≥ 115	Severe hypertension	Refer for immediate evaluation

Client Goals

- to maintain blood pressure within normal range
- to reduce or eliminate risk factors contributing to hypertension
- to be free from complications associated with hypertension
- to develop habits, such as weight reduction and sensible exercise, that can reduce blood pressure

Interventions

- Assist client in identifying and implementing strategies that can reduce risk factors:
  - weight reduction
  - smoking cessation
  - restricting sodium intake
  - avoiding alcohol ingestion
  - developing an exercise program
  - reducing and effectively managing stress
- Support and teach client and caregivers/coach treatment plan:
  - medications: proper administration, side effects, adverse effects, importance of taking even if asymptomatic
  - diet modifications: sodium restriction, reduced saturated fats, reduction/elimination of alcohol, increasing potassium-rich foods
  - recognition of complications (e.g., congestive heart failure, retinopathy, myocardial infarction, altered mental status)
- Reinforce importance of strict compliance with treatment plan to avoid complications.
- Teach client and caregivers/coach proper method for measuring blood pressure.
- Discuss impact of antihypertensives on sexual function. Encourage client to report sexual dysfunction to physician and explore possibility of alternative medication or treatment.
- Encourage activity, which can aid in reducing blood pressure. Help client develop individualized exercise program; consult with physical therapist as needed.
- Encourage client to eat potassium-rich foods, which have been shown to lower systolic and diastolic blood pressures.
- Discuss safe use of fish oil supplements. Studies have shown fish oil to reduce blood pressure in hypertensive people, while not affecting blood pressure in persons with normal blood pressures (Morris et al., 1993).
- Instruct client to wisely use hawthorn berries and garlic, which have shown evidence of lowering blood pressure and cholesterol after a several months' trial (Auer et al., 1990).
- Caution about use of the herbs ginseng and licorice, which can raise blood pressure.
- Discuss use of calcium magnesium, bioflavonoids, the amino acid taurine, niacin, and vitamins A, C, and E (do not use vitamin E in high doses).

- Instruct client to use progressive relaxation, guided imagery, music, biofeedback, meditation, yoga, and other stress reduction measures. (A small study showed that the combined use of yogic relaxation, meditation and biofeedback, along with a galvanic skin response meter, enabled most hypertensive individuals to reduce or discontinue their medications (Patel, 1973).
- Offer and teach caregivers to give slow, stroking massages, which can cause a temporary reduction in blood pressure (Yates, 1990).
- Use aromatherapy with essential oils of ylang ylang, marjoram, or lavender.
- Consult with acupuncturist regarding the benefits of treatment for the client.
- Refer client to resources for additional information and support (see Box 9-7).

BOX 9-7

Resources for Information About Hypertension

American Heart Association
7320 Greenville Avenue
Dallas, TX 75231
(800) 242-8721
www.amhrt.org/

Citizens for the Treatment of High Blood Pressure
1990 M Street NW
Suite 360
Washington, DC 20036
(202) 296-7747

High Blood Pressure Information Center
National Institutes of Health
4733 Bethesda Avenue
Bethesda, MD 20814
(301) 952-3260

Impaired Physical Mobility

Description

Impaired physical mobility is a state in which physical movement is limited. Although musculoskeletal disorders are usually considered responsible for impaired mobility, movement alterations can also result from sensory loss, fatigue, pain, depression, dementia, and any other condition that causes weakness, pain, bedrest restrictions, and altered neuromuscular activity. The multiple hazards associated with immobility (Box 9-8) necessitate active interventions to prevent complications.

Client Goals

- to increase mobility
- to reduce or eliminate factors that contribute to immobility
- to be free of complications associated with immobility

BOX 9-8	Negative Consequences of Impaired Mobility

Cardiovascular	**Musculoskeletal**
Increased workload on heart	Osteoporosis
Hypotension	Ease of bone fractures
Thrombosis	Muscle atrophy
Respiratory	Contractures
Reduced chest expansion	**Skin**
Increased effort for breathing	Pressure ulcers
Poor gas exchange	**Neurological**
Insufficient ventilation	Sensory deprivation
Ineffective coughing	**Metabolic**
Increased secretions	Decreased metabolic rate
Gastrointestinal	Reduced heat conduction, increased perspiration
Poor appetite	
Stress ulcers	Decreased production of adrenocortical hormones
Increased catabolic activity, negative nitrogen balance	**Psychological**
Constipation	Depression
Fecal impaction	Anxiety
Genitourinary	Increased stress
Urinary stasis, calculi	Feelings of helplessness and hopelessness
Urinary tract infection	
Overflow, functional incontinence	Altered role performance
	Negative self-image, body image

Interventions

- Assist client in identifying and reducing/eliminating factors contributing to immobility. Positive steps should include those listed below.
  - controlling pain
  - improving nutritional state
  - strengthening muscles
  - providing assistive device, mobility aids (Figure 9-3)
  - encouraging activity
  - eliminating environmental barriers
- Ensure that client maintains proper body alignment. Use footboards, bedboards.
- Unless contraindicated, advise client to sit or keep head of bed elevated; prevent shearing force.
- Encourage good nutrition.
- Monitor intake and output. Ensure good fluid intake.
- Encourage good nutrition by providing several small-portioned meals rather than fewer large ones.
- Identify and utilize ways to stimulate appetite.

FIGURE 9-3

Mobility Aids

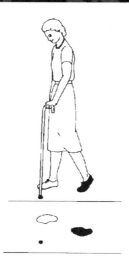

CANE
Ambulating with one cane or crutch. Shaded footprints and cane or crutch tips indicate where foot that bears weight is placed in each step. (This client has her right foot affected.) Client moves the cane forward, placing the tip on the floor just ahead of her unaffected, or stronger, leg and slightly out to the side of her foot. Then she takes one step forward with her affected leg. This brings the foot even with the cane or crutch.

Characteristics
- Assists balance by widening base of support; not intended for weight bearing
- Comes in a variety of styles
  Regular (straight): provides minimal assistance with balance
  Three- and four-point (quad): broader base of support, more cumbersome

Fit
- Length should approximate distance between greater trochanter and floor
- Elbow should be flexed slightly when cane rests 6 inches from side of foot

Use
- Use on unaffected side
- Advance when affected limb advances (i.e., if right leg is weak, the cane is held on the left and moved forward as the right leg steps)
- Hold close to body; do not move forward beyond toes of affected foot
- All canes should have suction grips to prevent slippage on floor

WALKER
A walker assists many clients to ambulate. (This client has her right foot affected.) **1,** Client uses both hands to lift the walker and set it in front of her. **2,** She steps ahead with the affected foot and leg. **3,** She steps forward with the unaffected foot and stands. Her hand supports her weight on the walker. She repeats this process.

Characteristics
- Broader base of support ; more stability than a cane
- Comes in a variety of styles

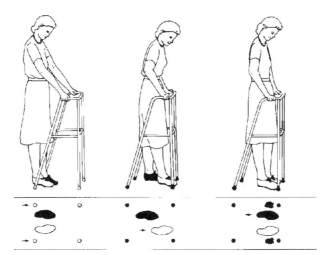

Pickup: assists with weight bearing

Rolling: pushed on wheels rather than lifted; reduces physical strain; often have seats to allow rest after several steps or propulsion from a sitting position

Fit

- Height equivalent to distance between greater trochanter and floor
- Elbows slightly flexed when hands on sides of walker

Use

- When weight bearing is allowed, advance walker and step normally
- When partial or no weight can be borne on one limb, thrust weight forward, then lift walker and replace all four legs on floor
- Always use both hands when transferring from chair or commode; back walker to seat and use arms of chair or commode to assist in standing

CRUTCHES

Shaded foot area and cane or crutch tips are indicated for weight-bearing foot for each step. Two-point gait can enable many clients to become more active in ambulation.

Characteristics

- Frequently difficult for older person to use because of inade-quate upper body strength, arthritic hands, and balance problems
- Not as stable as other mobility aids

Fit

- Individually sized
- Length should be equivalent to 2 inches below axilla to point on floor 6 inches in front of client
- Hand bars placement crucial because hands should bear total weight; elbow should be flexed, wrist slightly hyperextended; axillary pressure can cause radial nerve paralysis

Use

- Tailor gait to client's needs; consult with physical therapist
- Use good posture and pay particular attention to foot position on affected side (walking exclusively on ball of foot or toes can cause footdrop)
- General rule when climbing stairs: stronger foot goes up first, down last

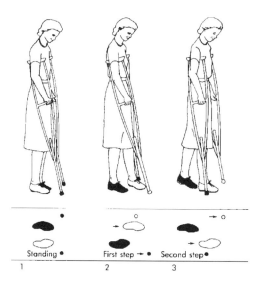

Standing •   First step → •   Second step •

1   2   3

Upstairs: step up with stronger foot; bring crutches to that step; raise affected foot
Downstairs: crutches to lower step; lower affected foot; follow with stronger foot
- Eliminate obstacles—waxed floors, throw rugs, extension cords, uneven surfaces, clutter

WHEELCHAIR

Characteristics
- Used when client's disability prohibits other walking aids
- Should not be used for convenience or speed of client or staff

Fit
- Individually prescribed based on height, weight, limb use, arm strength, and self-propulsion capacity

Use
- Prepare environment for wheelchair use: widen doorways and toilet stalls; plan a functional furniture layout with no rugs; lower mirrors, telephones, drinking fountains, counters; install ramps
- Use special pads and cushions to reduce pressure damage; shift weight and reposition frequently
- Lock chair and remove footrests when transferring to/from chair

From Hoeman S: *Rehabilitation/restorative care in the community,* St. Louis, 1990, Mosby.

- Prevent constipation.
- Evaluate environment for potential hazards; correct as needed.
- Assist client in increasing movement; plan individualized program using wide range of therapies, e.g., deep breathing, range of motion exercises (Figure 9-4), dance therapy, walking, yoga, physical therapy, stationary bicycling, tai chi, stretching, singing, water exercises, gardening. (See Chapter 5 for description of alternative therapies that can be used to increase movement.)

- Offer massages.
- Encourage caregivers/coach to motivate client to move through the use of diversional activities and promotion of maximum self-care.
- Observe for signs of complications and promptly correct.
- Recognize and reinforce gains in mobility.

FIGURE 9-4

Range of Motion Exercises

Joint	Normal range of motion
Shoulder	Free straight arm motion from relaxed position at side, forward and overhead to 160-degree angle
	Free straight arm motion backward to 30-degree angle with body

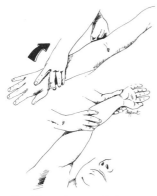

Shoulder in the extended position. Flexion occurs as the arm is lifted up and back.

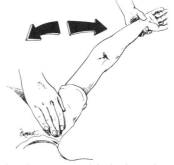

Sliding the arm toward the body produces shoulder adduction. Sliding the arm away from the body produces abduction.

Free straight arm motion laterally to 160-degree angle

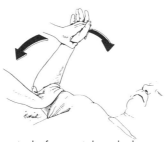

As the forearm is brought down, internal rotation occurs at the shoulder joint. As the forearm is brought up and back, external rotation occurs.

Joint	Normal range of motion
Elbow	From full-arm extension, hand should swing back to touch shoulder (160 degrees)

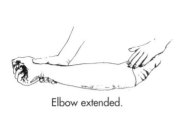

Elbow extended.

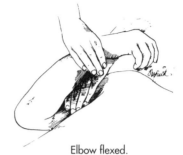

Elbow flexed.

Wrist   From perpendicular with ground, wrist should rotate 90 degrees to each side

From parallel to ground, wrist should flex downward 80 degrees, upward 70 degrees

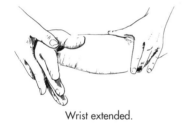

Wrist extended.

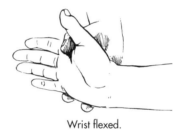

Wrist flexed.

From parallel with ground, wrist should move 10 degrees (thumbward), 60 degrees toward ulnar side

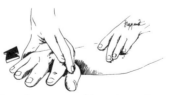

Lateral movement of the wrist produces radial and ulnar deviation.

Joint	Normal range of motion
Finger	Distal phalanx should flex 90 degrees (right angle with palm) and extend 30 degrees

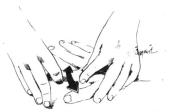

Fingers abducted away from the midline and adducted toward the midline (of hand).

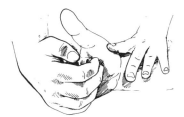

Fingers flexed as a group into a closed fist.

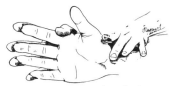

Finger extension is described as an open fist.

Thumb — Distal portion should bend 90 degrees (right angle)

Proximal portion should bend 70 degrees

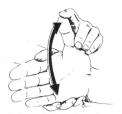

Thumb flexed toward and extended away from the fourth digit.

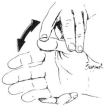

Thumb abducted and adducted in relation to the other fingers.

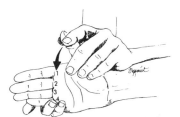

Thumb moved in opposition to the base of each of the other four digits.

Joint	Normal range of motion

Knee

From prone position: 100-degree

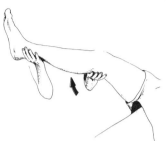

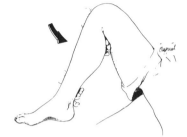

Movement of the lower leg upward produces knee extension. The hip is also in extension.

The knee and hip in a position of flexion.

Hip

From supine position, rising toward chin: 90 degrees with leg straight, 125 degrees with knee bent

From prone position: 5 degrees backward extension

From straight alignment with body: abduction of 45 degrees, adduction of 45 degrees

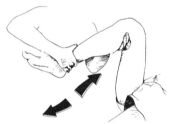

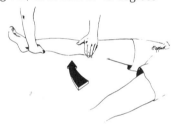

Caregiver can move the hip in flexion by sliding the leg back. Extension can be produced by sliding the leg forward.

Moving the leg away from the midline of the body abducts the hip.

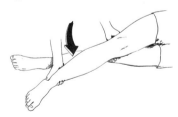

Moving the leg toward the midline of the body and crossing over it adducts the hip.

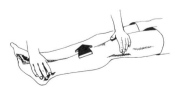

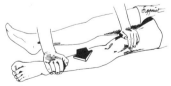

Rolling the leg inward causes the hip joint to rotate internally.

Rolling the leg outward causes the hip joint to rotate externally.

Joint	Normal range of motion
Ankle	Dorsiflexion (toward head) of 10 degrees, plantar flexion (toward floor) of 40 degrees Inversion of 35 degrees, eversion of 15 degrees

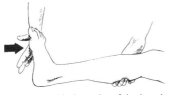

Pressure with the palm of the hand against the ball of the foot causes ankle dorsiflexion.

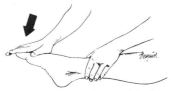

Pressure against the top of the foot causes ankle plantar flexion.

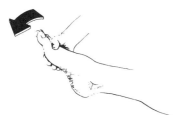

Turning the foot inward produces ankle inversion.

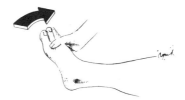

Turning the foot outward produces ankle eversion.

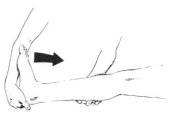

Heel cord stretching involves downward pull on the heel cord and dorsiflexion of the ankle.

From Dittmar S: *Rehabilitation nursing: process and application*, St. Louis, 1989, Mosby.

Arthritis

Description

Arthritis, an inflammation of the joints, is a major health problem and the number one chronic condition in persons over age 45 years. There are many types of arthritis (Table 9-5) and treatment varies depending on cause (Fig. 9-5 A, B).

TABLE 9-5

Arthritis Categorization by Cause

Type	Cause	Example
Cartilage degeneration	Breakdown of cartilage causing contact between ends of bones	Osteoarthritis
Synovitis	Inflammation of synovial membrane	Rheumatoid arthritis
Crystal arthritis	Small crystals deposited in joints	Gout
Joint infection	Bacteria in joint	Staphylococcus infections
Enthesopathy	Inflammation of tendons or ligaments	Ankylosing spondylitis

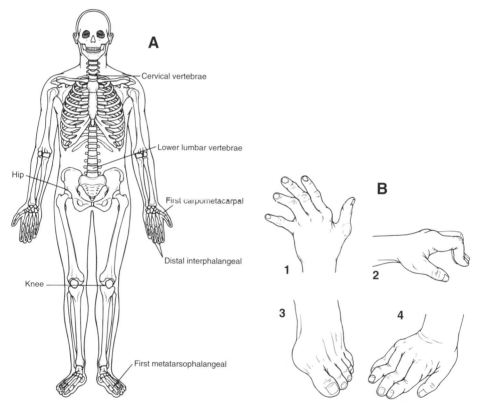

FIGURE 9-5A, B

A. Joints most frequently involved in osteoarthritis. B. Typical deformities of rheumatoid arthritis. 1, Ulnar drift. 2, Boutonniere deformity. 3, Hallux valgus. 4, Swanneck deformity.

From Lewis SM, Collier IC, Heitkemper MM: *Medical-surgical nursing: assessment and management of clinical problems*, ed 4, St. Louis, 1996, Mosby.

Client Goals

- to be free from pain
- to maintain optimal joint mobility and function
- to express understanding of disease and its management

Interventions

- Assist with diagnosis of type of arthritis, as needed, and development of appropriate treatment plan.
- Teach client and caregivers/coach about:
    - type of arthritis
    - medications: administration, safe use, side effects
    - exercise program
    - good body mechanics and positioning
    - dietary considerations
    - pain relief measures
    - use of assistive devices
- Assess impact of arthritis on ADL and IADL independence. Assist in improving independence, e.g., consult with physical and occupational therapists, arrange for assistive devices (Fig. 9-6).

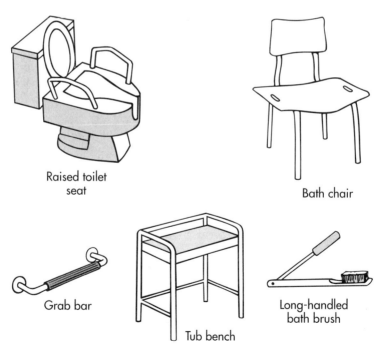

Raised toilet
seat

Bath chair

Grab bar

Tub bench

Long-handled
bath brush

FIGURE 9-6

Adaptive bath equipment commonly used in the home.

Modified from Ebersole P, Hess P: *Toward healthy aging: human needs and nursing response*, ed 5, St. Louis, 1998, Mosby.

- Assist client in identifying and, when possible, reducing factors that exacerbate condition, such as stress, weather changes, foods, overuse of joints.
- Assess pain and other symptoms related to arthritis. Ask client to rate symptoms (see Figure 4-1, page 51, for examples of methods client can use). Assist client in developing methods to manage pain, using nonpharmacological means first (Box 9-9).
- Assist with weight reduction if appropriate.
- Encourage good dietary intake, particularly fresh vegetables, fruits, nuts, and whole grains. Advise incorporation of cold water fish and other sources of fatty acids into diet, and reduction in fats and dairy products.
- Review diet for factors that could aggravate arthritis.
- For gout, teach low-purine diet (omission of organ meats, shellfish, yeast, herring, sardines, mackerel and anchovies; encourage client to eat alkaline-ash foods (e.g., milk, potatoes, citrus fruits) to reduce uric acid. Recommend use of supplements eicosapentaenoic acid (EPA), vitamin E, and quercetin (Pizzorno and Murray, 1989).
- Discuss safe use of supplements to improve joint flexibility: niacinamide, vitamins A, B_1, B_6, and E. Supplements with antiinflammatory actions include zinc, copper, selenium, manganese, pantothenic acid, flavonoids, tryptophan, sulfur, bee pollen, royal jelly, and evening primrose oil.
- Encourage and assist client in performing range of motion exercises.
- Advise and assist client to maintain good body alignment; teach proper use of splints and braces as indicated.
- Review impact of arthritis on sexual function. Counsel client as to ways to maximize sexual activity, e.g., taking analgesic prior to sexual activity, using different positions, incorporating massage into foreplay.
- Suggest herbal remedies as appropriate:
  - topical use of cream containing capsicum (chili peppers), which has been shown to reduce osteoarthritic pain and tenderness (McCarthy and McCarthy, 1992)
  - fish oil for rheumatoid arthritis pain (Belch et al., 1988)

BOX 9-9	Measures to Reduce Arthritic Pain
Individually planned exercise	Chiropractic treatment
Deep breathing	Acupuncture
Meditation	Herbs: yucca, devil's claw, hawthorn berries
Guided imagery	
Therapeutic touch	Shark cartilage
Application of heat and cold	Magnet therapy
Massage	Analgesic medications
Movement and posture re-education and improvement	

- for general alleviation of symptoms, meadowsweet, willow bark, black cohosh, prickly ash, celery seed, nettle, yucca, devil's claw
- Guide client in use of imagery to control symptoms.
- Recommend aromatherapy using essential oils of camphor, lemon, marjoram, and lavender.
- Advise client to use meditation, progressive relaxation, and other stress reduction measures.
- Consult with homeopathic practitioner regarding remedies for specific type of arthritis.
- Encourage client to express feelings and concerns.
- Refer client to resources for additional information and support (see Box 9-10).

BOX 9-10

Resources for Information About Arthritis

American Rheumatism Association
17 Executive Drive NE
Suite 480
Atlanta, GA 30329
(404) 633-3777
Arthritis Foundation
1314 Spring Street NW
Atlanta, GA 30309
(800) 283-7800
www.arthritis.org/

Association for People with Arthritis
Six Commercial Street
PO Box 954
Hicksville, NY 11802
(800) 323-2243
Rheumatoid Disease Foundation
5106 Old Harding Road
Franklin, TN 37064
www.mall-net.com/arth/

Osteoporosis

Description

Osteoporosis is a bone disorder characterized by a decrease in bone density due to a reduction in the mineral and protein matrix of bones. The resultant brittleness of the bones enables them to fracture under minimal stress. Osteoporosis is categorized as:

Type I (Postmenopausal): Primarily affects postmenopausal women between ages 55–75. Trabecular bone loss is greater than cortical bone loss. Fractures of the vertebrae and wrists are common.

Type II (Senile osteoporosis): Occurs between ages 70 and 80, affecting both sexes equally. Believed to be associated with low calcium. Both trabecular and cortical bone loss occurs. Fractures of the vertebrae, hip, and long bones are common.

A very small portion of osteoporosis can result from other conditions, such as hyperthyroidism, diabetes mellitus, immobility, and drugs (e.g., aluminum-based antacids, steroids, alcohol).

Client Goals

- to be free from fracture
- to maintain/improve mobility and activity
- to be free from additional loss of bone density

Interventions

- Ensure that client has received thorough diagnostic evaluation to determine type and confirm that no other disease (e.g., bone cancer) is present.
- Assist with and teach client and caregivers/coach about:
  - calcium-rich diet (men and women need at least 1000 mg/day, post menopausal women 1500 mg/day of calcium unless contraindicated)
  - exercise program, including weight-bearing exercise to prevent bone loss
  - good body mechanics
  - precautions to avoid fractures
  - proper use of estrogen
  - weight reduction measures, if indicated
- Reinforce importance of active state and avoidance of immobility. Explain that exercise can increase bone mass and strength.
- Consult with physician regarding estrogen replacement therapy.
- Advise client to limit foods that can promote calcium loss, e.g., carbonated drinks, caffeine, sugar, protein, sodium, alcoholic beverages.
- Encourage dietary intake of whole grains, legumes, fruits, green leafy vegetables, nuts and seeds, yogurt. Recommend vitamin D supplement.
- Discuss safe use of the calcium-rich herbs alfalfa and horsetail.
- Consult with homeopathic practitioner regarding use of remedies *Calcarea carbonica*, *Calcarea phosphorica*, *Calcerea fluorata*, and *Bufo rana*.
- Refer to resources for additional information and support (see Box 9-11).

BOX 9-11

Resources for Information About Osteoporosis

National Osteoporosis Foundation
1150 17th Street NW
Suite 500
Washington, DC 20036
(202) 223-2226
www.nof.org/

RESOURCES

Parkinson's Disease

Description

Parkinson's disease is a chronic, progressive disorder of the central nervous system that results from a deficiency of dopamine. Although the exact cause is not known, contributing factors include head injury, vascular damage to brain, drugs that interfere with dopaminergic function or that stimulate cholinergic activity, environmental toxins, and age-related changes to the brain.

Client Goals

- to demonstrate maximum self-care independence
- to satisfy ADL and IADL requirements
- to maintain joint motion within functional range
- to be free from injury and other complications of disease

Interventions

- Teach client and caregivers/coach about disease:
  - pathophysiology
  - signs and symptoms, factors that aggravate and improve them
  - medications
  - diet, including importance of maintaining stable diet and avoiding high protein intake as this can affect action of levodopa
  - exercise
  - skin care to control increased perspiration and oil production associated with disease
  - eye hygiene to prevent conjunctivitis from seborrhea scales accumulating on eyes and eyelash
  - emotional swings associated with disease
  - importance of recognizing unaltered intellectual function
  - importance of minimizing stress
  - prevention of complications (e.g., aspiration, falls, contractures)
  - use of assistive devices
- Recommend measures to assist with mobility, such as use of chairs with armrests to assist with rising from seated position and ambulation with wide-based gait.
- If swallowing or chewing is a problem, instruct client and caregivers to:
  - use semisoft foods
  - divide food into several smaller meals rather than three large ones
  - sit at 90-degree angle during ingestion of food and fluids and for approximately 45 minutes thereafter
  - flex head forward during swallowing (chin tuck)
  - keep head in midline
  - place food on uninvolved side (if paralysis is present)
  - ingest 1/2 to 3/4 teaspoon at a time
  - hold breath and then swallow
  - swallow again

- massage upward on laryngeal area to facilitate swallowing
- Suggest client wear garments with Velcro strips or zippers, rather than buttons and snaps.
- Encourage client to speak slowly and take a breath before beginning to speak to assist with dysarthria.
- Ensure that vitamin B_6 and vitamin B_6-rich foods (e.g., whole grains, raw nuts, bananas, potatoes, liver and fish) are not taken with levodopa. (This restriction is not necessary for levodopa combination drugs, like Sinemet.)
- Encourage use of vitamins C and E.
- Discuss safe use of the herb passion flower, which has antispasmodic and sedative effects.
- Advise client to use ginger if nausea occurs from antiparkinsonism medications.
- Suggest client use deep breathing, progressive relaxation, guided imagery, and other measures to reduce stress and relax.
- Evaluate environment for potential hazards, such as throw rugs, small objects in path.
- Monitor mental status; note signs of depression.
- Monitor intake and output; teach client to observe signs of urinary retention.
- Consult with physical and occupational therapists regarding measures to improve ADL independence.
- Encourage client to express feelings; provide support.
- Consult with neurologist regarding new technology to control symptoms, such as pulse generators that send electrical impulses that block tremor-causing brain signals and drug-infusion systems (Stodghill, 1997).
- Refer to resources for additional information and support (see Box 9-12).

BOX 9-12

Resources for Information About Parkinson's Disease

American Parkinson Disease Association
60 Bay Street
Suite 401
Staten Island, NY 10301
(800) 223-2732
www.the-health-pages.com/resources/apda/index.html

National Parkinson Foundation
1501 NW 9th Avenue
Miami, FL 33136
(800) 327-4545
www.parkinson.org/

Parkinson's Disease Foundation
c/o William Black Medical Research Building
650 West 168th Street
New York, NY 10032
(800) 457-6676

Parkinson's Educational Program
3900 Birch Street
Suite 105
Newport Beach, CA 92660
(800) 344-7872

Parkinson Support Group of America
11376 Cherry Hill Road
Suite 204
Beltsville, MD 20705
(301) 937-1545

United Parkinson Foundation
360 W. Superior Street
Chicago, IL 60610
(312) 664-2344
www.stepstn.com/nord/org_sum/102.htm

Multiple Sclerosis

Description

Multiple sclerosis is a progressive, degenerative disorder, in which a portion of the myelin sheath covering the nerves degenerates and is replaced with patches of sclerotic tissue; this results in interference with the conduction of impulses along the nerve. There is no predictable pattern to the symptoms; some people experience a few minor attacks over decades while others face rapid, steady deterioration.

Client Goals

- to display maximum independence in ADLs and IADLs
- to decrease frequency and severity of attacks
- to be free from complications associated with multiple sclerosis (e.g., aspiration, falls, burns)

Interventions

- Advise client to prevent fatigue, stress, and overexertion.
- Teach use of meditation, guided imagery, progressive relaxation, yoga, and other measures to manage stress and promote relaxation.
- Use touch therapy and massage.
- Encourage client to schedule regular rest periods.
- Assist client in developing individual exercise program. Consult with physical therapist.
- Encourage good nutrition. Promote diet to keep weight within ideal range and prevent constipation. Recommend a diet high in fatty acids and low in fat which has been shown to slow deterioration and lower death rates in multiple sclerosis (Swank and Dugan, 1990).
- Review safe use of nutritional supplements: essential fatty acids, niacin, zinc, magnesium, selenium, beta-carotene and vitamins C, B_6, and B_{12}.
- Assist client in identifying food sensitivities, which can decrease feelings of health and well-being.
- If swallowing problems are present, instruct client and caregivers to use semisoft foods, divide food into several smaller meals rather than three large ones, have client sit upright during eating, place food in back of mouth and tilt head forward when swallowing. (Refer to interventions discussed under *Potential for Aspiration*.)
- Instruct client and caregivers/coach in safe use of medications.
- Evaluate dental fillings for presence of mercury. Mercury toxicity can produce symptoms similar to multiple sclerosis; persons with multiple sclerosis have been found to have elevated mercury levels (Vimy, 1990). Consult with dentist regarding removing mercury fillings if indicated. Resources and the names of biologic dentists throughout the country can be obtained through Environmental Dental Association (800) 388-8124 and Foundation for Toxic-Free Dentistry (407) 299-4149.
- If indicated, prepare client for surgery, plasmapheresis, and other special procedures.

- Consult with speech therapist for assistance with speech problems.
- Recommend measures to compensate for deficits arising from disease, such as:
  - large print books for visual problems
  - carrying pencil and pad to make notes for memory deficit
  - bladder retraining or habit training for incontinence
- Consult with occupational and physical therapists regarding assistive devices, communication aids.
- Encourage client to express feelings and concerns.
- Refer to resources for additional information and support (see Box 9-13).

BOX 9-13

Resources for Information About Multiple Sclerosis

Multiple Sclerosis Association of America
601-05 White Horse Pike
Oaklyn, NJ 08107
(800) 833-4MSA
National Multiple Sclerosis Society
733 Third Avenue
New York, NY 10017
(800) 344-4867

www.nmss.org/
Swank Multiple Sclerosis Clinic
School of Medicine
Oregon Health Sciences University
3181 Sam Jackson Park Road
Portland, OR 97201
(503) 494-8370
www.ohsu.edu

Low Back Pain

Description

Back pain affects an estimated 80% of all people at some point in their lives and is the leading cause of disability for persons under age 45. Chronic back pain is pain that lasts greater than six months or recurs every three months to three years. Potential causes of low back pain include: injuries, inflammation, abnormal curvature, compression fracture, herniated disk, degenerative disk disease, obesity, congenital malformations, poor body mechanics, and psychological factors (e.g., stress, repressed anger).

Client Goals

- to have cause of back pain identified and corrected, if possible
- to verbalize elimination or reduction in pain
- to be free from complications secondary to back pain (e.g., pressure ulcers, pneumonia, falls, depression, negative self-image)
- to increase safe, appropriate mobility and exercise

Interventions

- Ensure that a thorough diagnostic workup has been done. Provide support and education through this process.

- Consult with physician and physical therapist regarding cause of back pain and recommended treatment plan (e.g., transcutaneous electrical nerve stimulator, medications, surgery).
- Establish mechanism for client to self-evaluate pain, such as describing pain on a scale of 0-10 (0 = no pain, 10 = most severe). (Refer to Chapter 4, Figure 4-1, for other examples of other tools to assess symptoms.)
- Assist client in utilizing most effective pain management measures for individual needs (Many of the same measures to manage arthritic pain, as described in Box 9-9, are applicable to low back pain.)
- Instruct client in proper body mechanics and posture.
- Instruct and support client in weight reduction if appropriate.
- Consult with physical therapist regarding exercises that are appropriate for client.
- Teach client safe use of analgesics.
- Discuss with client value of various alternative therapies for management of back pain:
  - Consult with chiropractor regarding chiropractic spinal manipulation, which has been demonstrated to reduce symptoms, disability, and time lost from work (Moore, 1993). (One-fifth of back pain sufferers have received chiropractic treatments [Eisenberg et al., 1993]).
  - Instruct client in yoga breathing exercises and postures to reduce stress and muscle tension.
  - Guide client in the use of imagery to visualize relaxation and pain relief.
  - Teach client to use biofeedback and progressive relaxation.
  - Provide massage; select method best suited for client's individual needs.
  - Use alternating hot (using water and hot apple cider vinegar) and cold application (10 minutes each). Reinforce safety precautions.
  - Refer to acupuncturist and acupressurist.
  - Consult with homeopathic practitioner regarding remedies such as *Arsenicum album, Arnica, Rhus toxicodendron, Calcarea fluorata, Natrum muriaticum, Ruta graveolens.*
  - Use aromatherapy: lavender, marjoram, rosemary and sage for muscle fatigue; black pepper, ginger, or birch for pain.

Diversional Activity Deficit

Description

Diversional activity deficit is the inability to occupy oneself in activities that pass time, entertain, or gratify. The individual experiences the environment as nonstimulating.

Chronic conditions can lead to physical limitations, lengthy treatments, frequent or long-term hospitalizations, financial burdens and other factors that interfere with participation in hobbies and other diversional activities. As a result, the individual can develop feelings of boredom, uselessness, restlessness, lethargy, anger, and isolation.

Client Goals

- to express satisfaction with quality and quantity of diversional activities
- to develop interest in/engage in at least one diversional activity weekly

Interventions

- Reduce or eliminate factors responsible for diversional activity deficit; e.g.:
  - control pain
  - help client obtain and learn to use assistive devices to maximize mobility and communication
  - arrange for transportation
  - refer for financial assistance
  - rearrange environment to promote activity
- Assist client in learning new hobbies, interests, games.
- Consult with occupational, physical, vocational, and recreational therapists.
- Encourage visitors. If acceptable to client, contact churches and community service organizations for volunteers to visit (in person or via telephone or e-mail) and participate in activities with client.
- Consult with librarian regarding talking books, music, and other available resources.
- Encourage client to express feelings.
- Offer positive reinforcement.

Self-Care Deficit

Description

A self-care deficit exists when the individual is partially or totally unable to bathe, groom, dress, toilet, or feed self. Chronic conditions can produce ongoing self-care deficits as a consequence of a disease, as occurs with a dementia, or periodic self-care deficits, as occurs when a disease exacerbates (e.g., multiple sclerosis) or a treatment (e.g., bedrest) or symptom (e.g., pain) limits self-care capacity. Self-care deficits can occur in the activities of daily living (Table 9-1) and instrumental activities of daily living (Table 9-2).

Client Goals

- to increase self-care independence
- to reduce or eliminate factors that interfere with self-care independence

Interventions

- Encourage client to be as independent as possible. Ensure that client is provided with ample time for self-care activities. Advise caregivers to allow client to do as much for self as possible. Instruct caregivers and coach to encourage and reinforce client's maximum independence.
- Set short- and long-term goals with client to increase self-care responsibility. Share these goals with caregivers and coach.
- Gradually increase self-care responsibilities.

- Provide assistive devices and mobility aids (Figure 9-3). Consult with occupational and physical therapists.
- Arrange for environmental modifications to accommodate client's disability and promote independence.
- Monitor intake and output, nutritional status, weight, vital signs, skin status, and general condition to ensure that no complications result from self-care deficits.
- Assist client in meeting ADLs as needed.
- Teach client and caregivers safety measures to prevent injury, such as proper transfer techniques, measuring bath water temperature, correct use of cane.
- Reinforce positive efforts.
- Refer to community resources for assistance, e.g.:
  Meals on Wheels
  homemakers services
  home health aide
  support group
  transportation services for the disabled

Cerebrovascular Accident (Nonacute Phase)

Description

A cerebrovascular accident (CVA), commonly called a stroke, is a sudden, severe decrease in cerebral circulation caused by a thrombus, embolus, or hemorrhage that results in a cerebral infarct. It is the third leading cause of death in the United States. Although persons of any age can experience a CVA, most strokes occur in people between ages 75 and 85 years of age. In addition to advanced age, sex and race influence risk, with males being more likely to suffer a CVA than females, and blacks more than other races. Other risk factors include hypertension, atherosclerosis, heart disease, high cholesterol levels, impaired glucose tolerance, cigarette smoking, obesity, alcohol abuse, and sickle cell anemia and other blood diseases. Symptoms can appear suddenly and profoundly or slowly and subtly and vary depending on the part of the brain affected (Box 9-14).

Client Goals

- to engage in activities of daily living with maximum independence
- to be free from complications secondary to CVA
- to express acceptance of altered roles and functions

Interventions

- Assess effects of CVA on ADL performance. Consult with multidisciplinary team regarding potential for recovery of function. Support treatment plan.
- Encourage mobility. Assist client with range-of-motion exercises and proper positioning. Instruct client and caregivers in techniques. Consult with physical therapist as needed.

BOX 9-14   Effects of Stroke

Right Hemisphere Lesion	Left Hemisphere Lesion
Left hemiplegia	Right hemiplegia
Individual unaware of deficits	Individual aware of deficits
Poor judgment	Judgment normal
Short attention span	Repetitious actions and speech
Memory deficits involving spatial information	Memory deficits involving language
Inability to quickly transfer learning	Impaired ability to read, write, speak
Performance affected, not comprehension	Comprehension affected
Fast, impulsive behaviors	Slow, cautious movements
Speech impairments, language intact	Speech and language impairments
Low likelihood of regaining prestroke function	Good potential to restore prestroke function

---

- Protect client from injury. Discuss with client and caregivers safety risks, such as poor coordination, altered sensations, diplopia; offer suggestions for reducing risks.
- Promote communication. Instruct caregivers/coach in helpful techniques, such as:
  - keeping statements short and simple
  - presenting one question or idea at a time
  - using short sentences
  - speaking on an adult level at a normal tone
  - eliminating distractions (radio or television in background)
  - limiting choices (e.g., rather than *What do you want to eat?* ask *Would you like chicken or fish for dinner?*)
  - allowing ample time for response
  - displaying patience and understanding; reducing stress in communication process
  - not reacting to client's frustrations and emotions
  - using communication boards and other assistive devices as needed
  - ensuring that client understands before progressing
  - offering positive reinforcement
- Explain to caregivers and coach emotional reactions client may display (e.g., anger, depression, crying) and their need not to personalize the reactions. Allow client to ventilate feelings.
- Encourage maximum participation in ADLs. Consult with occupational therapist regarding assistive/adaptive equipment that could benefit client (see Figure 9-3). Instruct caregivers in techniques.

- Observe for dysphagia. Consult with dietician regarding foods that could be easily swallowed (e.g., thick rather than thin liquids). Instruct client to eat slowly and thoroughly chew foods; advise caregivers and coach to reinforce this.
- Protect skin integrity. Use massage, protective padding, and frequent position changes.
- Assist with incontinence control (see *Altered Urinary Elimination: Incontinence,* pages 181–184).
- Recommend that client consult with acupuncturist. Acupuncture has been shown to improve neurological scores and increase maximum performance capacity in persons who have had CVA (Ehrlich and Haber, 1992; Hu et al., 1993).
- Refer client to speech therapist as appropriate.
- Guide client in use of imagery to visualize improved circulation.
- Refer client for/instruct in biofeedback. EMG biofeedback has been shown to improve gait, grip, grasping ability, and other hand functions in persons who have experienced a CVA (Schleenbaker and Mainous, 1993).
- Ensure that client with history of CVA or who is at high risk has adequate potassium intake. People with hypokalemia have a higher rate of stroke mortality than those with normal levels of potassium (Khaw and Barrett-Connor, 1987).
- Recommend vitamin E supplement. Vitamin E is believed to reduce platelet aggregation and, when combined with aspirin, has been shown to be more effective than aspirin alone in reducing morbidity and mortality associated with transient ischemic attacks (Steiner et al., 1995).
- Consult with physician regarding referral for hyperbaric oxygen therapy, which has been shown to improve motor power and spasticity in stroke victims (Walker, 1996). (Some sources of information about hyperbaric oxygen therapy are listed in Box 9-15.)
- Use essential oils of lavender, rosemary, and basil for massage of paralyzed parts of body unless contraindicated.
- Recommend use of ginkgo biloba to improve cerebral circulation and function. This herb has been shown to improve blood flow, memory, concentration, and depression (Kleijnen and Knipschild, 1992). Other herbs that could help the nervous system are lavender, rosemary, and Siberian ginseng.
- Refer to resources for additional information and support (see Box 9-16).

BOX 9-15

Resources for Information About Hyperbaric Oxygen Therapy

American College of Hyperbaric Medicine
4001 Ocean Drive
Lauderdale-by-the-Sea, FL 33308
(800) 552-0255
Ocean Hyperbaric Center
4001 Ocean Drive
Lauderdale-by-the-Sea, FL 33308
(800) 552-0255

Undersea and Hyperbaric Medical Society
10531 Metropolitan Avenue
Kensington, MD 20895
(301) 942-2980
www.uhms.org

BOX 9-16

Resources for Information About Cerebrovascular Accident

American Heart Association Stroke Connection
7320 Greenville Avenue
Dallas, TX 75231
(800) 553-6321
www.amhrt.org/hs97/strokeco.html
National Aphasia Association
PO Box 1887
Murray Hill Station, NY 10156
(800) 922-4622
National Institute of Neurological Disorders and Stroke
9000 Rockville Pike
Building 31, Room BA16
Bethesda, MD 20892
(800) 352-9424
www.ninds.nih.gov

National Stroke Association
8480 East Orchard Road
Suite 1000
Englewood, CO 80111
(800) STROKES
www.stroke.org
Stroke Clubs
805 12th Street
Galveston, TX 77550
(409) 762-1022

References

Anibarro B, et al.: Asthma with surfite intolerance in children: a blocking study with cyanocobalamin, *Journal of Allergy and Clinical Immunology* 90:103-9, 1992.

Auer W, et al.: Hypertension and hyperlipidemia: garlic helps in mild cases, *British Journal of Clinical Practice*, Supplement 69:3-6, 1990.

Belch JJF, et al.: Effects of altering dietary essential fatty acids on requirements for nonsteroid antiinflammatory drugs in patients with rheumatoid arthritis, *Annals of Rheumatic Disease* 47:96-104, 1988.

Davini P, et al.: Controlled study on L-carnitine therapeutic efficacy in post-infarction, *Drugs Under Experimental and Clinical Research* 18(8):355-65, 1992.

Eisenberg DM, et al.: Unconventional medicine in the United States: prevalence, costs, and patterns of use, *New England Journal of Medicine* 328:246-52, 1993.

Ehrlich D and Haber P: Influence of acupuncture on physical performance capacity and hemodynamic parameters, *International Journal of Sports Medicine* 13:486-91, 1992.

Epstein G, et al.: Alleviating asthma with mental imagery, *Alternative and Complementary Medicine* 5(1):42-52, 1997.

Foster S: *Passion flower*, Botanical Series 314. Austin, TX, 1993, American Botanical Council.

Hu HH, et al.: A randomized controlled trial on the treatment for acute partial ischemic stroke with acupuncture, *Neuroepidemiology* 12:106-13, 1993.

Jain SC, et al.: Effect of yoga training on exercise tolerance in adolescents with childhood asthma, *Journal of Asthma* 28(6):437-42, 1991.

Kamikawa T, et al.: Effects of coenzyme Q10 on exercise tolerance in chronic stable angina pectoris, *American Journal of Cardiology* 56:247-51, 1985.

Khaw KT, Barrett-Connor E: Dietary potassium and stroke-related mortality, *New England Journal of Medicine* 316:235-40, 1987.

Kleijnen J and Knipschild P: Ginkgo biloba for cerebral insufficiency, *British Journal of Clinical Pharmacology* 45:333-36, 1992.

McCarthy GM and McCarthy DJ: Effect of topical capsaicin in the therapy of painful osteoarthritis of the hands, *Journal of Rheumatology* 19:604-07, 1992.

Moore, JS: *Chiropractic in America*, Baltimore, MD, 1993, Johns Hopkins University Press.

Morris MC, Sacks F, and Rosner B: Does fish oil lower blood pressure? *Circulation* 88:523-33, 1993.

Patel CH: Yoga and biofeedback in the management of hypertension, *Lancet* 322:1053-55, 1973.

Pizzorno JE and Murray MT: *A textbook of natural medicine*, Seattle, 1989, John Bastyr College Publications.

Reilly D, Taylor MA, Beattie NGM: Is evidence for homeopathy reproducible? *Lancet* 344:1601-06, 1994.

Richter AA, Herlitz J, Hjalmarson A: Effect of acupuncture in patients with angina pectoris, *European Heart Journal* 12(2):175-78, 1991.

Schleenbaker RE and Mainous AG: Electromyographic biofeedback for neuromuscular reeducation in the hemiplegic stroke patient: a meta-analysis, *Archives of Physical Medicine and Rehabilitation* 74(12):1301-4, 1993.

Shahar E, et al.: Dietary n-3 polyunsaturated fatty acids and smoking-related chronic obstructive pulmonary disease, *New England Journal of Medicine* 331:228-33, 1994.

Skobeloff EM, et al.: Intravenous magnesium sulfate for the treatment of acute asthma in the emergency department, *Journal of the American Medical Association* 262:11210-13, 1989.

Steiner M, Glantz M, and Lekos A: Vitamin E and aspirin compared with aspirin alone in patients with transient ischemic attacks, *American Journal of Clinical Nutrition*, 62 (Supplement 6):1381S-84S, 1995.

Stodghill R: A jolt of relief from Parkinson's disease, *Business Week* March 24, 1997, p 34.

Swank RL and Dugan BB: Effect of low saturated diet in early and late cases of multiple sclerosis, *Lancet* 336:37-39, 1990.

Vimy MJ: Glomerular filtration impairment by mercury from dental 'silver' fillings in sheep, *Physiologist* 33:A94, August 1990.

Walker M: Reversal of residual stroke symptoms using hyperbaric oxygen therapy, *Alternative and Complementary Therapies* 2(1):24-31, January-February, 1996.

Yates J: A physician's guide to therapeutic massage: its physiologic effects and their application to treatment, Vancouver, BC, 1990, *Massage Therapists Association of British Columbia*.

Recommended Readings

Bach JR, ed: *Pulmonary rehabilitation: the obstructive and paralytic conditions*, St Louis, 1996, Mosby.

Batmanghelidj F: *How to deal with back pain and rheumatoid joint pain*, Falls Church, VA, 1991, Global Health Solutions.

Bresler DE: *Free yourself from pain*, Topanga, CA, 1992, The Bresler Center.

Charash BD: *Heart myths*, New York, 1992, Viking Penguin.

Cooper K: *Overcoming hypertension*, New York, 1990, Bantam.

Cranton E: *Bypassing bypass*, Troutdale, VA, 1992, Medex Publishers.

Edwards S: *Sally Edwards' heart zone training: exercise smart, stay fit and live longer*, Holbrook, MA, 1996, Adams Media Corp.

Finn KL: A family affair: coping with heart disease and other chronic illnesses, *USA Today* 123(2592):63-65, 1994.

Fishman TD, Freedline DPM, and Kahn D: Putting the best foot forward, *Nursing 96* 26(1):58-60, 1996.

Gaby A: *Preventing and reversing osteoporosis*, Roseville, CA, 1993, Prima Publishing.

Galsworthy TD and Wilson PL: Osteoporosis: it steals more than bone, *American Journal of Nursing 96* (6):26-34, 1996.

Gagnon D and Morningstar A: *Breathe free*, Wilimot, WI, 1990, Lotus Press.

Hench K and Pinals RS: When multiple illnesses complicate osteoarthritis, *Patient Care* 28(20):113-120, 1994.

Hickey T and Searle MS: Activity participation and well-being among older people with arthritis, *Gerontologist* 35(4):463-72, 1995.

Hoffman D: Heart-smart herbs: tonics to keep your ticker in tip-top shape, *Vegetarian Times* 224(4):102-105, 11996.

Ivker R: *Sinus survival*, Los Angeles, 1992, Jeremy P. Tarcher, Inc.

Jacobowitz RS: *150 most-asked questions about osteoporosis: what women really want to know*, Emmaus, NY, 1993, Hearst Books.

James DG and Studdy PR: *Color atlas of respiratory diseases*, ed 2, St Louis, 1992, Mosby.

Kerton CA: Assessing for ascites, *Nursing 96* 26(4):53, 1996.

Kerton CA: Assessing for breath sounds, *Nursing 96* 26(6):50, 1996.

Kerton CA: Assessing normal heart sounds, *Nursing 96* 26(2):56-57, 1996.

Kantrowicz F: *Taking care of arthritis*, New York, 1991, Harper Perennial.

Kwiterovich P: *The Johns Hopkins complete guide for preventing and reversing heart disease*, Rocklin, CA, 1993, Prima Publishers.

Lorrig K and Fries J: *The arthritis helpbook*, Reading, MA, 1990, Addison-Wesley Publishing Co.

Mansfield J: *Arthritis: the allergy connection*, Wellingborough, England, 1990, Thorsons Publishers Ltd.

McFadden N: Are you happy? *Real Living with Multiple Sclerosis* 1(9):10-13, 1994.

Meissner JE: Caring for patients with multiple sclerosis, *Nursing* 24(8):60-62, 1994.

Moore R: *The high blood pressure solution: natural prevention and cure with the "K" factor*, Rochester, VT, 1993, Healing Arts Press.

Ornish D: *Dr Dean Ornish's program for reversing heart disease*, New York, 1990, Ballantine.

Roth E and Streicher S: *Good cholesterol, bad cholesterol*, Rocklin, CA, 1993, Prima Publishers.

Rothfeld GS and LeVert S: *Natural medicine for back pain*, Emmaus, PA, 1996, Rodale Press.

Schatz MP: *Back care basics: a doctor's gentle yoga program for back and neck pain relief*, Berkeley, CA, 1992, Rodmell Press.

Russek LG and Schwartz GE: Energy cardiology: a dynamical energy systems approach for integrating conventional and alternative medicine, Advances, *Journal of Mind-Body Health* 12(4):4-24, 1996.

Swisher JW: Chronic bronchitis: how and whether to prescribe antibiotics for acute exacerbations, *Consultant* 36(1):47-53, 1996.

Walker M: Reversal of residual stroke symptoms using hyperbaric oxygen therapy, *Alternative and Complementary Therapies* 2(1):24-31, 1996.

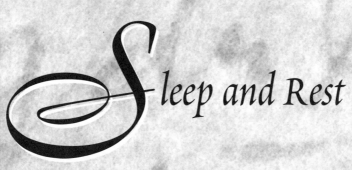

Chapter 10

Sleep and Rest

*P*eriods of retreat from activity and stimulation are necessary to refresh and renew the body, mind, and spirit. Sleep and rest enable us to maintain health, heal, and achieve a sense of balance and well-being. Sleep is a state of unconsciousness from which we can be aroused. During sleep the basal metabolic rate decreases, thereby slowing most bodily functions. There is reduced responsiveness to external stimuli and relaxation of skeletal muscles; blood pressure and pulse fall. Sleep is controlled by two specialized areas of the brain stem: the reticular activating system (RAS), which is associated with wakefulness, and the bulbar synchronizing region (BSR), which is most active during sleep. It is believed that these two systems intermittently activate and then suppress the brain centers, causing states of wakefulness and sleep.

There are two kinds of sleep: *REM (rapid eye movement) sleep* and *NREM (non-rapid eye movement or slow wave) sleep*. During REM sleep, in which the sympathetic nervous system dominates, the following occur:

- active dreaming
- irregular muscle movements (e.g., rapid eye movements, irregular pulse and respirations)
- depressed muscle tone
- restoration of mental function
- more difficult arousal than during NREM sleep

The deep or slow-wave sleep of NREM is characterized by:

- the absence of dreams
- slow, rolling eye movements
- profound restfulness
- decreased blood pressure, respirations, and metabolic rate

A normal sleep cycle consists of four stages of NREM sleep and a final stage of REM sleep (see Box 10-1). The length of each sleep cycle changes with age: although the actual number of hours slept does not change significantly throughout adulthood, with advanced age there is a decrease in the amount of deep sleep and an increase in light sleep.

Rest is a period of inactivity and peace. Throughout the day, periods of rest interspersed with activity are beneficial; however, inactivity does not necessarily equate to a restful state, and vice versa. A change in activity—for example, taking a walk or engaging in a hobby—can be refreshing and restful.

Chronic illnesses can disrupt sleep-rest patterns in a variety of ways (Box 10-2). Assessment should include a review of the effect of illnesses on sleep-rest patterns.

A variety of nonpharmacological and alternative therapies (Box 10-3) can be effective in promoting rest and sleep. Due to the potentially serious effects of medications, these alternatives should be considered before sedatives are used.

BOX 10-1   Sleep Cycles

Stage I NREM (Non-Rapid Eye Movement) Sleep

Light sleep from which sleeper can be easily awakened

Eyes roll from side to side

Heart and respiratory rates slightly decrease

Will advance to next stage within several minutes if left undisturbed

Sleep interrupted during any other stage will cause cycle to return to Stage I

Stage II NREM Sleep

Continued light sleep with higher state of relaxation

Sleep remains light and easily broken

Continued decline in temperature and heart and respiratory rate

Eyes are still

Stage III NREM Sleep

Early stage of deep sleep

Continued slowing of bodily processes

Relaxation of muscles

Moderate stimulation required to arouse sleeper

Stage IV NREM Sleep

Extreme relaxation, deepest stage of sleep usually reached in 20–30 minutes and lasting about 30 minutes

Decreased vital signs and body movements

Considerable stimulation required to arouse sleeper

This stage diminishes with age and may be absent in some older adults

It is believed that this stage is essential to physically restoring the body

REM (Rapid eye movement) Sleep

Deepest sleep level

Decreased tonus of head and neck muscles

Increased and possibly irregular vital signs

Electroencephalogram (EEG) resembles stage I

Sleepers drift into REM from stage IV about once every 90 minutes, four to five times each night

Can be disrupted by amphetamines, alcohol, barbiturates, or phenothiazine derivatives

Deprivation can result in irritability, anxiety, acute psychotic episodes

BOX 10-2   Effects of Chronic Illness that Can Interfere with Sleep

Pain

Coughing

Dyspnea, orthopnea

Muscle cramps

Poor peripheral circulation

Nocturia

Nightmares, hallucinations

Confusion

Anxiety, fear

Insufficient daytime activity

Effects of medications

BOX 10-3   Nonpharmacological Measures to Promote Sleep and Rest

Protein-rich or starch snack at bedtime

Nutritional supplements: melatonin, calcium, magnesium, B vitamins, chromium, L-tryptophan; niacinamide (vitamin B_3), one gram at bedtime

Increased exercise in late afternoon and early evening

Exposure to sunlight in early day

Avoidance of caffeine, alcohol

Meditation

Breathing exercises, progressive relaxation

Massage

Therapeutic touch

Guided imagery

Herbal teas: chamomile, lime blossom, valerian

Homeopathic remedies based on specific cause

Acupuncture

Environmental adjustment (lighting, sound, temperature)

Hot bath (105°F) approximately one hour before bedtime

Assessment Considerations

When assessing sleep, ask specific questions to gain insight into the actual quantity and quality of sleep and rest. Areas to review include:

- usual time for going to bed, falling asleep, awakening
- sleep inducers (e.g., music, drugs, bath)
- number of times awakened during the night, number of nighttime trips to the bathroom
- symptoms experienced during sleep (e.g., pain, coughing, dyspnea, nightmares)
- number of pillows, blankets used
- quality of sleep
- client's satisfaction with quality and quantity of sleep
- naps
- measures used for rest and relaxation
- recent changes in sleep-rest pattern
- energy level, fatigue
- complaints

Complaints pertaining to sleep need to be carefully explored. For instance, a client may complain of "insomnia" because she awakens at 3 a.m. every morning. However, if the client is napping frequently during the day and retires for bed at 9 p.m., her sleep quota may be fulfilled by 3 a.m. If awakening at 3 a.m. is distressful to the client, she could be advised to stay awake later or reduce daytime naps.

Without a complete history, there could be a risk that the client's complaint could be mislabeled as insomnia and a sedative prescribed unnecessarily.

Spouses or caregivers who are aware of the client's sleep pattern can be asked about observations concerning the client's sleep pattern. This can be beneficial in detecting signs consistent with sleep apnea (e.g., snoring and sudden awakening) because the client may not be aware of these signs. Likewise, family members and caregivers may report excessive daytime sleepiness that could be associated with conditions such as narcolepsy, whereas the client may not report this as a problem.

Clinical signs can give clues to sleep disturbances also. These signs could include the following: fatigue, apathy, irritability, restlessness, inattention, nodding off during the day, reddened conjunctiva, dark circles around eyes, swollen eyelids, poor coordination, headache, slurred speech, confusion, disorientation, and hallucinations.

Related Diagnoses

Sleep Pattern Disturbance

Description

Any disruption of sleep time that causes the client discomfort or interferes with lifestyle is a sleep pattern disturbance. It can be manifested by difficulty falling or staying asleep, daytime fatigue, nodding, and other physical signs, as well as the client's complaints.

Client Goals

- to achieve 6–8 hours of uninterrupted sleep nightly
- to feel rested during the day
- to be free from complications related to disturbed sleep

Interventions

- Assist client in eliminating underlying cause, if possible (e.g., control of pain or cough, readjusting medication schedule to avoid need for nighttime toileting, modifying diet, changing bedtime).
- Determine effective sleep inducers for the client and assist client in utilizing them (e.g., music, television, reading material, snack).
- Offer massages; teach caregivers massage techniques to promote relaxation.
- Encourage daytime activity and exercise.
- Assist client and caregivers in developing a balanced schedule of activity and rest throughout the day.
- Assist in controlling environmental interruptions to sleep. Suggest that lighting be dimmed and a nightlight provided, and room temperature be maintained between 70–75° F. Control noise; recommend a white-noise generator which produces soothing sounds while masking other noises.
- Review medications used by client for those that could disrupt sleep; examples of these drugs include Benadryl capsules, Nicoderm Nicotine

Transdermal System, Prozac, Seldane-D Extended Release Tablets, Theo-X Extended Release Tablets, and Xanax. Consult with physician regarding possible alternatives to the medication.

- Encourage use of nonpharmacological sleep inducers (see Box 10-3).
- Discuss use of melatonin, which has been shown to be effective in improving the quality of sleep and reducing sleep disturbances (Garfinkel et al., 1995; Petrie et al., 1993).
- If sedatives are absolutely necessary, suggest use of those that are least disruptive to the normal sleep cycle (e.g., flurazepam, diazepam, chlordiazepoxide).
- Refer to resources for additional information and support (see Box 10-4).

BOX 10-4

Resources for Information About Sleep Pattern Disturbance

American Sleep Disorders Association
1610 14th Street NW
Suite 300
Rochester, MN 55901
(507) 287-6006
www.asda.org

Narcolepsy Network
PO Box 1365
FDR Station
New York, NY 10150
(914) 834-2855; (415) 591-7884
www.websciences.org/narnet

Sleep Apnea

Description

Approximately 17 million Americans suffer from sleep apnea with the prevalence being more than two times greater in males. Sleep apnea syndrome consists of at least five apneic episodes (10 seconds or longer discontinuation of breathing) per hour of sleep. It is characterized by snoring and sudden awakenings, of which the client typically is unaware. There are three types:

central sleep apnea: caused by a defect in the central nervous system that affects the diaphragm;

obstructive sleep apnea: in which a blockage in the upper airway interferes with normal air flow; this is usually accompanied by snoring (Fig. 10-1); and

mixed: a combination of central and obstructive sleep apnea.

In each type, the client has decreased oxygen saturation through the night. Disrupted sleep, morning headache, altered mood and alertness, and daytime sleepiness and fatigue accompany sleep apnea.

Client Goals

- to eliminate or reduce episodes of sleep apnea
- to achieve adequate rest to participate in daily activities
- to be free from daytime sleepiness, fatigue

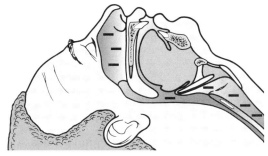

Patient predisposed to OSA

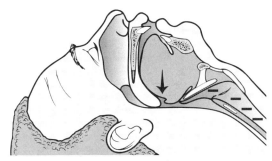

Apneic episode

FIGURE 10-1

In obstructive sleep apnea, a blockage in the upper airway interferes with normal air exchange. From Smolley LA: How to help patients with obstructive sleep apnea, *J Respir Dis* 11:723–732, 1990. Illustration by Robert Margulies.

Interventions

- Refer client to sleep clinic or other resource for evaluation of disorder. Support treatment plan, e.g.:
  - weight reduction
  - continuous positive airway pressure (CPAP): a form of respiratory therapy in which slightly pressurized air is pumped into the nose to counteract the negative pressure that causes the snoring, and airway narrowing and collapse. (Clients using CPAP should be advised to not discontinue using the CPAP unless under the direction of a physician as symptoms can return.)
  - surgery: removal of tonsils, realignment of bite, uvulopalatopharyngo-plasty.
- Assist client in modifying sleeping position to avoid lying on back, which allows the tongue to fall back and block the airway. One method is to sew or attach padding along the center seam of back of a pajama top to prevent rolling onto the back; placing rolled pillows in the center of the bed may help, also.

- Advise client to avoid alcohol and depressant medications, which can further aggravate the problem by decreasing respiratory drive and relaxing throat muscles.
- Advise client and caregivers to be alert to increased potential for injury as a result of daytime fatigue and inattentiveness. Studies have found that people with sleep apnea get into three times as many auto accidents as the rest of the population and are seven times more likely to have multiple accidents (Associated Press, 1997).
- Refer to resources for evaluation and additional information and support (see Box 10-5).

BOX 10-5

Resources for Information About Sleep Apnea

American Sleep Apnea Association
PO Box 66
334 D Pleasant Street
Belmont, MA 02178
(617) 489-4441
www.nicom.com/(asaa

RESOURCES

References

Associated Press, People with sleep disorders found more accident-prone, *The Baltimore Sun* May 22, 1997, p 7A.

Garfinkel D, et al.: Improvement of sleep quality in elderly people by controlled-release melatonin, *Lancet* 346:541-44, 1995.

Petrie K, et al.: A double-blind trial of melatonin as a treatment for jet lag in international cabin crew, *Biological Psychiatry* 33(7):526-30, 1993.

Recommended Readings

Davis S: Why we must sleep, *American Health* 15(3):76-79, 1996.

Dotto L: *Losing sleep*, New York, 1990, Quill.

Kaufman D and Goldberg P: *Everybody's guide to natural sleep*, Los Angeles, 1990, Jeremy P. Tarcher.

Lamberg L: Who me? Fall asleep at the wheel? *American Health* 15(5):84-87, 1996.

Cognitive and Perceptual Functions

*T*he reception, interpretation and expression of sensory stimuli and knowledge are essential for self-actualization and the promotion of health and healing. Normality in the cognitive-perceptual pattern implies that the individual is able to understand and use symbols, and acquire, process, use and store information. Cognition, the ability to obtain and use knowledge, is dependent on perception. Perceptual stimuli are received through:

- visual exteroceptors
- auditory exteroceptors
- cutaneous proprioceptors (pressure, temperature, pain)
- taste proprioceptors
- smell proprioceptors
- kinesthetic interoceptors (movement)
- static or vestibular interoceptors (position of body in space, regulation of bodily functions, sensual stimulation)

For the most part, these processes work without our conscious thought or effort and enable us to appropriately engage in daily activities, protect ourselves, and enjoy the pleasures of the world.

A variety of factors related to chronic conditions can affect sensory and thought processes. Some are obvious, such as the risks growing from diseases like dementias, schizophrenia, and cataracts. Other factors are related to the consequence or treatment of diseases, such as pain or adverse drug reactions.

Assessment Considerations

Cognitive and perceptual status are useful to assess as early in the client-clinician relationship as possible because these functions affect the quality and quantity of data obtained during all interactions thereafter. This assessment begins with the initial contact when the following clues can yield insights into cognitive and perceptual status:

Grooming and dress: Is clothing clean, presentable, appropriate for the season, and appropriately worn? Is client clean and odor-free? Is hair clean and combed? Are cosmetics and accessories excessive or bizarre?

Posture: Does client appear stooped and fearful? Is body alignment normal?

Movement: Are tongue rolling, twitching, tremors, or hand wringing present? Are movements hypoactive or hyperactive?

Facial expression: Is face masklike or overly dramatic? Are there indications of fear, pain, anger?

Level of consciousness: Does client drift into sleep and need to be aroused (i.e., lethargic)? Does client offer only incomplete or slow responses and need repeated arousal (i.e., stuporous)? Are painful stimuli the only type to which the client will respond (i.e., semiconscious)? Is there no response, even to painful stimuli (i.e., unconscious)?

Language: Does the client appear not to understand questions and comments? Are inappropriate words used? Does the client struggle to understand or express words or phrases?

Speech: Is rate and level appropriate? What is tone and inflection?

Hearing: Does client tilt head to favor one ear, appear to have difficulty hearing, ask to have words repeated, or ignore conversation? Is a hearing aid worn?

Sight: Does client wear glasses? Can client see printed material?

Pain: Does client show signs of discomfort or favor any body part?

Through effective questioning, specific problems can be unveiled; examples of questions could include:

Have there been any recent changes to your vision or hearing?

Can you taste different flavors, smell different scents?

Do you have any problem with dizziness or lack of balance?

Do you have any difficulty feeling the temperature of objects?

Do you have any pain or unusual sensations?

Have you noticed any changes in your thinking ability, memory, mental function?

Are you having any problems with relationships?

Do you ever feel nervous? Restless? Out of control?

Additional questions can be asked to assess cognitive function. A variety of reliable, validated tools can be used for cognitive testing, including the Short Portable Mental Status Questionnaire (Pfeiffer, 1975), the Philadelphia Geriatric Center Mental Status Questionnaire (Fishback, 1977), Mini-Mental Status (Folstein et al., 1975), and OARS (Duke University, 1978). In addition, many agencies have their own tools for general mental status assessment. Most of the tools test for the following:

- orientation to person, place, and time
- memory and retention
- ability to follow a three-stage command
- judgment
- calculation

Regardless of the tool used, it is important that it be used in a consistent manner. For example, suppose a client's orientation to place is assessed by one clinician using the question *What city are we in?* and the client answers correctly. If, several days later, another clinician assesses orientation using the question *What is the name of this facility?* and the client responds incorrectly, it would be difficult to determine whether there was a change in cognition because comparative data would be lacking. On the other hand, differences in responses to the same set of questions could yield insights into changes. Poor performance on cognitive testing should warrant further evaluation.

A complete physical examination, including a review of medications and laboratory evaluation of blood and urine, can assist in identifying causes of cognitive and perceptual disturbances. Additional diagnostic testing may be warranted for specific problems.

Related Diagnoses

Altered Thought Processes

Description

Altered thought processes occur when there is a disruption in mental activities, including thought, language competency, reality orientation, problem-solving, judgment, and comprehension. Persons with this diagnosis may appear bewildered, perplexed, disoriented, distracted, and speak and behave inappropriately. Altered thought processes can take either of the following forms:

- delirium: an acute, reversible alteration in cognition accompanied by an alteration in level of consciousness, or
- dementia: a progressive, irreversible deterioration of mental function.

Some chronically ill individuals may possess dementias, such as Alzheimer's disease and multiinfarct dementia as their primary diagnosis; others may develop dementias secondary to other chronic conditions, such as the dementias related to alcoholism, AIDS, and Parkinson's disease. At times, the consequences of many chronic diseases can lead to deliriums (Box 11-1). Because there are many similarities in the clinical manifestations of delirium and dementia (Table 11-1), it is important that clients be carefully assessed to differentiate the two and ensure appropriate treatment.

Client Goals

- to have causative factor identified and corrected, if possible
- to demonstrate normal cognition
- to be free from injury and complications related to altered thought processes

Interventions

- Assist in evaluation to determine underlying cause. Keep client calm and safe during process.
- Collaborate with psychiatrist, psychiatric nurse specialist, and other clinicians.
- Support treatment plan; explain to client and caregivers.
- Provide safe, calm environment:
  - control stimuli (noise, traffic flow, bright lights)
  - maintain room temperature between 70° to 75° F
  - remove clutter and potentially hazardous substances
  - keep area lighted with soft lights
- Promote orientation:
  - offer simple, basic explanations
  - remind of person, place and time
  - put clock and calendar in room
  - clarify misconceptions
- Provide consistency in caregivers and approaches.

BOX 11-1	Complications from Chronic Conditions That Can Cause Delirium

Anemia	Hypotension
Dehydration	Hypoxia
Drug toxicity	Malnutrition
Infection	Metabolic imbalance
Hyperthermia	Sensory deprivation or overload
Hypothermia	Sleep deprivation
Hypoglycemia	Stress

TABLE 11-1

Differences and Similarities Between Delirium and Dementia

	Delirium	Dementia
Onset	Sudden	Gradual, subtle
Cognition	Altered	Altered
Level of consciousness	Altered, hypervigilance to coma	No alteration
Cause	Disrupted cardiac, renal or respiratory function; malnutrition; dehydration; alcohol or drug toxicity; hypotension; hypoxia; hypoglycemia; infection; sleep deprivation; stress	Organic disease such as Alzheimer's disease, ischemic cerebral lesions, Wernicke's encephalopathy, Pick's disease, Jakob-Creutzfeldt disease, Parkinson's disease, Huntington's disease, hydrocephalus, AIDS, heavy metal toxicity
Prognosis	Good, reversible with prompt treatment	Poor; irreversible, progressive decline

- Monitor dietary intake, fluid intake and output, bowel elimination, and hygiene.
- Be alert to *sundowner's syndrome*, a condition characterized by a worsening of agitation, wandering, disorientation and other unusual behaviors in the early evening after "the sun goes down." Advise caregivers to try to reduce this by:
  - having room lighted before evening approaches to avoid light to dark change
  - using nightlights
  - placing client's personal possessions in view
  - checking on client and offering reassurance frequently

- offering toileting assistance
- using touch therapeutically
- If antipsychotic medications are prescribed, ensure that they are properly used. Monitor client's behaviors and reactions to medications. Teach client and caregivers adverse signs for which to observe.
- Consult with physical and occupational therapists.
- Advise clients to observe for signs of complications, such as infections, pressure ulcers, dehydration.
- Provide counseling and support to caregivers and family. Refer to local support groups as appropriate.
- Utilize relaxation measures as appropriate (e.g., music, deep breathing, massage, touch therapy).

Alzheimer's Disease

Description

Alzheimer's disease is a progressive, degenerative, irreversible cognitive disorder. An estimated four million adults suffer some form of dementia, most of which is Alzheimer's disease. When the disease strikes persons under age 60, it is referred to as presenile dementia; senile dementia of the Alzheimer type is that which occurs after age 60.

Organic changes associated with Alzheimer's disease include brain atrophy with widening of sulci, narrow convolutions, lateral ventricular enlargement, reduction in white matter, cortical neuronal loss, senile plaques, and neurofibrillary tangles in the cortex. It is believed that a genetic predisposition toward Alzheimer's disease exists; this belief is supported by the presence of several generations of persons with the disease within affected families. Also, a relationship has been shown between Alzheimer's disease and Down syndrome in that some symptomatology and the features of the brain (e.g., presence of nerve plaques and neurofibrillary tangles) on autopsy are similar. Although to date no conclusive evidence has been presented, there has been speculation that environmental toxins may have a role in the disease due to the elevated levels of aluminum and mercury found in the brain of Alzheimer's victims.

Although more research is needed in this area, there is evidence that the risk of Alzheimer's disease is significantly reduced in women who take estrogen after onset of menopause (Tang et al., 1996).

Symptoms develop gradually and progress at different rates among affected individuals. Often in the early stages of the disease, symptoms are subtle; the individual may be forgetful, oblivious to social graces, indecisive, and appear to have a disinterest in life. Significant cognitive deficits appear as the disease progresses, accompanied by inattention to grooming and hygienic practices. In the latter stages, communication is impaired, motor function deteriorates, and physical status declines. Incontinence, swallowing difficulties, impaired coordination, misinterpretation of the environment, and reduced ability to protect self from injury are among the problems that force the Alzheimer's victim to be dependent on others for care.

Alzheimer's disease can take a significant toll on the family of the affected client. Not only are they faced with significant caregiving responsibilities, but also must witness their loved one becoming a virtual stranger to them. The physical, emotional, social, and economic health of the entire family unit can suffer, emphasizing the importance of addressing the family's needs in the care plan.

Client Goals

- to participate in self-care activities to maximum extent possible
- to effectively communicate needs
- to be free from injuries and complications related to diagnosis

Interventions

- Ensure that proper evaluation has been conducted to rule out other possible causes of dementia. (Sometimes the diagnostic label "Alzheimer's disease" is used when the client shows signs of dementia, even when there has been inadequate diagnostic testing.)
- See interventions for Altered Thought Processes.
- Regularly assess self-care capacity and assist caregivers in adjusting activities to changes in client's level of independence. Encourage caregivers to promote as much independence as the client is capable of demonstrating.
- Use and advise caregivers to use calm speech and manner in care activities.
- Ensure that environment fosters maximum function e.g.:
  - control of stimuli
  - use of clocks and calendars
  - name or photograph on bedroom door
  - use of familiar/personal objects
- Monitor activities of daily living and general status for:
  - dietary and fluid intake
  - weight
  - bowel and urinary elimination
  - skin integrity and cleanliness
  - oral hygiene
  - sleep and rest pattern
  - mobility
- Consult with dietician regarding proper diet. Finger foods may be useful to offer as snacks to replace calories expended during wandering. Semi-soft foods may help reduce risk of aspiration when swallowing problems are present. Suggest adaptive utensils to assist client in feeding independence.
- Encourage exercise to decrease agitation and restlessness and to prevent complications.
- Advise caregivers to orient client to reality and not foster misperceptions.
- Use consistency in approaches, procedures, and caregivers.
- Recommend use of touch.

- Instruct caregivers to give simple, one-step directions to client and to reinforce positive behaviors.
- Evaluate environment for potential hazards and correct as necessary:
  - remove medications and noningestible substances from areas used by client
  - cap electrical outlets
  - attach safety rails in bathroom and stairways
  - adjust water heater to be no higher than 120° F
  - install alarms on doors
  - remove clutter and throw rugs
  - control access to stoves, irons and other potentially dangerous appliances and tools
- Discuss with the family the realities of the disease's progression and future plans for caring for the client.
- Ensure that the client is wearing an identification bracelet and that a recent photograph of the client is available in the event that the client wanders away.
- Discuss safe use of the herb ginkgo biloba. In a double-blind study of persons with early Alzheimer's disease, those who received 240 mg of ginkgo biloba daily demonstrated better memory, attention, and social function than the control group (Hofferberth, 1994).
- Encourage good intake or supplementation of folic acid, zinc, selenium, and vitamins B_6, B_{12}, C, and E.
- Monitor family's status. Discuss impact of caregiving on their health and the importance of their caring for themselves. Encourage caregivers to attend to their own needs (see Chapter 3) and assist them in obtaining information, support, and assistance for care of client. Provide them with the name of the local chapter of the Association for Alzheimer's Disease and Related Disorders. For additional resources, see Box 11-2.

BOX 11-2

Resources for Information About Alzheimer's Disease

Association for Alzheimer's Disease and Related Disorders
919 North Michigan Avenue
Suite 1000
Chicago, IL 60611
(800) 272-3900
www.alz.org/

Respite Programs for Caregivers of Alzheimer's Disease Hotline
(800) 648-COPE

Schizophrenic Disorders

Description

Schizophrenia is a brain disease that primarily affects the limbic system and its connections. Hereditary predisposition and early trauma are factors in the development of the disease; stress can aggravate the disease in vulnerable people. The disease most often strikes in late adolescence and early adulthood.

Normal perceptions become distorted to persons with this thought disorder. The diagnosis of schizophrenia is made when specific symptoms have been present for at least six months (Box 11-3). The symptoms must not be due to an organic disorder or mood disturbance. The DSM-IV categorizes schizophrenia into several types (American Psychiatric Association, 1994):

Catatonic: catatonic rigidity, stupor, waxy flexibility

Disorganized: flat affect, incoherence, silliness

Residual: absence of disorganized behavior, hallucinations and delusions

Paranoid: extreme suspiciousness, delusions of grandeur and persecution

Undifferentiated: mixture of symptoms associated with other types

The disease can affect individuals and progress in different ways, ranging from the exacerbation of active psychotic symptoms to the absence of all symptoms during a remission.

Schizophrenia becomes a chronic disorder for most of its victims. Symptoms generally last for at least six months and typically remain for a lifetime. Prior to the 1960s most people affected by schizophrenia spent a majority of their lives in psychiatric hospitals; however, now hospitalization primarily involves short stays during acute phases of the disease and community-based treatment. Many of these individuals survive in the community by living with their families. Often, the client's condition creates tremendous stress for family members, reinforcing the need for strong family support. Families need help in understanding that there can be periods of remission and exacerbation of the disease, and that residual effects (e.g., low energy, lack of interest in participating in family and social functions, blunted affect) can be present after an acute episode. Family members and caregivers should be assisted in identifying early signs of exacerbation, which could include altered sleep pattern, agitation, depression, and withdrawal.

Client Goals

- to have a reduction in symptoms
- to have an increased awareness of reality

BOX 11-3	Symptoms Associated with Schizophrenia	
Delusions		Hearing one's thoughts out loud
Hallucinations		Incoherent speech
Poor insight		Lack of demonstration of feelings
Illogical thinking		Absence of early waking
Inappropriate affect		

- to improve social skills
- to participate in activities of daily living, be free from complications associated with ADL deficits
- to take medications appropriately, be free from adverse effects of medications

Interventions

- Accept client and develop a trusting relationship. Convey respect for client's feelings.
- Without arguing or threatening the client, do not support delusions. Reinforce reality and focus on the here and now. Let the client know his or her feelings and views are respected, even if you do not share them.
- Assist client in learning effective strategies to relate to others.
- Educate client and caregivers in the safe use of medications (e.g., psychotropics). Reinforce that these drugs can effectively control symptoms if taken correctly. Review potential side effects (Box 11-4). Emphasize that medications should not be discontinued without medical supervision as symptoms are likely to recur when these drugs are stopped.
- If substance abuse is a problem, refer client for counseling and assistance.
- Help client, coach and caregivers recognize prodromal symptoms (signs of relapse) early. These symptoms vary from individual to individual and could include social withdrawal, altered sleep pattern, depression, and anxiety. As soon as these symptoms are noted, professional help should be sought to prevent relapse; an increase in medication may be necessary.
- Reinforce importance of avoiding stressful situations to aid in preventing relapse. Inform client of changes, prepare for procedures, and avoid fostering misperceptions.
- Encourage client to participate in activities; provide feedback on behavior.
- Teach caregivers strategies to help client with hallucinations, such as reducing stimuli, avoiding touching the client, distracting, reinforcing reality, and medicating as prescribed.
- Encourage client to participate in counseling and support therapist's recommendations. (Counseling for persons with schizophrenia tends to be supportive, rather than analytical, to assist client in coping and problem-solving skills.)
- Ensure that client ingests a good diet to promote physiological and psychological health.
- Encourage aromatherapy using lavender to aid in relaxation and creating a pleasant environment.
- Support caregivers and family. Provide education concerning the disease, care, medications, stress reduction, and prevention and recognition of relapse. Refer to counseling and support groups as needed (see Box 11-5).

BOX 11-4   Common Antipsychotic Drugs and Their Side Effects

Antipsychotic drugs can have profound effects in older adults. They can produce sedation, hypotension, and anticholinergic and extrapyramidal symptoms.

ANTICHOLINERGIC SYMPTOMS

Dry mouth	Restlessness	Short-term memory loss
Constipation	Fever	Hallucinations
Urinary retention	Confusion	Agitation
Blurred vision	Disorientation	Picking behaviors
Insomnia		

EXTRAPYRAMIDAL SYMPTOMS

Parkinsonism: tremors; postural unsteadiness; rigidity of muscles in limbs, neck, and trunk; pill-rolling motion with fingers; shuffling gait

Akinesia: decrease in spontaneous movement

Dystonia: holding neck or trunk in rigid, unnatural position, such as turned to one side or hyperextended

Akathisia: inability to sit still

Tardive dyskinesia: thrusting movements of tongue; lip smacking, puckering, or chewing movements; abnormal limb movements

Commonly prescribed antipyschotic drugs and their risk of side effects are listed below:

Generic Name	Brand Name	Sedation	Hypo-tension	Anti-cholinergic symptoms	Extra-pyramidal symptoms
Acetophenazine	Tindal	Mild	Mild	Moderate	Mild
Chlorpromazine	Thorazine	Marked	Marked	Marked	Mild
Fluphenazine	Prolixin	Mild	Mild	Mild	Marked
Haloperidol	Haldol	Minimal	Minimal	Mild	Marked
Loxapine	Loxitane	Mild	Mild	Moderate	Moderate
Mesoridazine	Serentil	Marked	Moderate	Mild	Minimal
Molindone	Moban	Mild	Mild	Moderate	Moderate
Perphenazine	Trilafon	Mild	Mild	Moderate	Moderate
Thioridazine	Mellaril	Marked	Marked	Marked	Mild
Thiothixene	Navane	Mild	Mild	Mild	Marked
Trifluoperazine	Stelazine	Mild	Mild	Mild	Marked

NURSING IMPLICATIONS

- Use antipsychotic medications only when absolutely necessary and for the management of specific target symptoms. The physician's order should describe the specific behaviors for which the drug should be used.
- Ensure that the smallest possible therapeutic dosage is administered initially. If desired results are not seen, the dosage can be gradually increased.
- Regularly assess client's behavior, intake and output, and side effects.
- Help client and caregivers understand that several weeks of therapy may be needed before the effectiveness of the drug is noticed.
- Consult with the physician to reduce the dosage and discontinue the drug as soon as clinically feasible.

Modified from Eliopoulos C: Restraint appropriate care, *Long-Term Care Educator* 2(Lesson 11):6, 1991.

BOX 11-5

Resources for Information About Schizophrenic Disorder

Schizophrenics Anonymous
c/o Mental Health Association
15920 West Twelve Mile
Southfield, MI 48076
(313) 557-6777

Impaired Verbal Communication

Description

Impaired verbal communication describes a condition in which there is an interference in the ability to use or understand language (Box 11-6). Problems in regard to speech (the mechanics of producing words) or language (the comprehension and expression of words) are included in this diagnosis (Figure 11-1). Impaired verbal communication can result from anatomical defects, neuromuscular disorders, altered cerebral circulation, cognitive deficits, hearing impairments, and linguistic differences secondary to cultural or ethnic identity.

Client Goals

- to develop a mechanism for communication
- to express understanding of verbal communication
- to communicate in a clear, appropriate manner
- to describe satisfaction with social interactions

Interventions

- Ensure that evaluation has been done to determine cause of impairment. Support treatment plan.
- Follow and reinforce recommendations of speech therapy.
- Educate client, coach, and caregivers about nature of impairment and effective communication strategies. Some suggestions could include:
  - use a calm approach
  - do not raise your voice (unless a hearing impairment necessitates)

BOX 11-6   Aphasia

Aphasia is the conventional term for organically caused losses or disturbances in language (i.e., reading, writing, understanding, and speaking, or use of symbolic signs and sounds) due to cerebral damage. These disorders can be classified as:
- *expressive:* inability to communicate through writing or speaking
- *receptive:* inability to comprehend written or spoken words
- *global:* loss of all forms of communication, involves comprehension and expression of communication

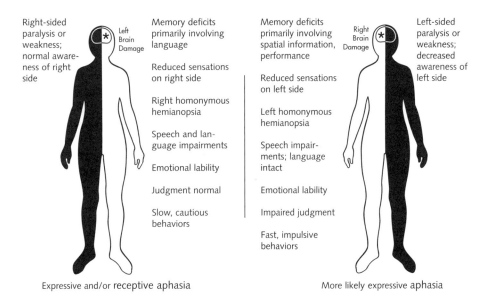

Right-sided paralysis or weakness; normal awareness of right side

Left Brain Damage

Memory deficits primarily involving language

Reduced sensations on right side

Right homonymous hemianopsia

Speech and language impairments

Emotional lability

Judgment normal

Slow, cautious behaviors

Memory deficits primarily involving spatial information, performance

Reduced sensations on left side

Left homonymous hemianopsia

Speech impairments; language intact

Emotional lability

Impaired judgment

Fast, impulsive behaviors

Right Brain Damage

Left-sided paralysis or weakness; decreased awareness of left side

Expressive and/or receptive aphasia

More likely expressive aphasia

FIGURE 11-1

The brain damage from a cerebrovascular accident (CVA) can impair speech in a variety of ways. Left brain damage can cause a repetitious speech and decreased vocabulary retention span. The person with right brain damage can be verbally fluent without the deficit being readily apparent. Anterior frontal lobe CVA can result in altered sentence structure and the uncontrollable or uncharacteristic use of profanity. With posterior frontal lobe CVA, confabulation or inappropriate grouping of words may be present.

- allow adequate time for communication to be processed, words to be formed
- give the client the opportunity to complete sentences without finishing them for client
- use questions that can be responded to with a nod or short answer
- speak slowly and clearly
- encourage client to ask for repetition or clarification
- use visual cues
- Assist client in obtaining and using assistive devices for communication, such as word boards, computers, flash cards, synthesizers. (Consult with speech and occupational therapists for recommendations.)
- Encourage socialization and diversion.
- Refer to support groups (e.g., Lost Chord Club) as appropriate.

Sensory-Perceptual Alteration

Description

Sensory-perceptual alterations exist when the usual and accustomed sensory stimuli are inaccurately experienced or recognized. The client experiences a change in the amount, pattern, or interpretation of incoming stimuli as a result of physiologic, sensory, motor, or environmental disruptions. These alterations can be caused by age-related changes, neurological disease, musculoskeletal conditions, medications (ototoxic drugs, sedatives, tranquilizers), environmental factors, trauma, physical or social isolation, or recurrent ear, eye, or upper respiratory infections.

Client Goals

- to accurately receive and interpret sensory stimuli
- to correctly utilize eyeglasses/hearing aid
- to be free from injury related to sensory deficit

Interventions

- Ensure that client has been thoroughly evaluated to identify underlying cause.
- Assist client in reducing or minimizing factors that contribute to sensory-perceptual alterations:
  - control noise
  - adjust lighting to prevent glare and shadows
  - encourage use of eyeglasses/hearing aid
  - prevent and correct sensory overload
  - promote physical health
  - consult with physician regarding medication change
- Educate client and caregivers in methods to stimulate senses, such as:
  - promoting orientation with use of clocks, calendars
  - providing client with room with window if possible
  - using a variety of colors and textures in decor
  - providing aromatherapy
  - incorporating flavorful foods in diet
  - playing music
- Advise caregivers to explain actions to client to avoid misperceptions.
- Protect client from injury:
  - maintain hot water temperature below 110°F
  - color-code faucet handles
  - keep stairways well-lighted
  - label liquids and other substances with large print
  - avoid storing noningestible substances near ingestible ones
  - ensure that home has smoke detectors
- Support treatment plan for specific condition.
- Refer to resources for information, referral and support (see Box 11-7).

BOX 11-7

Resources for Information About Sensory-Perceptual Alteration

Alexander Graham Bell Association for the Deaf
3417 Volta Place NW
Washington, DC 20007
(202) 337-5220
www.agbell.org

American Council of the Blind
1211 Connecticut Avenue, NW
Suite 506
Washington, DC 20036
(202) 833-1251
acb.org

American Humane Association Hearing Dog Program
1500 W. Tufts Avenue
Englewood, CO 80110
(303) 762-0342

Blinded Veterans Association
1735 DeSales Street NW
Washington, DC 20036
(202) 347-4010
www.bva.org

Design Center for the Deaf
Department of Environmental Design
Rochester Institute of Technology
Rochester, NY 14623
(716) 464-1653
www.rit.edu

Guide Dogs for the Blind
PO Box 1200
San Rafael, CA 94902
(415) 479-4000
www.guidedogs.com

Guiding Eyes for the Blind
250 East Hartsdale Avenue
Hartsdale, NY 10530
(914) 723-2223
www.guiding-eyes.org

Independent Living Aids
11 Commercial Street
Plainview, NY 11803
(516) 681-8288

Leader Dogs for the Blind
1039 S. Rochester Road
Rochester, MN 48063
(313) 651-9011
www.leaderdog.org

Lighthouse National Center for Vision and Aging
111 East 59th Street
New York, NY 10022
(800) 334-5497
www.social.com/health/nhic/data/hr2400/hr2458.html

National Association of the Deaf
814 Thayer Avenue
Silver Spring, MD 20910
(301) 587-1788
www.nad.org

National Association for Visually Handicapped
305 East 24th Street
New York, NY 10010
(212) 899-3141
www.navh.org

National Braille Association
654A Goodwin Avenue
Midland Park, NJ 07432
(201) 447-1484
alamo.digiweb.com/nfb/national_braille_assoc.htm

National Information Center on Deafness
Gallaudet University
T-6, 800 Florida Avenue NE
Washington, DC 20002
(202) 651-5109
www.gallaudet.edu

National Library Service for the Blind and Physically Handicapped
Library of Congress
1291 Taylor Street NW
Washington, DC 20542
(202) 287-5100
lcweb.loc.gov/nls

Recorded Periodicals
919 Walnut Street
Philadelphia, PA 19107
(215) 627-0600
www.libertynet.org/~asbinfo/mags.html

Recordings for the Blind
215 West 58th Street
New York, NY 10022
(212) 751-0860

Self-Help for Hard of Hearing People
PO Box 34889
Washington, DC 20034
www.shhh.org

Cataract

Description

A cataract is a slowly developing opacity of the lens or its capsule. All individuals have some degree of cataract formation as they age, causing this to be a common chronic condition among the elderly. Some individuals may be affected slightly (e.g., having sensitivity to glare), whereas others may have significant visual impairment.

Client Goals

- to have cataract removed
- to be free from injury related to cataracts

Interventions

- Ensure that the client has had recent ophthalmologic examination.
- Reduce glare with use of sunglasses and translucent coverings on windows to filter sunlight; use several soft lights rather than large harsh ones.
- Prepare client for surgical removal of lens. Explain follow-up treatment that will be necessary.
- Encourage good intake of vitamins A and C, which have been shown to reduce incidence of cataracts (Hankinson et al., 1992).
- Refer to local resources for education and support.

Glaucoma

Description

Glaucoma is a condition characterized by a rise in intraocular pressure caused by an increased production and/or decreased outflow of aqueous humor. It can be of two types:

Acute or closed-angle: sudden onset of eye pain, nausea, vomiting, blurring of vision; blindness results if not promptly treated

Chronic or open-angle: most common form; symptoms develop gradually; reduced peripheral vision, tired feeling in eyes, headaches, misty vision

Client Goals

- to maintain intraocular pressure within normal range
- to be free from injury related to impaired vision

Interventions

- Determine client's visual capacity; modify environment to accommodate visual field.
- Reinforce importance of regular ophthalmologic examination with tonometry.
- Teach client to avoid situations that increase intraocular pressure such as:
  - coughing, sneezing, aggressive nose blowing
  - strenuous exercise
  - straining during defecation

- emotional stress
- use of drugs that increase intraocular pressure (stimulants, blood pressure elevators, cold and allergy medications)
- Advise client to avoid eyestrain or overuse of eyes.
- Teach client and caregivers safe use of medications that may be prescribed for condition:
  - parasympathomimetics (miotics)
  - sympathomimetics
  - carbonic anhydrase inhibitors
  - hyperosmotic agents
- Advise client and caregivers to report acute symptoms immediately.
- Encourage use of assistive devices.
- Assist client in locating resources to assist with ADLs, IADLs, and diversional activities (e.g., Books on Tape).

Hearing Impairment

Description

An inability to receive or perceive sound is a hearing impairment. A hearing impairment can occur due to a conductive loss, in which sound is not transmitted satisfactorily, or a perceptive loss, in which there is a problem in the nerve's reception of the sound; some clients can have a combination of both types. Foreign objects and cerumen impactions also can be causes of hearing impairment.

Client Goal

- to effectively receive incoming auditory stimuli
- to establish effective mechanism for communication

Interventions

- Ensure that the client has been properly evaluated for hearing impairment; support treatment plan.
- Communicate and instruct caregivers/coach to communicate with client in manner that maximizes strengths:
  - approach client from front
  - face directly when speaking
  - gain client's attention before beginning to speak
  - speak slowly and distinctly
  - supplement words with exaggerated facial movements and body language
  - speak loudly without high-pitched yelling
  - ensure that the client has understood communication; encourage questions
  - write important information to promote client's understanding
  - at night:
    - touch client to gain attention prior to speaking

- • shine light on own face when speaking to client
- Regularly inspect ear canal for cerumen impaction which can further diminish hearing. If cerumen impaction is present, irrigate ears. Advise client to avoid using cotton-tipped applicators because this can pack cerumen in the ear canal and cause an impaction.
- Consult with speech and hearing therapist or occupational therapist for recommendations.
- Assist client in obtaining and using assistive devices (e.g., speaking tube, telephone amplifier, audioloop, alarms that blink lights rather than emit sounds).
- Encourage the client to engage in social activities; encourage family to include client
- Promote good nutritional status. Research has shown noise-induced hearing loss and tinnitus to be more prevalent in persons with vitamin B_{12} deficiencies (Shemesh et al., 1993).
- Refer to resources for education and support (see listing of resources under discussion of diagnosis of Sensory-Perceptual Alteration, page 263).

Chronic Pain

Description

Another impairment that develops with chronic pain is a decrease in the client's ability to perceive and respond to the environment because of the distraction caused by continual pain. Pain is a state in which the client experiences an uncomfortable sensation in response to a noxious stimulus. Unlike acute pain, which can be relieved and is time-limited, chronic pain has no predictable time limitations, and usually only limited relief is obtained by conventional analgesics. Examples of conditions that cause chronic pain include arthritis, shingles, phantom limb, migraine, and terminal cancer.

Client Goals

- to eliminate source of pain
- to experience reduction in or elimination of pain
- to utilize safe, effective pain relief measures
- to be free of pain enough to perceive and respond to positive stimuli in the environment

Interventions

- Assist in identifying underlying cause. (Keep in mind that although a serious medical problem exists that could cause pain, other factors could be responsible for pain, such as positioning, adverse drug reaction, anxiety.) Evaluate for referred pain (Figure 11-2). Support treatment plan.
- Recommend that client self-assess pain using a scale of 0-10, thermometer, scale, or speedometer (refer to Figure 4-1 in Chapter 4).
- Educate client and caregivers in supportive measures such as:
  - controlling environmental stimuli, reducing noise

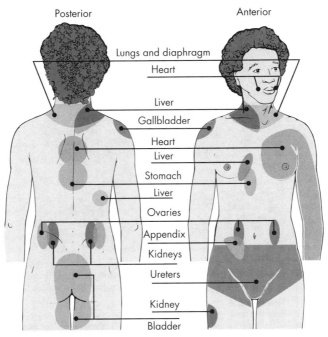

Posterior

Anterior

Lungs and diaphragm

Heart

Liver

Gallbladder

Heart

Liver

Stomach

Liver

Ovaries

Appendix

Kidneys

Ureters

Kidney

Bladder

FIGURE 11-2

Areas of referred pain. From Lewis SM, Collier IC, Heitkemper MM: *Medical-surgical nursing: assessment and management of clinical problems*, ed 4, 1996, Mosby.

- positioning body in proper alignment
- preserving energy
- Teach client pain control measures:
  - Self-hypnosis
  - Guided imagery
  - Biofeedback
  - Yoga (particularly effective for back pain, arthritis, migraine)
  - Topical capsaicin (chili peppers) for fibromyalgia, arthritic and nerve pain (Capsaicin Study Group, 1991; McCarthy et al., 1994)
- Offer massages and teach caregivers to massage client. Massage has been shown to provide pain relief for a variety of conditions ranging from soft tissue injury to inflammatory bowel disease (Joachim, 1983; Danneski-old-Samsoe et al., 1986).
- Use therapeutic touch.
- Refer client to acupuncturist for treatment. Many chronic pain victims have been helped by acupuncture.
- If analgesics are used, ensure that the client uses them correctly and monitors effects (Figure 11-3).
- Refer to resources for education and support (see Box 11-8).

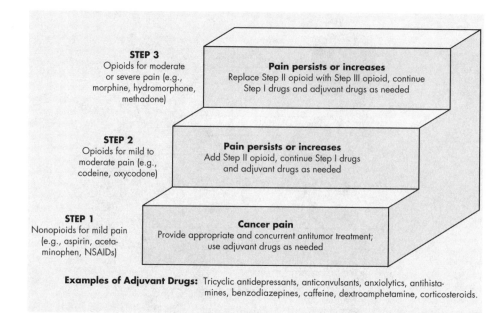

STEP 3
Opioids for moderate or severe pain (e.g., morphine, hydromorphone, methadone)

Pain persists or increases
Replace Step II opioid with Step III opioid, continue Step I drugs and adjuvant drugs as needed

STEP 2
Opioids for mild to moderate pain (e.g., codeine, oxycodone)

Pain persists or increases
Add Step II opioid, continue Step I drugs and adjuvant drugs as needed

STEP 1
Nonopioids for mild pain (e.g., aspirin, acetaminophen, NSAIDs)

Cancer pain
Provide appropriate and concurrent antitumor treatment; use adjuvant drugs as needed

Examples of Adjuvant Drugs: Tricyclic antidepressants, anticonvulsants, anxiolytics, antihistamines, benzodiazepines, caffeine, dextroamphetamine, corticosteroids.

FIGURE 11-3

The analgesic ladder proposed by the World Health Organization. (NSAIDs refers to nonsteroidal antiinflammatory drugs [e.g., ibuprofin, naproxen, ketorolac].)

BOX 11-8

Resources for Information About Pain Management

American Academy of Pain Management
3600 Sisk Road
Suite 2D
Modesto, CA 95356
(209) 545-2920
www.aapainmanage.org/index.html
American Chronic Pain Association
PO Box 850
Rocklin, CA 95677
(916) 632-0922
www.social.com/health/nhic/data/hr2400/hr2428.html

National Chronic Pain Outreach Association
7979 Old Georgetown Road
Suite 100
Bethesda, MD 20814
(301) 652-4948
neurosurgery.mgh.harvard.edu/ncpainoa.htm

Headaches

Description

Many chronic diseases can cause headaches that can be quite debilitating for clients. There are various types of headaches (Box 11-9), each differing in cause, frequency, duration, prodromal symptoms, and treatment. Situations, often those under the control of the client (e.g., skipping meals, sleeping excessively, tension, exposure to toxic fumes), can cause headaches and affect the client's coping and self-care capacity, as well as cognitive-perceptual ability.

Client Goals

- to identify and correct cause of headache
- to learn and utilize measures to prevent headaches
- to identify and utilize effective strategies for reducing/eliminating headache

Interventions

- Assist client in identifying characteristics associated with headache:
  - prodromal symptoms
  - frequency
  - time of day of onset
  - duration
  - location (one side of head, generalized)
  - nature/type of pain (throbbing, dull, sharp)
  - situations that improve or worsen headache
  - other symptoms (sinus drainage, blurred vision, fever, wheezing, paresthesias)
- Prepare and support client with diagnostic procedures.
- Determine the way in which the headache affects activities of daily living, self-care capacity.
- Assist client in identifying factors that trigger headache; these could include any one or more of the following:
  - fatigue
  - stress

BOX 11-9   Types of Headaches

Tension	Traction-inflammatory
Medical problems	Infection
Psychogenic problems	Arteritis
Vascular	Intracranial, extracranial
Migraine	Occlusive vascular structures
Cluster	
Hypertensive	

- hunger
- food (particularly those containing nitrates, monosodium glutamate, and tyramine; chocolate; yogurt; ripened cheeses; cured meats; marinated foods; pork; caffeine)
- alcohol
- changes in climate
- allergies
- menstruation
- Instruct client in avoiding trigger factors.
- Support treatment of underlying cause.
- Educate client in use of measures to prevent and treat headache:
  - Promotion of rest and relaxation, regular sleep pattern, stress management
  - Regular exercise
  - Good diet
  - EMG biofeedback has been shown to have higher success rates for treating headaches than medical or psychological treatments (Andrasik, 1990)
  - Guided imagery
  - Herbs: Ginkgo biloba has shown some benefit for reduction of headaches (Kleijnen and Knipschild, 1992); feverfew has been proven effective in the prevention of migraines (Johnson et al., 1985)
- Consult with homeopathic practitioner regarding use of homeopathic remedies. Incidence and intensity of migraines has been shown to decrease with homeopathic treatments (Brigo and Serpelloni, 1991).
- Refer to acupuncturist. Although acupuncture has had mixed results in the relief of tension headaches, it has been effective in the management of migraines (Vincent, 1989; Baischer, 1995).
- Educate client in the proper use of analgesics. Advise client not to take ergot preparations if pregnant; these drugs can stimulate uterine contractions.
- Encourage client to express feelings and stressors, which can contribute to headaches. Refer for counseling if indicated.
- Refer to resources for education and support (see Box 11-10).

BOX 11-10

Resources for Information About Headaches

American Council for Headache Education (ACHE)
875 Kings Highway
Suite 200
Woodbury, NJ 08096
(800) 255-ACHE
www.achenet.org

National Headache Foundation
5252 North Western Avenue
Chicago, IL 60625
(800) 843-2256
www.headaches.org

Herpes Zoster

Description

Herpes zoster, commonly known as shingles, is a disease caused by the varicella virus (the same organism that causes chickenpox). It occurs as a reactivation of the viral infection that lies dormant after a primary case of chickenpox. Advanced age, lymphomas, Hodgkin's disease, and cancer are among the conditions that compromise the immune system and ease the path for the reactivation of the infection. Because post-herpetic pain can last months after the infection, prevention and early treatment of shingles are important. Without these, post-herpetic pain can turn into chronic pain and result in the same cognitive-perceptual impairments.

Client Goals

- to be free from recurrence of herpes zoster
- to utilize measures to boost immune function
- to be free from impairments of cognition/perception

Interventions

- Educate client in ways to stimulate immune function:
  - *Relaxation exercises.* Relaxation training was shown to significantly increase natural killer cell activity and decrease levels of herpes virus (Kiecolt-Glaser et al., 1985).
  - *Stress management.* Stress has been demonstrated to be a factor in the development and recurrence of herpes (Kiecolt-Glaser, 1985).
  - *Good diet.* Client should avoid excessive consumption of refined carbohydrates.
  - *Multivitamins.* Persons taking multivitamins have been shown to have fewer infections than those using placebos (Chandra, 1992).
  - *Vitamin E.* This vitamin has been particularly useful in boosting immune response in the elderly (Meydani, 1995).
  - *Herbs.* Echinacea has been proven to have a positive effect on immune function (Melchart et al., 1994).
- Recommend use of capsaicin cream (made from chili peppers) for the relief of shingles pain. A controlled trial of capsaicin cream demonstrated it to be effective in relieving post-herpetic neuralgia (Bernstein et al., 1989).
- Consult with homeopathic practitioner regarding use of remedies: *Arsenicum album, Rhus toxicodendron, Sepia, Natrum muriaticum, Hepar sulphurus calcareum, Caladium seguinam.*
- Assist client in management of pain (see diagnosis " Chronic Pain," pages 266–268).
- Educate client and caregivers in preventing spread of infection. People who have not had chickenpox are at risk of developing the disease after exposure to someone with a shingles infection. Strict isolation may be necessary to prevent spread of infection through airborne routes and direct contact during the time that the lesions are draining. Reinforce importance of good handwashing.
- Refer to sources of support and additional information (see Box 11-11).

BOX 11-11
Resources for Information About Herpes Zoster

Herpes Resource Center
PO Box 13827
Research Triangle Park, NC 27709
(919) 361-8488
www.social.com/health/nhic/data/hr1400/hr14
74.html

Knowledge Deficit

Description

A knowledge deficit implies a state in which the individual possesses a deficiency in cognitive knowledge or psychomotor skills that alters or risks altering health maintenance and self-care.

The diagnosis of a chronic illness carries the potential for the client to possess knowledge deficit as the client and caregivers must learn about the disease process, diagnostic tests, treatments, adverse effects, and self-care adjustments. Even with the provision of information, clinicians cannot assume the client possesses knowledge because a variety of factors can interfere with learning, such as visual impairment, poor hearing, low motivation, poor attention span, anxiety, denial, cognitive deficit, language differences, and cultural orientation. The clinician must assess knowledge and skills possessed by the client to ensure that the client is equipped to manage and live with the illness. The clinician cannot assume that the client possesses adequate or correct knowledge about the condition based on the fact that the client is not newly diagnosed; there is no guarantee that knowledge was effectively taught or learned.

Client Goals

- to restate knowledge about condition and its care
- to demonstrate required self-care practices related to condition

Interventions

- Evaluate client's and caregivers' knowledge and skills to identify deficits, priorities, and client's concerns.
- Determine learning ability:
  - intellectual capacity
  - educational level
  - psychomotor skills
  - emotional state, motivation
  - physical capacity
- Develop teaching plan and describe purpose and outline of presentation.
- Select a time that will capitalize on client's ability to learn (e.g., time of day when energy is high, pain controlled, no visitors are present).

- Select an environment conducive to learning (quiet, no distractions, private, relaxing, controlled temperature).
- Utilize a variety of teaching methods that are appropriate to the client's abilities and needs.
- Pace teaching according to client's learning rate and needs.
- Allow ample time for questions and return demonstrations.
- Provide written material for the client to keep for reinforcement of teaching and reference.
- Obtain feedback from client, coach, and caregivers to evaluate effectiveness of education.
- If agreeable to client, arrange visit with another client who possesses the same condition to discuss the condition and its care from the client's perspective.
- Recommend that the client obtain educational materials from organizations and special interest groups pertaining to condition (e.g., Heart Association, Parkinson's Disease Association).

Developmental Disability

Description

Developmental disability, formerly known by the term *mental retardation,* refers to subaverage general intellectual functioning with deficits in adaptive behavior that begin to manifest during the developmental period. There are a variety of causes, including Down's syndrome, Tay-Sach disease, drug abuse, injury during labor and delivery, high fever, head trauma, and oxygen deprivation. The American Association of Mental Deficiency and American Psychiatric Association recognize five levels of developmental disability (Box 11-12). Increasing numbers of developmentally disabled children are surviving into middle and late adulthood and may develop other chronic conditions as they age.

Client Goals

- to participate in self-care to maximum degree capable
- to be free from complications secondary to self-care deficits

Interventions

- Determine self-care independence; reinforce to caregivers importance of allowing client to be maximally independent.
- Suggest routine schedule and pattern of activities be followed.
- Assist client in obtaining assistive devices to increase self-care capacity.
- Give simple, one-stage directions.
- Monitor/advise caregivers to monitor diet, intake and output, skin status.
- Identify risk factors in environment and recommend measures to reduce risks.
- Consult with special education teachers and physical, occupational, and speech therapists; support recommendations.

BOX 11-12 **Levels of Developmental Disability**

Level 0: Borderline

IQ range of 68-83

potential adult mental age of 10 years, 11 months to 13 years, 3 months

usually capable of being self-supporting and maintaining basic life style

Level 1: Mild or Educable

IQ range 52-67

potential adult mental age 8 years, 6 months to 10 years, 10 months

capable of holding employment in highly structured setting with close supervision

usually can live in a community setting

Level 2: Moderate

IQ range 36-51

potential adult mental age 6 years, 1 month to 8 years, 5 months

may be able to hold employment at sheltered workshop or neighborhood jobs

Level 3: Severe

IQ range 20-35

potential adult mental age 3 years, 9 months to 6 years

may be able to perform basic self-care with assistance

may be able to perform limited tasks in sheltered workshop

Level 4: Profound

IQ below 20

potential adult mental age 3 to 8 years or lower

incapable of self-care, may require total assistance

- Offer support to caregivers. Encourage them to express feelings and concerns. If appropriate, introduce discussion of other care options to ensure that plans exist in the event caregivers are no longer available. Refer to local support groups and organizations that can supply additional information and support (see Box 11-13).

BOX 11-13
Resources for Information About Developmental Disability

The ARC
500 East Border Street
Suite 300
Arlington, TX 76010
(817) 261-6003
TheArc.org/welcome.html
Association for Birth Defect Children
827 Irma Street
Orlando, FL 32803
(800) 313-2232
www.birthdefects.org/MAIN.HTM
Learning Disabilities Association of America
4156 Library Road
Pittsburgh, PA 15234
(412) 341-1515
www.ldanatl.org

National Down Syndrome Congress
1605 Chantilly Drive
Suite 250
Atlanta, GA 30324
(800) 232-NDSC
members.carol.net/~ndsc
People First
PO Box 648
Clarkston, WA 99403
(509) 758-1123
www.irccv.org/i&r/iris/g90xytk7.htm
Sibling Information Network
62 Washington Street
Middletown, CT 06457
(203) 344-7500
www.social.com/health/nhic/data/hr2100/hr21
58.html

References

Andrasik F: Psychologic and behavioral aspects of chronic headache, *Neurologic Clinics* 8(4):961-76, 1990.

American Psychiatric Association: *Diagnostic and statistical manual of mental disorders*, ed 4, Washington, D.C., 1994, American Psychiatric Association.

Baischer MD: Acupuncture in migraine: long-term outcome and predicting factors, *Headache* 35(8):472-474, 1995.

Bernstein JE, et al.: Topical capsaicin treatment of chronic postherpetic neuralgia, *Journal of the American Academy of Dermatology* 21:265-70, 1989.

Brigo B and Serpelloni G: Homeopathic treatment of migraines: a randomized double-blind controlled study of sixty cases, *The Berlin Journal on Research in Homeopathy* 1(2):98-105, 1991.

Capsaicin Study Group: Treatment of painful diabetic neuropathy with topical capsaicin, *Archives of Internal Medicine* 151:2225-29, 1991.

Chandra RK: Effect of vitamin and trace-element supplementation on immune responses and infections in elderly subjects, *Lancet* 340:1124-27, 1992.

Danneskiold-Samsoe B, Christiansen E, Andersen RB: Myofascial pain and the role of myoglobin, *Scandinavian Journal of Rheumatology* 15:175-78, 1986.

Duke University Center for the Study of Aging: *Multidimensional functional assessment: the OARS methodology*, Durham, NC, 1978, Duke University.

Fishback DB: Mental status questionnaire for organic brain syndrome, with a new visual counting test, *Journal of the American Geriatrics Society* 25(2):167, 1977.

Folstein MF, Folstein S, and McHugh PR: Minimental state: a practical method for grading the cognitive state of patients for the clinician, *Journal of Psychiatry Research* 12:189, 1975.

Hankinson SE, et al.: Nutrient intake and cataract extraction in women: a prospective study, *British Medical Journal* 305:335-39, 1992.

Hofferberth B: The efficacy of EGb 761 in patients with senile dementia of the Alzheimer type: a double-blind, placebo-controlled study on different levels of investigation, *Human Psychopharmacology* 9:215-22, 1994.

Joachim G: The effects of two stress management techniques on feelings of well-being in patients with inflammatory bowel disease, *Nursing Papers* 15(5):18, 1983.

Johnson ES, et al.: Efficacy of feverfew as prophylactic treatment of migraine, *British Medical Journal* 291:569-73, 1985.

Kiecolt-Glaser JK, et al.: Psychosocial enhancement of immunocompetence in a geriatric population, *Health Psychology* 4(1):25-41, 1985.

Kleijnen J and Knipschild P: Ginkgo biloba for cerebral insufficiency, *British Journal of Clinical Pharmacology* 45:352-58, 1992.

McCarthy DJ, et al.: Treatment of pain due to fibromyalgia with topical capsaicin: a pilot study, *Seminars in Arthritis and Rheumatism* 23(6), Supplement 3:41-47, 1994.

Melchart D, et al.: Immunomodulation with echinacea: a systematic review of controlled clinical trials, *Phytomedicine* 1:245-54, 1994.

Meydani M: Vitamin E, *Lancet* 345:170-75, 1995.

Pfeiffer E: A short, portable mental status questionnaire for the assessment of organic brain deficit in elderly patients, *Journal of the American Geriatrics Society* 23(10):433, 1975.

Shemesh Z, et al.: Vitamin B_{12} deficiency in patients with chronic tinnitus and noise-induced hearing loss, *American Journal of Otolaryngology* 14:94-99, 1993.

Tang MX, et al.: Effect of estrogen during menopause on risk and age of onset of Alzheimer's disease, *Lancet* 348:429-432, 1996.

Vincent CA: A controlled trial of the treatment of migraine by acupuncture, *Clinical Journal of Pain* 5(4):305-12, 1989.

Recommended Readings

Andreasen NC: Symptoms, signs, and diagnosis of schizophrenia, *Lancet* 346(8973):477-82, 1995.

Barilla J: Pain, pain, go away . . . natural remedies show effectiveness, *Health News and Review* Summer 1995, p. 7.

Bazargan M and Hamm-Baugh VP: The relationship between chronic illness and depression in a community of urban black elderly persons, *The Journal of Gerontology* Series B, 50(2):S119-128, 1995.

Bresler D: *Free yourself from pain*, Topanga, CA, 1992, The Bresler Center.

Cobb JL, D'Agostino RB, and Wolf PA: Norms for the mini-mental state examination, *Journal of the American Medical Association* 270(18):2178, 1993.

Cooper JW: Managing disruptive behavioral symptoms: today's dos and don'ts, *Nursing Homes* 42(1):35-38, 1993.

Dossey B: Helping your patient break free from anxiety, *Nursing 96*, 26(10):52-54, 1996.

Fisher S and Greenberg RP: Prescriptions for happiness? *Psychology Today* 28(5):32-38, 1995.

Fletcher RJ and Poindexter AR: Current trends in mental health care for persons with mental retardation, *Journal of Rehabilitation* 62(1):23-27, 1996.

George M: Art for health's sake, *Community Care* 1102(2):26, 1996.

Greenberg M: A real head case: physical symptoms can indicate psychological distress, *Muscle and Fitness* 54(2):58-60, 1993.

Hall LL: The biology of mental disorders, *Journal of the American Medical Association* 269(7):844, February 17, 1993.

Johnson RS: Keeping secrets: why Black men are still reluctant to seek therapy, *Essence* 26(7):91-95, 1995.

Karpen M: Tinnitus: the sound only the patient hears, *Alternative and Complementary Therapies* 2(3):145-152, 1996.

Kelleher KJ and Wolraich ML: Diagnosing psychosocial problems, *Pediatrics* 97(6):899-92, 1996.

Kendler KS and Roy MA: Validity of a diagnosis of lifetime major depression obtained by personal interview versus family history, *American Journal of Psychiatry* 152(11):1608-25, 1995.

Keville K: Boost your brain power: herbs to improve your memory and mental acuity, *Vegetarian Times* 223(3):94-98, 1996.

Kroll D: Alternative therapies for chronic pain management, *Alternative and Complementary Therapies* 2(1):5-8, 1996.

Kumasaka L and Miles A: My pain is God's will, *American Journal of Nursing* 96(6):45-47, 1996.

Laporte JR and Figueras A: Placebo effects in psychiatry, *Lancet* 344(8931):1206-1210, 1994.

Lewis R: Evening out: the ups and downs of manic-depressive illness, *FDA Consumer* 30(5):26-30, 1996.

Lewis DC: Substance abuse and mental health, *Brown University Digest of Addiction Theory and Application* 13(3):12, 1994.

Liberman J: *Light: medicine of the future*, Santa Fe, NM, 1993, Bear and Co. Publishing.

Lipton R, Newman L, and MacLean H: *Migraine: beating the odds*, Reading, MA, 1992, Addison-Wesley.

McGuffin P, Owen MJ, and Farmer AE: Genetic basis of schizophrenia, *Lancet* 346(8976):678-83, 1995.

Michels R and Marzuk PM: Progress in psychiatry, *New England Journal of Medicine* 329(8):552-561, 1993.

Mizsur GL: Depression and paranoia: is your patient at risk? *Nursing* 25(2):66-68, 1995.

Okpaku SO, Sibulkin AE, and Schenzler C: Disability determinations for adults with mental disorders: Social Security Administration vs independent judgments, *American Journal of Public Health* 84(11):1791-1796, 1994.

Olfson M, et al.: Psychological management by family physicians, *Journal of Family Practice* 41(6):543-51, 1995.

Ornstein R and Sobel D, editions: *The healing brain: a scientific reader*, New York, 1990, The Guilford Press.

Robbins L and Lang SS: *Headache help: a complete guide to understanding headaches and the medicines that relieve them*, Boston, 1995, Houghton Mifflin Co.

Simonton C, Simonton S, and Creighton J: *Getting well again*, Los Angeles, 1978, Jeremy P. Tarcher.

Spitzer RL, et al.: Health-related quality of life in primary care patients with mental disorders: results from the PRIME-MD 1000 study, *Journal of the American Medical Association* 274(19):1511-18, 1995.

Starr C: Mental illness therapy takes a few steps forward, *Patient Care* 29(17):6, 1995.

Thara R: A family burden, *World Health* 47(2):10-12, 1994.

Tinterow MM: *Hypnosis, acupuncture and pain*, Wichita, KA, 1989, Bio-Communication Press.

Van Os J and Neeleman J: Caring for mentally ill people, *American Journal of Nursing* 96(1):36-38, 1996.

Warren T: *Beating Alzheimer's*, Garden City Park, NY, 1991, Avery Publishing Group, Inc.

Weber S: The effects of relaxation exercises on anxiety levels in psychiatric inpatients, *Journal of Holistic Nursing* 14(3):196-205, 1996.

Wilkinson G: Can suicide be prevented? Better treatment of mental illness is more appropriate aim, *British Medical Journal* 309(6958):860-2, 1994.

Windle RC, Scheidt DM and Miller GB: Physical and sexual abuse and associated mental disorders among alcoholic inpatients, *American Journal of Psychiatry* 152(9):1322-1329, 1995.

Self-Perception and Self-Concept

*O*ur views of ourselves are highly personal and individual, based on a variety of experiences and impressions (Figure 12-1). Self-concept begins its formation early in life and evolves through our lifetimes. Early in life, much of our self-concept develops as a result of interactions pertaining to our basic physiologic needs. For example, if our needs for food, cleanliness, and comfort are satisfied, we feel loved, secure and worthy; if these needs are not met, we ultimately may develop perceptions about the world and ourselves that result in low self-worth. As we mature into adulthood, the physical needs, although important, may affect self-concept to a lesser degree than psychosocial factors, such as our occupation, attractiveness, social contacts, and normalcy.

A variety of factors affect the impact of chronic illness on self-concept (Box 12-1). The perception of self as a whole, "normal" individual can be threatened as the chronically ill individual faces lifestyle modifications, occupational restrictions, altered relationships, changes in appearance, impaired bodily functions, reduced energy, dependency, and added demands imposed by the illness. The unfortunate dilemma is that a negative self-concept is not only at risk of developing as a result of the consequences of a chronic illness, but also the possession of a negative self-concept can interfere with the successful management of the chronic illness. The anxiety, depression, hopelessness and powerlessness that can grow from a poor self-concept weaken the capacity to cope and enjoy the highest possible quality of life attainable. Yet another burden is added to the already existing ones that may be faced. Clinicians are challenged to help chronically ill persons reconstruct their self-concept, finding purpose, meaning, and satisfaction within the revised self-concept created by the illness. The yin-yang nature of life implies that there is a positive element to every negative experience; clinicians need to help chronically ill clients understand this reality of the human experience and seek an awareness of the gifts their lives may have been given despite the sometimes harsh realities of living with a chronic illness.

Assessment Considerations

The client's appearance and behavior can give clues to self-concept. These clues can come from any of the following aspects of behavior:

- level of consciousness
- posture
- gait
- eye contact
- facial expression
- speech pattern
- appropriateness of dress
- grooming and hygiene

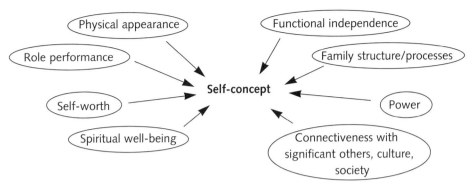

FIGURE 12-1

Influences on self-concept.

BOX 12-1	Factors Influencing the Impact That Chronic Illness May Have on Self-Concept
Age	Occupation
Type of illness	Dependents
Societal familiarity and attitudes toward illness	Financial status
	Lifestyle
Physical manifestations of illness	Availability of caregivers
Stability of illness	Faith
Self-care ability	Motivation
Support system	Coping and problem-solving skills
Attitude of spouse/significant other toward illness and care demands	

These observations are then supplemented by the interview, in which specific questions like the following are asked.

How has this disease affected your life? Your family's life?

Has this illness caused you to make any major changes in your work, lifestyle or other aspects of life? How?

Have people treated you differently since you have been diagnosed? How?

Do you engage in social activities in the same manner as before you were diagnosed?

How has this illness changed the way in which you engage in social activities?

Are you ever "moody" because of the illness and what it does to you? Describe.

How has this illness caused you to look at life differently?

Has anything positive come from this experience?

Do you ever have feelings of extreme sadness? anger? anxiety? What makes you feel this way and how do you cope with the feeling?

Do you ever take actions that are harmful to you or that are not in your best interest? Describe.

Where or from whom do you get your strength?

How do you feel about the future?

A mental status evaluation is beneficial in gaining insight into self-concept and self-perception.

Related Diagnoses

Anxiety

Description

Anxiety is a state in which the client feels uneasy, apprehensive, and a sense of impending doom. Anxiety differs from fear in that with fear there is a reaction to an identifiable threat, whereas that is not necessarily true with anxiety.

Symptoms associated with anxiety fall on a continuum (Figure 12-2). Physical, cognitive, and emotional symptoms (Box 12-2) can accompany anxiety and, in addition to creating significant discomfort and health risks, can reduce self-care capacity, further heightening anxiety and other reactions.

Anxiety can occur periodically as a result of the effects of chronicity, such as the threat of losing one's job, concern over the ability to care for one self, and anticipation of a worsening of the condition; specific crises or an exacerbation in the illness can promote temporary anxious states. Anxiety also can be a chronic condition in itself.

Client Goals

- to eliminate/reduce level of anxiety
- to cope effectively with anxiety
- to be free from complications secondary to anxiety (e.g., sleep deprivation, malnutrition, injury)

Interventions

- Assist in identifying factors causing or contributing to anxiety. (Be aware that even if anxiety is a long-term problem, new factors can be present that worsen the condition, and these new factors could possibly be correctable.) Monitor symptoms in relation to activities, events, and contacts. Consult with the health care team regarding interventions to eliminate or reduce causative/contributing factors.
- Support treatment plan. Encourage client to engage in prescribed therapies.
- Identify the level of anxiety the client is experiencing (Figure 12-2); ask client to self-assess level of anxiety using symptom scale (see Figure 4-1).

CONTINUUM OF ANXIETY			
Mild	**Moderate**	**Severe**	**Panic**
• Increased alertness and awareness • Increased hearing sensitivity and eye movements • Heightened ability to react and respond	• Inattention and reduced awareness of environment • Decreased ability to think clearly	• Drastically decreased perceptual field • Altered thought patterns • Difficulty focusing on more than one detail at a time	• Significant misperceptions of environment • Inability to clearly review or understand a situation • Unpredictable or inappropriate responses • Abnormal behaviors

FIGURE 12-2

Continuum of anxiety.

BOX 12-2   Symptoms Associated with Anxiety

Physiologic
Rapid pulse, increased blood pressure
Chest pain
Increased psychomotor activity, trembling, aching muscles
Headaches
Dizziness
Sleep disturbances
Change in appetite
Change in bowel elimination pattern
Dry mouth
Indigestion, nausea
Urinary frequency
Heavy perspiration
Dyspnea, hyperventilation

Cognitive
Difficulty concentrating, focusing
Confusion
Poor memory
Rumination, asking same question repeatedly
Orientation to past rather than present or future

Emotional
Apprehension
Irritability, angry outbursts
Loss of control, helplessness
Crying
Nervousness
Fears, phobias

- Develop plan with client to reduce level of anxiety, using specific symptom scale. (If client is rating anxiety on a scale of 0-10 in which 0 = no anxiety, identify current level of anxiety on scale, for example "8", and jointly develop goal with client to reduce anxiety to "2–3" by the end of one month.)
- Reduce environmental stimuli such as noise, extreme temperatures, glare, bright lights, distractions, and busy traffic flow.
- Ensure that client understands safe use of antianxiety drugs. Review and discuss with physician conditions that could contraindicate use of antianxiety drugs such as alcohol intoxication, myasthenia gravis, blood dyscrasias, acute narrow-angle glaucoma, and severe pulmonary, hepatic, or renal disease. Assist client in preventing complications associated with common side effects such as:

Side effect	Potential complication
Drowsiness, ataxia, weakness, unsteady gait	Falls
Sleep disturbances	Fatigue, falls, self-care deficit
Gastrointestinal upset	Poor nutritional status
Constipation	Fecal impaction, anorexia
Impaired bladder control	Urinary incontinence, impaired skin integrity

- Advise caregivers/family members to establish and maintain consistent routines with client and to reduce uncertainty.
- Review client's diet. Recommend elimination of caffeine-containing products.
- Monitor client's mental status, weight, elimination pattern.
- Instruct client in stress reduction techniques such as progressive relaxation, meditation, and imagery.
- Teach and encourage client to practice tai chi and yoga.
- Use music therapeutically to promote relaxation.
- Offer back massages; train caregivers, coach, and significant others to give massages to client. Various studies have supported the belief that therapeutic massage is effective in reducing anxiety (Field et al., 1992; Ferrell-Torrey and Glick, 1993). Massaging with Roman chamomile added to the massage oil has been shown to reduce anxiety to a greater extent than the use of other herbal oils (Wilkinson, 1995).
- Use therapeutic touch, which has been demonstrated to be more effective than casual touch or conversation in reducing anxiety levels (Kramer, 1990).
- Recommend the use of the herb valerian, which has been shown to have potent anti-anxiety and sedative effects (Leathwood et al., 1982; Lindahl and Lindwall, 1989).
- Be available and encourage client to express feelings and discuss coping strategies.
- Refer to local support groups and other sources of additional information (see Box 12-3).

BOX 12-3

Resources for Information About Anxiety

ABIL Inc.
1418 Lorraine Avenue
Richmond, VA 23227
(804) 266-9409
Anxiety Disorders Association of America
6000 Executive Boulevard
Suite 513
Rockville, MD 20852
(301) 231-9350
www.aada.org

Council on Anxiety Disorders
PO Box 17011
Winston-Salem, NC 27116
(919) 722-7760
Phobics Anonymous
PO Box 1180
Palm Springs, CA 92263
(619) 322-COPE

Disturbance in Self-Concept

Description

Disturbance in self-concept is a state in which the individual experiences negative feelings about self. This can result from a change in body image, self-esteem, functional status, role performance, or personal identity.

Client Goals

- to demonstrate/express positive views of self

Interventions

- Identify factors contributing to disturbance in self-concept and assist client in eliminating/reducing them (e.g., obtaining prosthetic device, joining support group, job retraining).
- Discuss potential new roles with client and encourage a process of self-discovery in establishing modified lifestyle.
- Encourage socialization.
- Identify accomplishments of client and offer positive reinforcement.
- Encourage client to express feelings.
- Advise caregivers, coach, and significant others to focus on client's capabilities rather than limitations and to reinforce client's efforts at independence and normalcy.
- Advocate for client's empowerment. Ensure that client is given opportunity to make decisions on own behalf and is not treated in a paternalistic manner.
- Support client with grieving of losses (e.g., function, appearance, roles).
- Encourage client to reminisce about past in order to gain perspective on life (Box 12-4).
- Allow client to express feelings without judgment.
- Assist client in learning new skills and developing new roles. Refer to occupational and recreational therapists and vocational counselors.
- Refer to counseling as needed.

BOX 12-4   Guiding Clients through Reminiscence

Reminiscence is a therapeutic review of one's past life to:
- Resolve current conflicts
- Illuminate the individual's past
- Organize and understand significance of past events
- Cope with the present and future
- Maximize use of long-term memory when short-term memory is poor
- Offer a comfortable mechanism for expressing self more comfortably
- Maintain identity and self-esteem

Use reminiscence to assess:
- Individual accomplishments, needs
- Self-esteem
- Cognitive function
- Emotional stability
- Unresolved conflicts
- Coping ability
- Expectations for the future

GROUP PROCESS

Use questions to initiate and guide reminiscence. Strategies could include:
- Listening actively and with interest to discussions of clients' lives
- Helping clients compile poems, oral histories, or scrapbooks of their lives
- Asking clients to share information about their past. Questions could include "What was it like to leave Europe and come to America?" "How did you celebrate holidays as a child?" "What were your parents and grandparents like?" "Did you have any pets when you were young?" "How did you spend your time as a teenager?" "What was the factory like when you started working there?"
- Playing old songs and showing old photos, newspapers or magazines, and asking what was happening in the client's life at that time
- Structuring intergenerational activities in which the old can share their past with the young
- Respecting clients' privacy so that periods of silent reminiscing are not disturbed
- Asking clients to talk about a specific event or time (e.g., "Tell me how it was to be a girl in Germany." "What was your first job like?" "What was the city like when you were a teenager?")
- Using questions to help clients explore emotional responses to past events (e.g., "How did you feel when your town was invaded during the war?" "How difficult was it for you as a young widow?" "Were you disappointed at having to quit school?")
- Gently redirecting the conversation if clients' responses are repetitious or aimless (e.g., "you mentioned that before . . .did that event have a special meaning for you?" "Let's get back to how you began your career." "How do you feel about the problems you describe between yourself and your family?")
- Listening to clients' responses; this is the most important function in reminiscence
- Informing clients of time constraints and enforcing them; if appropriate, ask clients to summarize or identify the lesson/theme of the conversation

From Eliopoulos C: *Manual of gerontologic nursing,* ed 2, St. Louis, 1999, Mosby, pp. 367-368.

Depression

Description

The mood alteration referred to as depression is a feeling of extreme sadness, self-depreciation, hopelessness, helplessness, and disinterest in activities of daily living. Suicide is a very real risk.

Depression occurs more frequently among women than men. A prior episode of depression, family history of the disorder, weak or nonexistent support system, abuse of drugs or alcohol, use of certain medications (Box 12-5), medical comorbidity, and reduced levels of norepinephrine, serotonin, or their metabolites are risk factors for depression. A chronic illness and the demands it imposes can create added stress in the client's life and be the risk factor that triggers serious depression; therefore, clinicians should observe for symptoms (Box 12-6) of this problem during their regular contact with chronically ill clients.

Depression affects not only the emotional aspects of the client, but also the cognitive, physical, social, and spiritual dimensions. When depressed, the client is less able to meet the demands imposed by chronic illnesses and may suffer a worsening of the condition or decrease in functional independence as a result; this, in turn, can cause the client to feel more depressed, and thus, a vicious cycle is established (Figure 12-3). Effective treatment of depression is essential to protecting the client from harm, but also to strengthen self-care capacity to meet the demands imposed by other chronic conditions.

BOX 12-5	**Drug Groups That Carry A High Risk for Inducing Depression**
Analgesics	Appetite suppressants
Antianxiety agents	Cardiovascular agents
Antibiotics	Nonsteroidal antiinflammatory agents
Antihypertensives	Sedatives
Antiparkinsonians	Steroids, hormones
Antipsychotics	

BOX 12-6	**Symptoms of Depression**
Isolation, withdrawal	Decreased interest in sex
Extreme sadness	Poor concentration and judgment
Negativism	Inability to make decisions
Verbalization of hopelessness, pessimism, guilt	Disinterest in self-care
Self-depreciation	Increased dependency
Fatigue	Noncompliance with treatments, care plan
Altered sleep pattern	Suicidal thoughts or plans
Altered nutritional state	

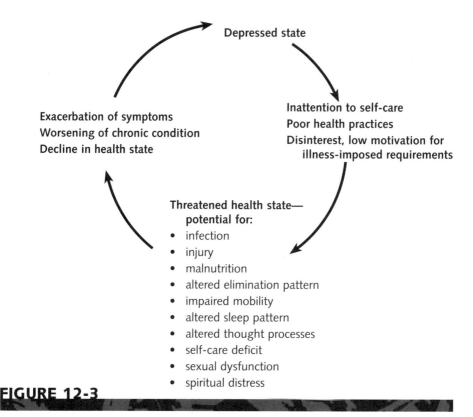

FIGURE 12-3

The vicious cycle of depression and chronic illness.

Client Goals

- to express feelings
- to identify and reduce/eliminate cause of depression
- to be free from injury
- to consume adequate diet to meet metabolic needs
- to be oriented to person, place and time
- to have reduction in symptoms
- to be free from complications secondary to effects of depression (e.g., constipation, fatigue, sleep deprivation, malnutrition, impaired skin integrity)
- to express feelings of hope, self-worth

Interventions

- Review factors that could contribute to depression. Even if depression is a long-term condition, look for other factors that could worsen mood. Consult with psychiatrist and other health team members for effective treatment plan; support treatment plan.
- Educate client, caregivers, and coach about depression and its treatment.
- Establish regular, frequent contact with client. Encourage expression of feelings without judgment. Sit in silence if client does not feel like talking.

- Use touch to convey empathy.
- Encourage participation in activities or volunteer work to build self-esteem.
- Empower client. Provide maximum opportunities for decision-making and control over activities unless contraindicated.
- Display hope in potential for improvement.
- Assist client in forming short-term goals and finding opportunities for success.
- Ensure that client understands safe use of antidepressant drugs; monitor effects. Reinforce that at least one month of therapy is necessary before effects of antidepressants are realized. Encourage client to continue taking medication as prescribed, even when mood improvements are achieved.
- Develop a contract with client regarding suicide prevention that includes agreement that client will:
  - report thoughts of suicide
  - discuss suicidal ideas or plans
  - accept clinician's judgment of need for suicidal precautions
- Monitor physical status (e.g., elimination pattern, weight, hygiene).
- Encourage physical exercise. Studies have supported the fact that exercise and physical activities improve mood and decrease symptoms of depression (Ross and Hayes, 1988) and that running is as effective as psychotherapy in relieving symptoms of depression (Griest et al., 1978).
- Encourage client to use the herb St. John's wort, which has been shown to be as effective as antidepressant drugs in treating depression (Ernst, 1995). Advise client to be careful of exposure to sunlight when taking this herb as it can cause photosensitivity.
- Offer and encourage client to obtain massages. Research supports that a 30-minute daily massage is effective in reducing symptoms in persons being treated for depression (Field et al., 1992).
- Discuss use of light therapy which has been shown to improve mood, particularly in individuals with seasonal affective disorder (Gutfield, 1993).
- Refer client to local support groups and sources of additional information (see Box 12-7).

BOX 12-7
Resources for Information About Depression

Depressed Anonymous
1013 Wagner Avenue
Louisville, KY 40217
(502) 569-1989
depanon@aol.com
Depressives Anonymous
(212) 689-2600
National Depressive and Manic-Depressive Association
730 North Franklin

Suite 501
Chicago, IL 60610
(800) 826-3632
www.ndmda.org
National Organization for Seasonal Affective Disorder (NOSAD)
PO Box 40133
Washington, DC 20016
www.nyx.net/~lpuls/sadorg.html

Hopelessness

Description

Hopelessness is a state in which the client sees no positive options for the future and believes nothing can be done to change the situation.

Hope is the force that fuels us to face an unknown future. It motivates us to attempt to achieve goals and change situations. It instills a belief that there will be better tomorrows. Hardships and discomforts can be better endured if one has hope that the future will be happier or easier.

The diagnosis of a chronic illness initially can trigger feelings of depression and hopelessness. The image the client holds of self and the future is now colored by the variables associated with a disease. As time goes on, the client understands the realities of the disease, including the limitations that are real and those that are unlikely; this enables a revised image of the future to be constructed, accompanied by new goals, plans and actions. That which is hoped for may need to be changed, but the condition of hope is present.

Hopelessness can interfere with the healing process and rob clients of the resources required to face the challenges of chronic illness. Clinicians need to assist chronically ill clients in nurturing the critical elements of hope (Box 12-8) to promote effective coping with chronic conditions and a high quality of life.

Client Goals

- to reduce feelings of hopelessness
- to identify elements of life that can inspire hope

Interventions

- Establish a trusting relationship with client. Encourage expression of feelings.

BOX 12-8   Critical Elements of Hope

Mutuality and affiliation: sharing, caring, trust in others
Sense of the possible: believing goals and plans are achievable
Avoidance of absoluting: not viewing situations as all or nothing
Anticipation: having expectations for future
Action: establishing and achieving goals
Psychologic well-being and coping
Purpose and meaning in life
Freedom: power, self-determination
Reality surveillance: search for clues that confirm feasibility and value of hope
Optimism
Mental and physical energy

Adapted from Miller JF: Inspiring hope. In Miller JF: *Coping with chronic illness: overcoming powerlessness*, ed 2, Philadelphia, 1992, F.A. Davis.

- Assess family dynamics to identify behaviors of significant others that contribute to hopelessness. Counsel as needed and offer strategies for promoting hope (e.g., providing maximum opportunities for client to be in control of self and activities, making plans for future events, continuing/developing intimate relationship, focusing on small delights of daily life).
- Assist client in developing realistic short-term goals; reflect on goal achievement.
- Engage in life review and reminiscence to assist client in identifying past successes in meeting challenges and link to current situation.
- Assist client in enjoying the pleasures of the here and now.
- Encourage an environment that promotes relaxation and happiness (e.g., presence of flowers, pets, stimulating colors, pleasant scents).
- Unless inappropriate or offensive for client, reinforce the hope offered by God and scriptures (Box 12-9), and assist client in satisfying spiritual needs. Refer to clergy as needed.
- Develop affirmations that client can use and prescribe that client repeat them daily. If possible, script a personalized audiotape for the client.
- Recommend that the client maintain a personal journal to promote self-understanding and personal growth. Journal writings can consist of:
  - current random thoughts and feelings
  - observations about personal behaviors and reactions
  - reflections of past relationships, behaviors
  - descriptions of dreams
- Use humor therapeutically. Engage in playful interactions.
- Assist client in participating in diversional activities. Consult with recreational and art therapists.
- Teach client to use progressive relaxation and guided imagery.
- Use music therapeutically. Consult with music therapist for selections that promote optimism and hope.
- Refer client to support group and/or link with person who has similar condition.

Powerlessness

Description

Powerlessness is a state in which the client feels a lack of personal control over certain events or situations. It occurs when the client perceives that his or her actions have no significant effect on outcome.

A history of experiencing events over which one has no control can foster feelings of powerlessness. The development of a chronic disease, progressive worsening of the condition, and exacerbation of symptoms that occur despite one's efforts foster feelings of powerlessness; thus, this diagnosis is a high-risk one for persons with chronic conditions (Box 12-10). Clients who feel powerless are less able to cope with their conditions, learn poorly, and may suffer knowledge deficits, low self-esteem, anxiety, depression, and a host of other complications.

BOX 12-9   Scriptural References to Hope

But for me, I will always have hope;
I will praise you more and more.
My mouth will tell of your righteousness,
of your salvation all day long,
though I know not its measure.
I will come and proclaim your mighty
acts,
O Sovereign Lord;
I will proclaim your righteousness,
yours alone.
Since my youth, O God, you have
taught me,
and to this day I declare your mar-
velous deeds.
Even when I am old and gray,
do not forsake me, O God,
till I declare your power to the next
generation,
your might to all who are to come.
Your righteousness reaches to the
skies, O God,
you who have done great things,
Who, O God is like you?
Though you have made me see troubles, many and bitter,
you will restore my life again;
from the depths of the earth
you will bring me up.

Psalm 71: 14-20

...we who have fled to take hold of
the hope offered to us may be
greatly encouraged.
We have this hope as an anchor for
the soul, firm and secure.

Hebrews 6: 18-19

May those who fear you rejoice when
they see me,
for I have put my hope in your word.
I know, O Lord, that your laws are
righteous,

and in faithfulness you have afflicted
me.
May your unfailing love be my comfort,
according to your promise to your
servant.

Psalm 119: 74-76

And we rejoice in the hope of the
glory of God.
Not only so, but we also rejoice in
our sufferings,
because we know that suffering produces perseverance;
perseverance, character; and character, hope.
And hope does not disappoint us,
because God has poured out his love
into our hearts...

Romans 5: 2-5

You are my refuge and my shield;
I have put my hope in your word.

Psalm 119: 114

Against all hope, Abraham in hope
believed and so became the father
of many nations,
just as it had been said to him, "So
shall your offspring be.
Without weakening in his faith, he
faced the fact that his body was as
good as dead,
since he was about a hundred years
old, and that Sarah's womb was
also dead.
Yet he did not waiver through unbe-
lief regarding the promise of God,
but was
strengthened in his faith and gave
glory to God, being fully per-
suaded that
God had power to do what he had
promised.

Romans 4: 17-21

Though outwardly we are wasting
away, yet inwardly we are being
renewed day by day.
For our light and momentary troubles
are achieving for us an eternal
glory

that far outweigh them all. So we fix
our eyes not on what is seen, but
on what is unseen.
2 Corinthians 4: 16-18

Don't be afraid; just believe.
Mark 5: 36

BOX 12-10   Indications of Powerlessness

Expressed feelings of having little or
no control over situation
Indecisiveness
Apathy
Depression

Aggressive behavior, acting out
Anxiety
Passivity
Noncompliance

Client Goals

- to identify reasons for feelings of powerlessness
- to describe ways to increase sense of self-control

Interventions

- Assist client in identifying factors contributing to powerlessness and in eliminating or reducing these factors (e.g., teach self-care techniques, obtain assistive devices, increase knowledge).
- Refer for professional counseling if appropriate.
- Encourage maximum decision-making and participation in care activities.
- Respect client's preferences (e.g., diet, schedule).
- Prepare client for procedures; offer explanations.
- Encourage client to express feelings openly.
- Assist client in setting realistic goals and developing means to meet them.
- Assist client to maintain internal locus of control by indicating how outcomes have been determined by his or her own actions.
- Avoid reinforcing manipulative behavior. Provide feedback to client about manipulative behaviors and offer suggestions for alternative means to get needs met.
- Educate client regarding chronic condition and its care.
- Reinforce/teach assertiveness skills.
- Advise client to develop and use affirmations that reinforce client's ability to determine and control events.
- Guide client in the use of imagery to enhance perception of self as being in control of life and chronic condition.

- Reinforce to caregivers importance of allowing client to have maximum decision-making and participation in activities.
- Advise coach to reinforce and promote client's self-determination and assertiveness.
- Refer to support groups.

References

Ernst E: St. John's wort, an antidepressant? A systematic, criteria-based review, *Phytomedicine* 2(1):67-71, 1995.

Ferrell-Torrey AT and Glick OJ: The use of therapeutic massage as a nursing intervention to modify anxiety and the perception of cancer pain, *Cancer Nursing* 16(2):93-101, 1993.

Field T, et al.: Massage reduces anxiety in child and adolescent psychiatric patients, *Journal of the American Academy of Child and Adolescent Psychiatry* 31(1):125-131, 1992.

Griest J, et al. Antidepressant running: running as treatment for nonpsychotic depression, *Behavioral Medicine* 5:19-24, 1978.

Gutfield G: The new science of rays and rhythms: cutting edge light therapies that can brighten your health, *Prevention* 45(2):67-71, 116-123, 1993.

Kramer NA: Comparison of therapeutic touch in stress reduction of hospitalized children, *Pediatric Nursing* 16(5):483-85, 1990.

Leathwood PD, et al.: Aqueous extract of valerian root improves sleep quality in man, *Pharmacology, Biochemistry and Behavior* 17:65-71, 1982.

Lindahl O and Lindwall L: Double blind study of a valerian preparation, *Pharmacology, Biochemistry and Behavior* 32:1065-66, 1989.

Ross CE and Hayes D: Exercise and psychological well-being in the community, *American Journal of Epidemiology* 127:762-71, 1988.

Wilkinson S: Aromatherapy and massage in palliative care, *International Journal of Palliative Nursing* 1(1):21-30, 1995.

Recommended Readings

Charmaz K: The body, identity, and self: adapting to impairment, *Commuter-Regional Airline News* 13(50):657-81, 1995.

Erdal KJ and Zautra AJ: Psychological impact of illness downturns: a comparison of new and chronic conditions, *Psychology and Aging* 10(4):570-78, 1995.

Kahn S: *The nurse's meditative journal*, Albany, NY, 1996, Delmar Publishers.

Lorig K, et al.: *Living a healthy life with chronic conditions*, Palo Alto, CA, 1994, Bull Publishing Co.

Miller JF: *Coping with chronic illness: overcoming powerlessness*, ed 2, Philadelphia, 1992, FA Davis Co.

Wood C: Is hope a treatment for cancer? Advances, *Journal of Mind-Body Health* 12(3):67-71, 1996.

Woog P, editor: *The chronic illness trajectory framework: the Corbin and Strauss nursing model*, New York, 1992, Springer Publishing Co.

Roles and Relationships

pecific behaviors and expectations, defined by self and others, are associated with the roles we fill. Our perceptions of roles are developed early in life through our socialization process and are reinforced throughout our lives. These socially recognized patterns of behavior establish our identity and position in society.

The ego-identity, self-esteem, and relational processes established through the mastery of roles may not be appreciated until our roles are threatened; this can result from the effects of chronic diseases. Chronic illness can alter roles by causing:

- a forfeiture of roles (having to resign from job or cease volunteering)
- inadequacy of role performance (being unable to engage in sex or care for children)
- adoption of new role (help-seeker, dependent, disease victim)

Clients may require assistance in adapting to and coping with role changes. Likewise, significant others in the clients' lives also may need support and guidance in adapting to clients' altered roles and preserving roles that can be maintained.

Assessment Considerations

Through interviews with the client and significant others, insight can be gained into both the client's usual roles as well as threats or actual changes to roles as a result of the chronic condition. Areas to review include:

- family structure and relationships
- friendships
- employment
- social activities
- interests
- volunteer activities

Identified role changes should be discussed with the client to determine the necessity of the alteration and reactions.

Demands imposed by the chronic illness that could alter roles should be discussed, including:

- client's willingness to accept help
- incorporation of treatments and other care activities into lifestyle
- management of symptoms

Assessment of the general physical and mental status of the client can reveal symptoms and changes in functional status that affect role performance.

Related Diagnoses

Altered Family Processes

Description

Altered family process is a state in which normal roles and functions within the family are inadequately fulfilled. Chronic illness can temporarily disrupt family processes, as can happen when the client is adapting to a new diagnosis or when symptoms exacerbate. A chronic illness can also cause permanent alterations, exemplified by a homemaker needing to return to the labor force due to the inability of her husband to continue working or an adult child needing to care for a dependent parent.

Client Goals

- to express satisfaction with family processes
- to develop effective coping strategies for altered family processes
- to be free from complications secondary to altered family processes (e.g., abuse, threatened health of caregiver, depression)

Interventions

- Establish trusting relationship with family; encourage open, honest communications.
- Recommend and assist with family conference.
- Review realities of situation. Guide family to view impact of client's illness on family unit and acknowledge realities.
- Assist family in identifying strengths and weaknesses in providing care, coping with client's illness and role changes, and readjusting lifestyle.
- Assist family in organizing activities and mobilizing resources to continue family activities as normally as possible.
- Refer to home health agency, respite care, counseling, support groups and other resources as needed.
- Assess family's knowledge of chronic condition; provide education accordingly.
- Monitor family's well-being on regular basis.

Grieving

Description

Grief is a state of emptiness and sadness following a loss.

Many losses can result from a chronic disease (e.g., health, function, limb, independence, job, status); therefore grieving is not an unusual state among chronically ill clients. Chronically ill persons can also experience anticipatory grief, in which they have emotional reactions to thoughts of the potential or impending losses that may arise from their conditions. As clients adapt to their illnesses, their grief should be expected to subside and not interfere with their ability to meet the demands of daily living. Clients need to be supported through their grieving to promote resolution and to ensure that their well-being is not threatened.

Client Goals

- to verbalize feelings about losses
- to utilize effective coping mechanisms
- to be free from complications secondary to grief (e.g., malnutrition, altered sleep pattern, suicide)

Interventions

- Develop trusting relationship with client.
- Encourage open expression of feelings without forcing client to confront issues for which he or she isn't ready.
- Display consistency in care activities and a nonjudgmental attitude.
- Utilize reminiscence and life review (see Chapter 12) to resolve old conflicts and put current losses into the perspective of the entire lifespan.
- Provide information and education as needed; answer questions honestly.
- If client is interested in seeking other opinions about diagnosis and treatment, assist in locating reputable practitioners.
- Utilize measures to instill hope (refer to interventions under Hopelessness in Chapter 12).
- Guide client in use of imagery to visualize self in a peaceful place.
- Be aware and advise caregivers and coach that client may fluctuate between various stages of grief (e.g., depression, acceptance, anger, bargaining, denial); encourage patience and understanding, and offer interventions that can be helpful for each stage, such as:
  - anger: avoiding defensiveness and counter-anger; having contact with client despite uncomfortable aspects of situation; accepting client's behaviors
  - denial: listen but avoid reinforcing unrealistic views or plans
  - depression: encourage expression of feelings; accept silence; do not avoid client, have contact; use touch therapeutically
- Monitor client's health status to ensure that complications secondary to grief are not developing (e.g., malnutrition, immobility, self-harm).
- Ensure that symptoms are under control; consult with physician and other health care practitioners for changes in treatment plan as needed.
- Refer to support groups, counseling, therapy as needed.

Altered Parenting

Description

Altered parenting is an interruption in the ability to nurture a child. A chronic illness can rob a parent of time and the physical and emotional energy required to care for, participate in activities with, and be available for a child.

Client Goals

- to identify capabilities and limitations in parenting role
- to adjust to necessary changes in parenting role
- to ensure that child's growth and development needs are fulfilled

Interventions

- Assess the impact of the client's illness on the parenting role. Discuss deficits and client's feelings about them.
- Review client's effectiveness at managing the chronic illness; increase self-care capacity where possible.
- Assist client in identifying alternate means for fulfilling parenting responsibilities (e.g., household help, Big Brother or Big Sister program, assistive devices, increased role of other family members).
- Reinforce existing parenting functions.
- Introduce to another parent who has dealt with similar problems who can share advice.
- Provide support and counseling to spouse and child as needed.
- Refer to social services, family therapist, psychologist, play therapist, support groups and other resources as needed.

Social Isolation and Impaired Social Interaction

Description

Social isolation implies a separation from satisfying social interactions and activities. Impaired social interaction is a state in which there is an interference with contact with other people.

Pain, fatigue, disabilities, disfigurement, financial limitations, and other effects of chronic illness can contribute to the client not desiring or being able to engage in social relationships. In turn, the physical and functional effects of the illness may discourage others from being socially involved with the client.

In addition to reports of impaired social interactions and social isolation, other signs can give clues to these problems, including: sleep disturbances, appetite disturbances, depression, anxiety, restlessness, anger, poor concentration, indecisiveness, attention-seeking behaviors, and expressions of boredom, hopelessness, or uselessness.

Client Goals

- to reestablish or establish meaningful social contacts
- to maintain or develop supportive, nurturing relationships
- to increase social activities

Interventions

- Identify factors contributing to problem and assist in correcting them as possible (e.g., obtaining assistive device, incontinence control, prosthesis, financial aid, transportation, therapy, information on local groups and activities).

- Encourage client to verbalize feelings.
- Assist client in adapting to new roles and activities.
- Encourage client to have a pet. The direct interactions with the pet are not only therapeutic, but also can be a stimulus for socialization and the development of new relationships.
- Explore alternative housing arrangements that could facilitate socialization, such as house sharing or relocation to sheltered living environment.
- Introduce client to concept of using computer networking for social encounters.
- Consult with families and coach regarding encouraging friends and family to visit.
- Consult with music, art, dance and recreational therapists regarding development of new interests.
- Refer to community support groups, adult day care, and other resources.

Recommended Readings

Charmaz K: The body, identity, and self: adapting to impairment, *Commuter-Regional Airline News* 13(50):657-81, 1995.

Doherty DS: Keeping body and soul together, *Journal of Christian Nursing* 13(3):36, 1996.

Lorig K, et al.: *Living a healthy life with chronic conditions*, Palo Alto, CA, 1994, Bull Publishing Co.

Mechanic D: Sociological dimensions of illness behavior, *Social Science and Medicine* 41(9):11207-17, 1995.

Michael SR: Integrating chronic illness into one's life, *Journal of Holistic Nursing* 14(3):251-267, 1996.

Miller JF: *Coping with chronic illness: overcoming powerlessness*, ed 2, Philadelphia, 1992, FA Davis Co.

Partners in Caregiving: Life after diagnosis, Winston-Salem, NC, 1995, Wake Forest University

Thompson M: Nurturing hope: a vital ingredient in nursing, *Journal of Christian Nursing* 11(4):10-17, 1994.

Zauszniewski JA: Self-help and help-seeking behavioral patterns in healthy elders, *Journal of Holistic Nursing* 14(3):223-236, 1996.

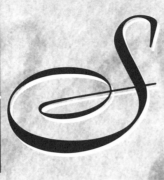

Sexuality and Reproductive Functions

*T*he capacity to enjoy and engage in sexual activity and the ability to procreate are basic components of adult health. Sexuality entails more than participation in and obtaining pleasure through physical sex acts; it includes one's sexual identity, roles, and expectations. To some women, attractiveness, the ability to dress stylishly, and modesty are part of femininity; to some men, a muscular body, being the bread-winner, and potency are viewed as essential for masculinity. Some individuals prize the intimacy of sharing romantic evenings and hugging as much as the act of intercourse; others prefer experimentation with a wide range of sexual aids and positions; some individuals seek gratification through masturbation, while still others engage in same-sex relationships. Patterns of sexuality vary widely, and clinicians are cautioned to remember this diversity when addressing sexuality issues.

Chronic illnesses can have profound effects on sexual identity and function (Table 14-1). Pain, limited mobility, fatigue, lack of sensation, dyspnea, and other physical consequences of chronic diseases can interfere with the ability to engage in sexual acts. The effects of treatments and medications can disrupt sexual function (Table 14-2). Depression, anxiety, lack of privacy, and stress are among the psychosocial problems that can produce sexual dysfunction. The reactions of sexual partners (e.g., fear over causing pain, repulsion at symptoms or disfigurement, guilt) can interfere with sexual relationships. The impact over alterations of sexual function can contribute to negative self-concept, poor self-esteem, altered relationships, depression, anxiety, grieving, and other disturbances.

Assessment Considerations

Questions pertaining to sexual history and current sexual function can aid in surfacing sexual dysfunction associated with chronic illness. Topics to review include:

For women:
- menstrual history
- pregnancy history, desire for future pregnancies
- pattern of gynecological care
- ability to engage in sexual activities, barriers
- ease of intercourse
- availability and attitude of partner
- knowledge of breast self-examination
- feelings about, satisfaction with current sexual function

For men:
- ability to engage in sexual activity, barriers
- availability and attitude of partner
- interest in having children
- knowledge of testicular self-examination
- feelings about, satisfaction with current sexual function

TABLE 14-1

Effects of Chronic Conditions on Sexuality and Sexual Function

Chronic condition	Potential effect on sexual function
Alcoholism	Decreased potency, delayed orgasm (female)
Atherosclerosis of lower extremity	Erection difficulties
Arthritis	Limited mobility, pain from position or activity
Cancer	Pain, fatigue, altered body image
Cardiovascular disease	Dyspnea, fatigue, fear of heart attack during sexual activity
Cerebrovascular accident	Decreased libido, impaired mobility
Diabetes mellitus	Decreased vaginal lubrication, impotency
Hypothyroidism	Decreased libido, decreased vaginal lubrication, erection difficulties
Liver disease	Impaired erection, decreased libido
Multiple sclerosis	Increased or decreased libido
Parkinsonism	Decreased libido, impotency
Prostatitis	Discomfort, interference with ejaculation
Renal disease	Decreased libido, lubrication, erection difficulties

TABLE 14-2

Examples of Sexual Dysfunction Resulting from Medications

Medication	Potential impact on sexual function
Androgens and anabolic steroids	Changes in libido, clitoral enlargement, testicular atrophy, vaginitis
Anticholinergics	Reduced vaginal lubrication, impotence
Antidepressants	Impotence, decreased libido
Antipsychotics	Change in libido, impaired ejaculations
Chlorpromazine	Decreased potency
Diuretics (high doses)	Altered libido, impotence
Estrogens	Altered vaginal discharge, breast tenderness
Ganglionic blockers	Impotence
Guanethidine	Retrograde ejaculation, decreased libido
Methyldopa	Decreased potency, reduced vaginal lubrication, decreased libido
Phenoxybenzamine	Inhibition of ejaculation
Propranolol	Impotency, decreased libido
Reserpine	Decreased libido, impotency

Physical examination supplements the sexual history. Males' genitalia should be inspected and prostate palpated. Females should have a complete gynecologic examination, including breast examination. The general appearance of clients should be noted to detect alterations in body structure or function, self-care deficits, or symptoms that could contribute to sexual dysfunction.

A review of the client's diagnosis and medications can assist in highlighting potential sources of sexual problems.

Related Diagnosis

Sexual Dysfunction

Description

Sexual dysfunction is an impairment in the ability to experience sexual pleasure. It can result from the physical and psychosocial effects of a chronic disease, medications, altered appearance, stress, misconceptions as to the effects of sexual activity on health state, or lack of privacy.

Client Goals

- to express satisfaction in fulfilling sexual needs

Interventions

- Establish open, accepting, nonjudgmental climate for discussion of sexual issues. Encourage honest expression of feelings. If helpful, interview client and partner separately.
- Determine factors contributing to sexual dysfunction (e.g., medications, misconceptions, pain); where possible, correct contributing factor.
- Educate client and partner about effects of chronic illness and treatments on sexual function. Clarify misconceptions. (Various organizations dedicated to specific health issues, such as the American Heart Association, offer literature pertaining to the impact of specific health problems on sexual function; obtain these resources for client.)
- Offer tips for improving appearance if necessary (e.g., wigs for alopecia, use of cosmetics, clothing styles to camouflage disfigurement).
- Advise client on measures to control symptoms during sexual activity (e.g., scheduling of medications to enhance respirations, taking warm bath to relax joints and muscles, use of vaginal lubricants).
- Review safe use of the herb ginkgo biloba for men with impotency due to arterial flow problems. Research has shown some improvement in blood flow and restoration in potency in men who were given ginkgo biloba for several months (Sikora et al., 1989).
- Discuss safe use of the herb Siberian ginseng, which is believed to have aphrodisiac effects. This herb also been shown to increase penile blood flow in a group of men who had not responded to traditional drug therapy (Brown, 1991).
- Refer client to acupuncturist to discuss benefit of treatment for increased

energy flow to sexual organs.

- Discuss alternative techniques for sexual expression (e.g., masturbation, massage, imagery, different positions); refer for sexual counseling as needed.
- Recommend aromatherapy using essential oils of sandalwood, jasmine, rose, and ylang ylang. Instruct partner to offer massages using these essential oils.
- Guide client in the use of imagery, biofeedback, and progressive relaxation.
- Consult with physician regarding use of Viagra in men.
- Respect privacy of client and partner; assist client and partner in obtaining private time and place.
- Refer to support groups, marriage counselor, and sex therapist as needed.

References

Brown DJ: Literature review: ginkgo biloba; Phytotherapy review and commentary, *Townsend Letter for Doctors* December 1991.

Sikora R, et al.: Ginkgo biloba extract in the therapy of erectile dysfunction, *Journal of Urology* 141:188A, 1989.

Recommended Readings

Bechtel S: *The sex encyclopedia*, New York, 1993, Fireside.

Bricklin M: The herb for the prostate, *Prevention*, 47(8):19-22, 1995.

Gillian F: *What's wrong with my hormones?* Newcastle, CA, 1992, Desmond Ford Publications.

Kamen B: *Hormone replacement therapy, yes or no: how to make an informed decision*, Novto, CA, 1993, Nutrition Encounter.

Murray MT: Natural approaches to impotence, *Let's Live* 63(7):42-48, 1995.

Ojeda L: *Menopause without medicine*, ed 2, Alameda, CA, 1992, Hunter House, Inc.

Weed SS: *Menopausal years*, New York, 1992, Ash Tree Publishing.

*C*oping and Stress Tolerance

*S*tress can result from anything that disturbs our normal physical or mental function. Sources of stress can be unpleasant factors, such as losing a loved one or experiencing pain, or positive factors, such as getting married or hearing good news about the results of a diagnostic test.

Stresses of Being Chronically Ill

Chronic illnesses certainly produce consequences that can disrupt physical and emotional equilibrium and cause stress. For instance, physical symptoms alone—such as pain, dizziness, and fatigue—can be a constant source of annoyance and frustration, in addition to producing physical discomfort. On top of all that, physical effects of the disease can reduce the body's ability to cope with other life stresses.

In addition to these physical effects, chronic diseases carry the risk of many emotional losses that can be highly stressful. There can be a loss of control as the illness requires adjusting future plans, lifestyle, and job. Second, some loss of independence can occur as disabilities imposed by the disease heighten the need to depend on others. Next, changes in appearance and roles can result in a loss of the self-image with which one had become comfortable. And finally, if social activities need to be changed because of the effects of a chronic illness and healthy friends find they have less in common with the chronically ill individual, there can be a loss of relationships. Of course, forfeiture of finances, home, hobbies, and status are but a sampling of the losses that can be experienced as a result of chronic illness.

Any one potential effect can be quite stressful in itself. But the reality is that the person with a chronic disease often faces several symptoms, changes, and losses that can cause a significant, and even dangerous, level of stress.

Effects of Stress

When first confronted by stress, the body mobilizes its defenses and prepares for "fight or flight." The sympathetic nervous system is aroused and stimulates the pituitary gland, which in turn releases ACTH (adrenocorticotropic hormone). The amount of adrenaline in the body increases, causing a rise in the state of alertness, breathing rate, heart rate, and muscle activity. As blood is sent to the muscles, the person's hands, fingers, and toes become cold. Pupils dilate, and hearing becomes more acute. Glycogen converts to glucose, blood clotting activity increases, and immune reactions are suppressed. Some of the physiologic, emotional, and intellectual symptoms associated with stress are listed in Box 15-1. The body's reactions to stress allow it to manage the additional demands it faces. As stress is eliminated or adapted to, bodily functions return to a normal or near normal level.

Typically, the average person experiences episodic stress: something occurs to cause stress, the body reacts, the stress is eliminated or diminished, and the body returns to normal. However, there are situations in which stress continues over a long period of time, as can occur for the person living with a chronic disease.

BOX 15-1   Symptoms of Stress

Physiologic	Emotional	Intellectual
Increased heart rate	Irritability	Forgetfulness
Rise in blood pressure	Depression	Poor judgment
Dryness of mouth and throat	Angry outbursts	Poor concentration
Sweating	Emotional instability	Reduced creativity
Tightness of chest	Disinterest in activities	Less fantasizing
Headache	Withdrawal	Errors in arithmetic and grammar
Nausea/vomiting	Restlessness	Preoccupation
Indigestion	Anxiety	Inattention to details
Diarrhea	Increased use of sarcasm	Reduced productivity
Trembling, twitching	Blocking	
Grinding of teeth	Tendency to cry easily	
Insomnia	Nightmares	
Anorexia	Suspiciousness	
Fatigue	Jealousy	
Slumped posture	Decreased involvement with others	
Tightness in neck and back muscles	Bickering	
Urinary frequency	Complaining, criticizing	
Missed menstrual cycle	Tendency to be easily startled	
Reduced interest in sex	Increased smoking	
Accident proneness	Use of alcohol and drugs	

Chronic stress causes the body to fatigue, have lowered resistance to illnesses, and manage episodic stress less effectively. An unhealthy cycle can develop in which the reduced ability to manage stress can increase the ill effects of stress, such as gastrointestinal disturbances, increased susceptibility to viral infections, and some forms of mental illness. The high risk for chronic stress highlights the importance of incorporating daily stress management measures into the daily lives of individuals who possess chronic illnesses.

Reducing Stress

Stress is known to contribute to illnesses, so it stands to reason that effective stress management can promote a healthy state that:

- strengthens the ability to maintain control of and cope with a chronic disease
- helps the body resist factors that can cause complications
- promotes a sense of well-being
- facilitates healing

Effective stress management is a positive health practice for all individuals, but it should be an essential part of the care plan for individuals with chronic diseases.

Stress management begins by getting in touch with one's body. The client should be guided to learn about the body's reaction to and manifestation of stress. Do palms become sweaty? Is there a tightening of the muscles in the neck and back? Does the heart pound so strongly that it feels that it will beat through the chest? Does the mouth feel as dry as cotton? Each individual needs to become aware of the way in which stress shows itself uniquely within him or her. By recognizing signs of stress early one can initiate stress-relieving exercises that can keep the effects of stress from escalating.

Controlling situations as much as possible is helpful in preventing some stress in one's life. This can begin by implementing sensible scheduling to avoid having too many changes or events happen at the same time. For example, a move to a new apartment shouldn't be planned during the holiday season, and it would be wise not to consider hosting a party during the same week that a new treatment is started. Noise, room temperature, and lighting can be controlled so that the environment is conducive to relaxation rather than overstimulation.

Some stress can be reduced by *avoiding unfulfilling or burdensome relationships*. Be they chronic complainers, gossips, pessimists, or favor-seekers, some people are a drain for the client and a source of stress. It is not only acceptable, but in many circumstances necessary for the client's health to change, when possible, or avoid these relationships. The client can be advised to discuss the problem with the offending person to assist in bringing about a necessary change that can salvage the relationship. For instance, the client might directly state to a coworker who spends lunch times incessantly complaining about work, *"I get upset rehashing work problems over lunch and would like to talk about our families, hobbies, or something else that is positive instead."* This action politely, but clearly, informs the coworker of the problem and its effect and offers a suggestion for change. If change is unachievable, the client may find it necessary to refuse to have social contact with stress-producing individuals and work on developing relationships with more positive people.

Setting limits is another important means of stress control. This may require the client to develop assertiveness skills so that the client's rights can be protected while respecting the rights of others. Examples of assertive and nonassertive ways of managing situations are discussed in Chapter 4.

Changing the way a stressor is viewed can reduce the amount of stress it causes. Rather than exaggerating the significance of a problem, the client can be encouraged to realistically evaluate the problem's importance or consequences in order to put it in proper perspective and help it to become manageable. For instance, suppose that a client with diabetes is told that he will need to inject himself daily with insulin rather than use oral medications. It's not hard to see that he could become stressed by thinking of the negatives *(Will I be able to inject myself? How much will this change my daily routine? Are the injections going to be painful? Does this mean I'm taking a turn for the worse?),* or he could decide to have a more constructive attitude *(There are thousands of people like me who inject themselves with no difficulty. The insulin will give me better control of my disease and help me to enjoy life more. A daily injection is a small price to pay for feeling good. Insulin injections enable many people to survive to advanced ages with diabetes.)* Likewise, to avoid worrying about a problem can minimize the stress caused by the problem. The client may need to be encouraged to repeat the old serenity prayer and learn to live by it: *God grant me the serenity to accept the things I cannot change, the courage to change the things I can, and the wisdom to know the difference.*

Considerable stress can be prevented by reducing the "shoulds" and "should nots" imposed on oneself. For example, the client may think:

- *I really am exhausted, but I shouldn't refuse to drive the carpool.*
- *I should clean the house because my mother-in-law is visiting.*
- *I shouldn't offend my coworker by telling her I don't want to discuss my illness at work.*
- *I really should make homemade cookies for the holidays.*
- *I shouldn't let my family know I'm not feeling my best today.*

Life imposes ample burdens on people who have chronic illnesses; they don't need to carry unnecessary loads on their shoulders. It is reasonable, legitimate, and healthy for the client to express needs and do what is best for himself or herself. The clinician should reinforce that there is nothing wrong with the client being selfish in this regard. The client needs to understand that most people are understanding and tend not to hold the same expectations of the client that the client may place on himself or herself. The best shoulds and shouldn'ts that the person with a chronic illness can follow are: *I should take care of my own needs and I should not worry about what others may think.*

Following good health practices also strengthens the ability to cope and manage stress. This includes eating a sound diet (as described in Chapter 7) and avoiding caffeine, simple carbohydrates, and food additives. It can be beneficial for the client to consider supplementation of the diet with vitamins that replace those lost during stressful periods and that increase the body's ability to manage stress; these include vitamins A, C, E, and the B-complex group.

Regular exercise is another good health practice that aids in stress reduction. Exercise programs must be individualized depending on the client's body type, general health state, and tolerance, and could range from walking to weight-lifting. Prior to engaging in any exercise program the client should be evaluated by a physician.

Getting ample rest and sleep, having a pet, listening to soft music, and building leisure activities into one's day are other effective stress-reduction health practices that can be encouraged. In addition, acupuncture, therapeutic massage, guided imagery, progressive relaxation, meditation, and yoga are among the *alternative therapies* that could prove useful for stress reduction (see Chapter 5 for descriptions of these practices.) The client can be advised to use specific herbs to promote relaxation and strengthen the body's ability to resist the ill consequences of stress (Box 15-2). Echinacea and ginseng can be recommended for use to protect the body from the long-term effects of stress.

Aromatherapy can assist in creating a calming environment. Some of the essential oils particularly useful include chamomile, lavender, citronella, and mandarin.

Some of these, and other general measures that could prove useful in stress management, are summarized in Box 15-3.

BOX 15-2	Herbs That Offer Protection from Stress

Ginseng	Lady's slipper
Echinacea	Catnip
Chamomile	Valerian
Hops	St John's wort

BOX 15-3	General Measures for Stress Reduction

- Identify sources of stress and attempt to change them.
- Eat a well-balanced diet; avoid "junk foods."
- Instead of coffee and cigarette breaks, enjoy breaks in which you do short relaxation exercises, recline in a quiet area, or listen to relaxing music.
- Exercise regularly.
- Take naps; allow ample time for sleep.
- Engage in an activity after work to unwind before going home.
- Schedule leisure activities into your life; develop a hobby.
- Take vacations and breaks from your routine work.
- Recognize your unique responses to stress and initiate stress-reduction measures when you detect them.
- Build meditation and relaxation exercises into your life.
- Engage in activities that put you in touch with nature.
- Minimize contact with people who add more stress than joy to your life.
- If subjected to chronic or high levels of stress, use ginseng and Echinacea to protect your body.
- Develop a sense of balance among your physical, mental, and spiritual parts.

Assessment Considerations

Symptoms of stress (Box 15-1) should be noted during the interview and physical examination. It could prove useful to question the client on a regular basis regarding stress management and coping. Insights can be gained by interviewing the client's coach and caregivers. After each assessment, any changes in the client's physical, emotional, social, and economic status should be reviewed, and interventions to compensate for them planned to prevent or minimize resultant stress.

Related Diagnoses

Ineffective Family Coping

Description

Ineffective family coping exists when a family member (or significant other) provides an inadequate quality or quantity of support to the client. This can be reflected in a variety of ways (Box 15-4). Not only does ineffective family coping reduce the support and assistance available to clients, but also can add stress to the client's life.

Client Goals

- to identify effects of family dynamics on self and family members
- to establish effective coping mechanisms within family

Interventions

- Encourage family to openly express feelings, concerns, needs, and frustrations. Help family identify dynamics and behaviors contributing to problem; aid in developing constructive coping strategies such as:
  - defining roles and responsibilities
  - setting clear limits
  - establishing consistent patterns of interaction
  - learning and using assertiveness skills
  - encouraging direct expression of needs
  - developing "win-win" methods of resolving conflict
  - listing and prioritizing problems and possible solutions

BOX 15-4   Indications of Ineffective Family Coping

- Lack of communication between family member* and client
- Family member describes lack of knowledge regarding client's condition
- Family member expresses inability to cope or fulfill caregiving demands
- Family member demonstrates preoccupation with effects of client's condition on family member
- Withdrawal of family member from activities with client
- Client describes insufficient support or assistance from family member
- Family member promotes unnecessary dependency of client
- Frequent arguments among family members
- Abusive actions by family member toward client
- Psychosomatic complaints of family member
- Decline in client's health status secondary to inadequate caregiving or effects of family member's behavior

* Family member implies any significant other in client's life

- • setting mutual goals
- • scheduling regular family conferences
- Identify need for education or skills development and provide instruction accordingly.
- Assess amount of personal private time family members have; assist them in developing schedules to have private time for self; locate resources to provide assistance or respite to family if necessary.
- Teach family members stress management techniques.
- Monitor for signs of abuse of client or other family members (Box 15-5); provide interventions to protect family members.
- Refer to family therapist, psychologist, financial counselor, social worker, and other sources of support as needed.

Ineffective Individual Coping

Description

Ineffective individual coping exists when the individual has deficits in fulfilling roles and responsibilities due to maladaptive behaviors or impaired problem-solving abilities. The effects and multiple losses associated with a chronic illness can produce sufficient stress to threaten an individual's ability to cope with normal life demands.

Client Goal

- to identify and utilize effective coping strategies

Interventions

- Assist in identifying and correcting underlying cause (improving physical status, obtaining financial aid, arranging home health care, teaching).

BOX 15-5   Examples of Abuse Within the Family

Physical injury: bruises, fractures, lacerations
Omitting necessary care
Humiliating victim
Instilling guilt in victim
Limiting victim's contact with people outside family
Accusing victim of forcing abuser to behave inappropriately
Threatening to abandon or take children away
Destroying possessions meaningful to victim
Denying victim access to money, food, or basic resources
Forcing victim to take harmful action or not comply with care plan
Making decisions for victim
Forcing unwilling client into sexual acts

- Aid client in identifying and eliciting assistance of significant other who can serve as chronic care coach. Provide education and support to coach as needed.
- Encourage client to openly express concerns and needs.
- Assist client in improving communication and problem-solving skills.
- Ensure that client has adequate knowledge about condition and care requirements.
- Explain procedures; encourage client to participate in care and make decisions to maximum degree possible.
- Teach client to use meditation, progressive relaxation, yoga, and imagery for stress reduction.
- Support client in making necessary lifestyle adjustments.
- Refer to support groups, counseling and other resources as needed.

Alcoholism

Description

Alcoholism is the abuse, dependency, or addiction to alcohol that threatens physical, emotional, and social health. Alcoholism decreases the ability to cope with the demands and effects of a chronic condition and can complicate the chronic condition (e.g., interfering with medications, decreasing immunity).

Alcohol differs from most other abused substances in that it is a legally sanctioned, easily accessible, socially acceptable product. This, along with the immediate pleasurable sensations derived from drinking, presents unique challenges in treating someone with alcoholism.

Chronic alcoholism can cause a variety of ill effects, including the development of other chronic diseases; some of these include:

- cirrhosis (Box 15-6; also refer to care plan in Chapter 7, page 162), alcoholic hepatitis
- hypertension, cardiomyopathy, coronary artery disease
- decreased immunity to infection
- polyneuropathy, pain, weakness
- anorexia, peptic ulcer, esophageal varices, chronic gastritis
- decreased libido, diminished sperm count, gynecomastia
- brain damage, dementia, Wernicke's encephalopathy
- depression, labile moods, attention deficit
- increased incidence of certain cancers (mouth, esophagus, liver, larynx)

In addition, alcoholism can create a host of psychosocial problems, such as altered family processes, job loss, accidents, and impaired social interactions.

Client Goals

- to abstain from alcohol
- to improve general health status
- to be free from complications associated with alcoholism

BOX 15-6	Facts About Cirrhosis

Cirrhosis is a progressive disease of the liver characterized by tissue scarring that ultimately results in severe liver failure and death. Cirrhosis increases in incidence in mid-life. Long-term ingestion of alcohol overworks the hepatic cells, eventually destroying them. Scar tissue develops and causes interference with circulation to the liver; this in turn destroys remaining cells. Destroyed cells cannot be replaced, but fortunately, damaged hepatic cells can heal, and the damaged liver can regenerate (although the remaining cells will need to work harder to compensate for the lost cells).

Early signs and symptoms of cirrhosis include dull abdominal ache, anorexia, altered bowel elimination, indigestion, nausea, and vomiting. As the disease progresses, other problems can develop, such as:

portal hypertension	abnormal pigmentation
pleural effusion	spider angiomas
bleeding tendencies	jaundice
testicular atrophy	palpable liver and spleen
menstrual irregularities	encephalopathy
gynecomastia	peripheral neuritis
severe pruritus	hallucinations
extreme dryness	paranoia
poor skin turgor	coma

Treatment measures include abstinence from alcohol, special diet to promote liver regeneration, avoidance of sodium and fats, cautious use of medications (due to reduced ability to detoxify drugs), regular medical follow-up, and counseling for alcoholism.

Interventions

- Review drinking history and pattern; note each of the following: amount, frequency, type of alcoholic beverage, factors precipitating alcohol use, effects of alcohol, behavior, and tolerance.
- Assess reactions of significant others (distressed over drinking, facilitators, denying reality).
- Assess for symptoms of complications (e.g., jaundice, altered cognition, pain, edema).
- If client is actively abusing alcohol and desires to withdraw, ensure that detoxification is done under close medical supervision; death from cardiac or respiratory failure can occur from delirium tremens.
- Guide client in confronting the diagnosis. The client's acknowledgement of the disease is the crucial first step toward recovery.
- Advise client to take vitamin and mineral supplement.
- Refer client to nutritionist to improve nutritional status.
- Ensure that client uses medications wisely as diseased liver is less able to detoxify. Be alert to and caution client and caregivers about interactions of alcohol with medications:

- alcohol interacts with analgesics, antibiotics, anticoagulants, anticonvulsants, antidepressants, antihistamines, barbiturates, digitalis, diuretics, insulin
    - alcohol can cause a tolerance to barbiturates, hypnotics, sedatives, and tranquilizers
- If client is taking disulfiram (Antabuse), monitor closely and provide education on precautions. Disulfiram acts as an alcohol antagonist by blocking its breakdown of acetaldehyde, which leads to acute physical distress within five to ten minutes of ingesting alcohol. (This is called acetaldehyde syndrome and is characterized by flushing, throbbing headache, nausea, vomiting, muscular aches, weakness, dyspnea, and chest pain.) It usually takes about five days for disulfiram to be eliminated from the body; the client needs to be cautioned about this.
- Recommend that client consult with an acupuncturist. Studies have shown acupuncture effective in the treatment of alcoholism, even with populations of alcoholics with minimal social and personal resources (Culliton and Kiresuk, 1996).
- Teach client to relax by using progressive relaxation, yoga, meditation, and the herbs hops, St. John's wort, and valerian.
- If client is so oriented, assist in strengthening spiritual and religious beliefs. Studies have shown lower rates of alcoholism among people who attended church, read the Bible, and prayed regularly as compared with those who did not (Koenig et al., 1994; Matthews and Larson, 1995); one prospective study spanning nearly 20 years showed the strongest predictor of future alcoholism among medical students to be the lack of religious affiliation (Moore et al., 1990).
- Discuss safe use of herbs with liver tonic and protecting effects, such as ginseng, licorice, and milk thistle.
- Ensure that client is referred for treatment of coexisting psychiatric disorders. (Sometimes alcohol is used by clients for the relief of anxiety, depression and other emotional problems.)
- Refer client for assistance in giving up alcohol (e.g., Alcoholics Anonymous, counseling); refer client and family members for counseling and support as needed (see Box 15-7).

BOX 15-7

Resources for Information About Alcoholism and Family Support

Adult Children of Alcoholics Worldwide Services Organization
PO Box 3216
Torrance, CA 90510
(310) 534-1815
www.recovery.org/acoa/acoa.html

Al-Anon Family Group Headquarters
PO Box 862
Midtown Station
New York, NY 10018
(212) 302-7240, (800) 356-9996
www.Al-Anon-Alateen.org

Alateen
PO Box 862
Midtown Station
New York, NY 10018
(212) 302-7240, (800) 356-9996
www.Al-Anon-Alateen.org
Alcohol and Drug Problems Association of North America
444 North Capitol Street NW
Suite 706
Washington, DC 20001
(202) 737-4340
Alcoholics Anonymous World Services
PO Box 459
Grand Central Station
New York, NY 10163
(212) 686-1100
www.alcoholics-anonymous.org
National Clearinghouse for Alcohol and Drug Information
11426-28 Rockville Pike
Suite 200
Rockville, MD 20852
(800) 729-6686
www.health.org
Women for Sobriety
PO Box 618
Quakertown, PA 18951
(800) 333-1606
www.mediapulse.com/wfs

References

Culliton PD and Kiresuk TJ: Overview of substance abuse: acupuncture treatment research, *Journal of Alternative and Complementary Medicine* 2(1):149-159, 1996.

Koenig HG, et al.: Religious practices and alcoholism in a southern adult population, *Hospital and Community Psychiatry* 45(3):225-31, 1994.

Matthews DA and Larson DB: *The faith factor: an annotated bibliography of clinical research on spiritual subjects*, Rockville, MD, 1995, National Institute for Health Care Research.

Moore RD, Mead L, and Pearson T: Youthful precursors of alcohol abuse in physicians, *American Journal of Medicine* 88:332-6, 1990.

Recommended Readings

Bennett HJ: *The best of medical humor*, ed 2, St. Louis, 1996, Mosby.

Bosker G: *Medicine is the best laughter*, St. Louis, 1995, Mosby.

Brewer KD: *The stress management handbook*, Shawnee Mission, KS, 1995, National Press Publications.

Charmaz K: The body, identity, and self: adapting to impairment. *Commuter-Regional Airline News* 13(50):657-81, 1995.

Erdal KJ and Zautra AJ: Psychological impact of illness downturns: a comparison of new and chronic conditions, *Psychology and Aging* 10(4):570-78, 1995.

Goleman D and Gurin J: *Mind/body medicine: how to use your mind for better health*, New York, 1993, Consumer Reports Books.

Greenberg M: A real head case: physical symptoms can indicate psychological distress, *Muscle and Fitness* 54(2):58-60, 1993.

Gordon J: *Stress management*, New York, 1990, Chelsea House Publishers.

Hochwald L: Natural stress solutions, *Natural Health* 26(3):68-81, 1996.

Kelleher KJ and Wolraich ML: Diagnosing psychosocial problems, *Pediatrics* 97(6):890-92, 1996.

Kuhn CC and Driscoll C: Humor yourself II: more lessons on laughter, *Real Living with Multiple Sclerosis* 1(5):12-15, 1994.

Miller JF: *Coping with chronic illness: overcoming powerlessness*, ed 2, Philadelphia, 1992, FA Davis Co.

Natelson EJ: Beating stress naturally, *Vegetarian Times* 198(2):86-89, 1994.

Peper E and Holt C: *Creating wholeness: a self-healing workbook using dynamic relaxation images and thoughts*, New York, 1993, Plenum.

Windle RC, Scheidt DM and Miller GB: Physical and sexual abuse and associated mental disorders among alcoholic inpatients, *American Journal of Psychiatry* 152(9):1322-1329, 1995.

Values and Beliefs

To view a chronic illness as a gift could be a difficult image to accept. In reality, most people would choose a disease-free, unimpaired life over that which must be lived with the inconveniences, self-care demands, discomforts, and limitations imposed by an illness. However, possessing a chronic disease can constructively alter our views of ourselves and life in general and provide the stimulus for many positive changes.

A chronic illness can shatter the fallacy that many of us possess that we are invincible and immortal. In many sometimes subtle and sometimes profound ways, we realize that there are forces beyond our control that change our lives and disrupt the best laid plans. That which was important yesterday seems irrelevant today.

Persons who possess chronic illnesses need to clarify their values in terms of that which is truly important in their lives. Recognizing how precious and uncertain life is can cause chronically ill persons to journey down new paths and avoid the wasteful detours taken by those unaffected by illness. For this reason, being affected by a chronic disease can cause people to live more meaningful lives that maximize that which each new day offers.

Many people affected by serious illnesses find considerable comfort in strengthening the spiritual foundations of their lives. This can take the form of active participation in a church or synagogue, or meditating alone in a garden. Spiritual beliefs provide the strength to accept the uncertainty and finiteness of our physical existence on earth. Bonding with a superior being or force can provide the nourishment for the soul that is necessary for healing.

Assessment Considerations

Areas to review to gain a perspective on the client's values and beliefs include:
- sense of self-worth
- feelings of being loved and loving others
- thoughts on perception of how others view him or her
- goals
- values
- beliefs about life
- spirituality
  - views, beliefs
  - religious practices
  - restrictions
  - meaningful religious objects
  - Sabbath days
  - dress or personal habits that have religious connotations
  - impact of illness on beliefs and practices

- name of religious or cultural leader who could be involved in healing and care
- sources of hope, strength

Spirituality, Religion, and Faith

Spirituality describes our search for meaning and purpose, including our beliefs about and relationship with God or a higher power in the universe. Spirituality differs from religion in that religion refers to a specific type of belief system, often associated with a certain philosophy and certain practices; religion is one part of spirituality.

When people have a positive, harmonious relationship with God or a higher power, they feel a sense of spiritual well-being, characterized by feelings of:
- being loved and valued despite their imperfections or errors
- love for others
- connectedness with other people, nature, the environment, and God or a greater power
- joy, hope, and peace, and
- a sense of purpose to their lives and the situations they experience.

Since the beginning of time, people have gained strength, purpose, hope, and the ability to face life's challenges through faith in a power greater than themselves. Now, scientific evidence supports the therapeutic benefits of faith. Of over 200 studies examining the role of faith in health and healing, most demonstrated a positive benefit of religious commitment (Matthews and Larson, 1995); for example:
- In a survey of caregivers of persons with cancer and Alzheimer's disease, religious faith was positively associated with a healthy emotional state (Rabins et al., 1990).
- An inverse relationship between religious commitment and depression was found among a group of urban blacks (Brown et al., 1990).

In a prospective study of older adults, religiosity was inversely related to subsequent disability and directly related to improved functional ability (Idler and Kasl, 1992).
- Persons with cancer who demonstrated apparent spiritual well-being were found to experience fewer anxiety states than those with spiritual distress (Kaczorowski, 1989).
- Among a group of 2679 people of various denominations studied, frequent church attenders had lower rates of psychopathology than infrequent attenders (Koenig, 1994).

Even intercessory prayer has shown benefit. In a study of nearly 400 patients in a coronary care unit, those who received intercessory prayer from a prayer group had a more favorable outcome and lower incidences of congestive heart failure, pneumonia, antibiotic use, intubation, and cardiac arrest than those who did not (Byrd, 1988).

Most people believe that prayer has a role in healing. A *Time* magazine poll of Americans disclosed that (Kaplan, 1996):

82% believed in the healing power of personal prayer

73% believed their illnesses could be cured or helped by the prayers of others

77% believed God sometimes intervenes to cure people who have serious illnesses

Further, 64% of those individuals surveyed believed health care professionals should join clients in prayer if clients so request. This is not to imply that clients or health care workers should be forced into religious activities against their wills, but rather that when the care provider and client are willing participants, prayers could be incorporated into caregiving activities. Examples of basic prayers that could be used are shown in Box 16-1. The psalms also provide wonderful foundations for prayers. (If unfamiliar with psalms, ask clergy for advice for specific psalms to use for certain needs.)

BOX 16-1   Examples of Prayers For Use With Clients

Heavenly Father, we thank you for Your kindness and mercy. We pray that you will protect (client) during this time and give (client) peace and strength to face the challenges ahead.

Dear God. Thank You for knowing and loving (client). We know that You are a loving, forgiving, merciful God on whom we can depend and trust. Please watch over (client), provide (client) with the inner resources to manage this illness, and help (client) find some beauty and joy in each day.

Our Father. As (client) faces these diagnostic tests/treatments, give (client) comfort, peace, and an awareness that you are by (client's) side during this time.

Father, comfort (client) during this time. Help (client) and (client's) loved ones to cope with this disease, gain the skills they need to manage it, and have peace with the knowledge of your presence.

Dear God, please protect (client) and help (client) to feel well enough to care for his condition.

Our Lord, please provide (client) with patience during this difficult time. Guide (client) toward actions that will promote health and healing. Help (client) understand that You have plans for all Your children, and to remember that our time on earth is but one part of the total plan that You have for him/her.

Related Diagnosis

Spiritual Distress

Description

Spiritual distress is a state in which beliefs or value systems are disturbed or at risk of being disrupted. Coping with chronic illness and its effects, facing losses, confronting one's own mortality, and wrestling with possible conflicts between prescribed treatments and religious beliefs are among the factors that can promote spiritual distress. The client may question the reason for God allowing the situation to happen or show signs of spiritual distress more subtly or indirectly (Box 16-2). The restoration or establishment of spiritual well-being is essential to providing the motivation and strength to enable the client to face the challenges of chronicity and achieve a satisfying quality of life.

Client Goals

- to maintain religious practices to maximum degree possible
- to discuss spiritual distress and conflicts
- to identify sources of support for achieving spiritual well-being

---

BOX 16-2   Signs of Spiritual Distress

Questioning belief system: "Why did God do this to me?" "I've tried to be a decent person and live a good life; why would something like this happen to me?" "What is the purpose of going on like this?" "Can there really be a God?"

Anger

Anxiety, bewilderment

Crying, depression

Guilt

Cynicism, sarcasm

Complaints, criticism of caregivers

Resentment toward those who are well

Withdrawal, social isolation

Refusal to make plans

Displaying a morbid sense of humor

Low self-esteem

Powerlessness

Hopelessness

Suicidal thoughts or plans

New or increased desire to attend religious services or visit with clergy

Physical symptoms: fatigue, poor appetite, sleep disturbances

---

Interventions

- Assist client in identifying factors contributing to spiritual distress (e.g., pain, loss of significant other, interference in church participation due to hospitalization, conflict between treatment and religious practice) and reducing or eliminating these factors (e.g., utilizing more effective pain relief measures, helping client establish new social contacts, arranging for client to be taken to service in hospital chapel, referral to clergy).
- Learn about client's religious practices and implications for care (Box 16-3); ensure that all caregivers respect client's beliefs and practices.
- Respect client's beliefs and use of items that are part of belief system such as cross, crystals, angels, amulet (charm or item believed to possess magical powers to ward off evil spirits), incense, icons, candles, and use of shaman, native healers, and voodoo.
- Assist client in maintaining religious practices:
  - provide Bible, special religious articles
  - obtain religious music, acquaint client with religious programs on television and radio
  - arrange visit from clergy
  - assist with preparation for attendance/participation in religious service
  - respect and assist client with rituals
  - read scripture
  - request caregiver or coach to read scripture and assist with religious activities
- Pray with and for client (see Box 16-1) if desired by client; if uncomfortable or unwilling to assist client in this manner, refer to other health care professional who can assist client with this need.
- Provide client with time and privacy for meditation and prayer.
- If client approves, refer client's needs to prayer group or individual for intercessory prayer.
- Respect client's desire not to be visited by clergy or participate in religious activities; ensure that others do not force these activities on client; be open and accepting of client's change of mind in desiring these activities at a later time.
- Do not try to convert client or challenge religious beliefs.
- Refer to clergy, native healer, support group, and other resources as needed.

Facing Death

A chronic illness heightens awareness of mortality and often begins a process of evaluating the life one has lived and the significance of the time that remains. Even if death is not imminent, chronically ill individuals may experience reactions as they come to terms with the finiteness of their lives. Some clients may feel bitterness and resentment that they won't have the quantity or quality of life to enjoy their later years or share experiences with children and grandchildren; others may

BOX 16-3	Major Religions: Implications for Clinicians

CHRISTIANITY

Christianity, the largest religion in the world, is based on the teachings of Jesus. It is believed that God manifested himself through his Son Jesus, who lived on earth and died on the cross as an atonement for the sins of humanity. Christmas is celebrated as the birth and Easter as the resurrection of Jesus. The Bible is the chief literature of Christianity. Christianity is divided into various groups with different practices: the traditional religions of the Roman Catholic and Eastern Orthodox churches and the reform religions of Prostestantism and various independent churches.

Catholic   Believe in the Pope as the head of the church on earth. Express their faith mainly in formulated creeds, such as the Apostles' Creed. Observe the sacraments of Mass, baptism of infants, confirmation, penance, matrimony, holy orders, and extreme unction (anointing individuals just before death). Attend Mass on Sundays and holy days and confess their sins to a priest at least once yearly. Fast from meat on Ash Wednesday and Good Friday; fasting during Lent and on Fridays is optional, although it is observed by some. Accept modern medical treatment. May want to have visit by priest when ill for confession and communion.

Eastern Orthodox   Includes Greek, Serbian, Russian, and other orthodox churches. Believe in Divine Liturgy, symbolism of bread and wine for body and blood of Christ. Recognize Jesus as head of church. Reject authority of the Pope; believe Holy Spirit proceeds from Father (rather than Father and Son). Priests do not need to practice celibacy. Church services are usually longer than other religions and performed in language of local people. Use icons (sacred pictures) to decorate church; sacraments are performed behind a screened area. Follow different calendar for religious feasts (e.g., Easter may fall on different date than that observed by other Christian groups). Fast during Lent and before Communion. Accept modern medical treatment. Holy unction administered to sick but not always as last rites. Pray for the dead and believe that the dead look after those on earth.

Protestant   Divided into several different churches that have various practices. Began as revolt with Catholic Church; reject authority of the Pope. Lutherans, Methodists, and Presbyterians support modern medical treatment, practice communion and last rites. Presbyterians believe worship of God should be done in simple, dignified way.

Baptists and Pentecostals view illness as a form of punishment or an act by Satan. They are baptized as adults. Against consumption of alcohol, coffee, tea, pork, or tobacco. Some may display some resistance to modern medical treatment and instead prefer divine healing through laying on of hands.

Episcopalians may abstain from meat on Fridays and fast during Lent and before Communion. May practice spiritual healing as adjunct to modern medicine. Practice confession, Communion, and last rites.

Other Christian Religions   Christian Scientists (Church of Christ, Scientist) observe a religion based on the use of faith for healing and may oppose traditional medical treatments such as medications, intravenous lines, transfusions, and special therapies. Believe sickness and sin are not real but only appear to humans; therefore it is possible to heal humans of sickness, sin, and limitations. Utilize Christian Science practitioners who devote their lives to healing. May be less likely to accept disease as incurable.

(continued)

Friends (Quakers) believe God is personal and real, not a figment of imagination, true religion is experiential, and any believer can achieve communion with Christ without the use of trained clergy or church rituals. There is no clerical hierarchy. Do not use alcohol. May oppose the use of medications. Do not believe in an afterlife.

Jehovah's Witnesses take most ideas from the New Testament Book of Revelation. Believe Christ will return when there will be a great battle at Armageddon between him and the forces of evil; the evil will be defeated and for the next 1000 years Christ will reign on earth. Worship in Kingdom halls rather than churches. There are no special ministers; each member is considered to be a minister of the gospel and must house visit and distribute their literature every month. Believe other churches are controlled by the devil. Do not eat meats containing blood unless blood has been drained; do not consume alcohol or tobacco. Oppose modern medical treatments, such as transfusions.

Mennonites believe in nonviolence, a simple and plain dress style, and a simple life-style. They are baptized as adults. They may resist medications.

Mormons (Church of Jesus Christ of Latter Day Saints) have no professional clergy; believe any male member can lead service. Do not consume coffee, tea, or alcohol or use tobacco; may restrict meat intake and fast once each month. Believe illness results from violation of God's commandments or failure to follow laws of health. May oppose modern medical treatment and use divine healing through laying on of hands.

Seventh-Day Adventists advocate principles of healthful living through diet, exercise, and philanthropic outlook. Saturday, the seventh day of the week, is their holy day. Treatment may be opposed on the Sabbath. May practice divine healing. Oppose consuming coffee, tea, or alcohol; may not eat meat and shellfish. May desire baptism or communion when seriously ill.

Unitarians represent a highly liberal branch of Christianity. Believe in God as a single being rather than belief in the doctrine of the Trinity. Accept modern medical treatment. Believe individuals are responsible for their own health status.

Christians may vary widely on whether to accept cremation.

JUDAISM

Judaism, a religion that has been practiced since the time of Moses (1500-1200 BC), recognizes one universal God (Yahweh) and believes that Jews were specially chosen to receive God's law. Jews observe their Sabbath from sundown Friday to nightfall Saturday, during which there is attendance at the synagogue and a Sabbath meal. On the Sabbath, Orthodox Jews will not work (testimony to God having created the universe in six days and having rested on the seventh) and may refuse nonemergent medical treatment. Religious services are led by a rabbi who acts more as a teacher than a traditional minister.

There are three branches of Judaism. Orthodox Jews believe in the divinely inspired five Books of Moses, also known as the Torah, and strictly adhere to the traditions of Judaism. Within this branch are the Hasidic Jews who subscribe to a traditional dress style. Reform Jews are more liberal; they call synagogues temples and may ordain female rabbis. Conservative Jews are between Orthodox and Reform Jews; they attempt to apply Jewish laws to daily life.

Essential to Jewish practice is the observance of laws and customs. These include observance of dietary restrictions that only kosher (fit) foods be eaten; pork and shellfish are forbidden, as is the mixing of dairy and meat products at the same meal. Meat must be butchered according to special rabbinical rituals. Circumcision is another practice of Jews and consists of cutting off the foreskin of the penis; this gives special identity to Jews and welcomes the infant into the religious community.

Besides the Sabbath observance, Jews observe other special celebrations. These are viewed as not merely memorials to ancient events, but as opportunities for Jewish people to relive and renew their connection with the spiritual/historical events that make up their heritage; these include the following:

Rosh Hashanah (New Year): Two-day celebration that occurs in September or October (based on the Jewish lunar calendar); a time when Jews examine their lives

Yom Kippur (Day of Atonement): considered the most holy day, in which Jews fast from food and water and repent their sins of the previous year; Orthodox Jews may not wash, engage in sex, bathe, or wear leather shoes

Sukkoth (Feast of Tabernacles): celebrated 5 days after Yom Kippur; week-long feast commemorating God's providence during Israelites' sojourn in the desert; families often build tentlike structures decorated with harvest fruits in which they may eat and sleep

Hanukkah (Festival of Lights): celebrated in December; commemorates restoration of the Temple after it had been desecrated by the Syrians in 160 BC; during this celebration a candelabra holding eight candles is used in which an additional candle is lighted each day of the celebration

Purim: occurs in February or March; celebrates the deliverance of the Jewish people from a plot to annihilate them through the reading of the Book of Esther; Jews may fast on day preceding

Pesach (Passover): occurs in spring; celebrated through the seder, a ceremonial meal in which wines, unleavened bread (matzo), and other special foods are used symbolically during the reading of the Haggadah, the story of the Jews' escape from Egypt

Shavous: Two-day holiday, 7 weeks after Passover, that celebrates the receiving of the Torah on Mt. Sinai

Jews support modern medical treatments. On death, the body is washed and burial occurs as soon as possible thereafter. During the time of death and burial, mourners show their sorrow by wearing a torn garment or a symbolic black cloth. After burial, mourners enter a 7-day period of shiv'ah in which they avoid work and social functions.

Jews believe that after death the person stands in judgment before God and is punished or rewarded, depending on the life he or she has lived on earth.

ISLAM (MUSLIM)

Islam is the world's third largest monotheistic (belief in one God) religion. It was founded by the prophet Mohammed, who was born in Mecca about 570 AD. Mohammed was a human messenger or prophet who was used by God to communicate God's word. Muslims believe Jesus was another prophet, who will return at the end of the world to guide the faithful. The Koran represents the Word of God and is the scripture followed by Islamics. There is no organized priesthood. Friday is the Sabbath.

Islam is divided into two groups: the Sunni muslims, who represent most Islamics, and Shi'ite muslims.

(continued)

Islamics eat no pork and abstain from alcohol. Cleanliness is an important part of their practice. They may pray five times daily, facing toward Mecca. They accept medical treatments if these do not violate religious practices. Illness is seen as God's will.

Dying Islamics may want to confess. On death, the family prepares the body and the body must face Mecca. Organ donation, cremation, and autopsy (unless required by law) are prohibited.

BUDDHISM

Buddhism is an offshoot of Hinduism and has many followers in the East. Buddhists believe enlightenment is found through individual meditation rather than communal worship. Buddhists see the root of all suffering in life as an outgrowth of desire for false selfhood and other desires. They strive to achieve a form of liberation and enlightenment known as nirvana. The moral code that leads to nirvana is the Eightfold Path:

Right understanding: life is understood as changing and painful

Right thoughts: thoughts of goodwill and nonharming

Right speech: avoidance of lies, slander, gossip, harsh words

Right action: refraining from killing, stealing, harmful sexual behavior

Right means of livelihood: healing morally with tasks of daily life, avoidance of jobs involving weapons, intoxicating drinks, slaughter of animals

Right effort: resisting impulses that generate greed and violence

Right mindfulness: attention to what is being done at the moment and the changing realities of life

Right concentration: concentration on right goals and thoughts through the use of meditation

Buddhists are vegetarians and abstain from alcohol and tobacco. They may oppose medications and refuse treatments on holy days. Euthanasia is allowed in hopeless situations. Illness may be viewed as a test of strength that aids in one's development; meditation may be an important part of the healing process.

HINDUISM

Hinduism may be the world's oldest religion and is the religion of most of India's inhabitants. Hinduism has no scriptures, no fixed doctrines, and no common worship. Most Hindus believe everything is part of one reality, although some worship many Indian gods.

Two key concepts of Hindu belief are karma (belief that every person is born into a position in life based on deeds of previous life) and samsara (reincarnation). Among Hindus there can be different types of beliefs such as the protection of cows (symbolizes human obligation to protect the weak or oppressed) and nonviolence.

Health and dietary practices parallel those of Buddhists. Illness may be viewed as a result of sin from another life. Cremation is supported.

From Eliopoulos C: Understanding religious differences, *Long Term Care Educator* 4(12), 1993. Health Education Network, 11104 Glen Arm Road, Glen Arm, MD 21057.

feel guilty about the burden they will place on their loved ones; teenagers fear that they'll not enjoy the normal joys of marriage and parenthood because of their illnesses. Reactions will vary depending upon health status, diagnosis, age, support system, values, and attitudes and experiences with death.

Clinicians need to support chronically ill individuals as they come to terms with their mortality and prepare for death. Realistic explanations of the disease and symptom management may be useful. The client should be made aware of hospice programs, support groups, and other sources of assistance during the dying process. The Hospice Link, (800) 331-1620, can aid in locating hospice programs and providing general information on hospice care. The process of life review should be conducted to aid the client in coming to terms with the life that has been lived, resolving conflicts, and preparing for death. The client can be guided to clarify values, consider realistic goals, and develop strategies for fulfilling goals, as possible (Figure 16-1). Imagery, progressive relaxation, meditation and the therapeutic use of touch can have important roles in providing the comfort that aids the client in preparation. Assistance with financial and legal plans may be offered. The support and care of significant others should not be overlooked.

The reality of death may be beyond control, but the manner in which death is approached is not. A chronic illness can be a "wake-up call," serving as a warning that life is precious and should not be taken for granted. It can motivate an individual to resolve conflicts with significant others, express feelings to loved ones, take actions to realize plans, and separate the important from the superfluous. In some ways a chronic illness can be a gift, reinforcing the yin-yang nature of the human experience that teaches us that within every negative experience is some positive seed.

The client can be asked to list on one side of the scale those aspects or activities of life that are important and on the other side, list those that have been or are being realized. The client then can be asked to list ways to achieve more goals so that the scale can be better balanced.

Goals
Leave legacy for family by organizing family photos and writing family history
Read Bible daily
Write to friends to express that I care
Take grandchildren to Disney World

Achievements
Made travel arrangements for trip to Disney World
Read Bible daily

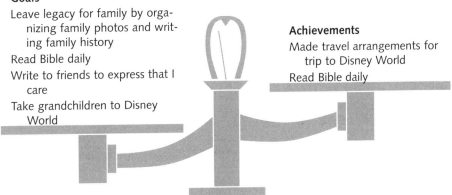

FIGURE 16-1

Helping the client to clarify goals.

References

Brown DR, Ndubuisi SC, and Gary LE: Religiosity and psychological distress among blacks, *Journal of Religion and Health* 29(1):55-68, 1990.

Byrd RB: Positive therapeutic effects of intercessory prayer in a coronary care unit population, *Southern Medical Journal* 81:826-9, 1988.

Idler EL and Kasl SV: Religion, disability, depression, and the timing of death, *American Journal of Sociology* 97(4):1052-79, 1992.

Kaczorowski JM: Spiritual well-being and anxiety in adults diagnosed with cancer, *Hospice Journal* 5(3):105-116, 1989.

Kaplan M: Ambushed by spirituality, *Time*, June 24, 1996, p. 62.

Koenig HG, et al.: Religious practices and alcoholism in a southern adult population, *Hospital and Community Psychiatry* 45(3):225-31, 1994.

Matthews DA and Larson DB: *The faith factor: an annotated bibliography of clinical research on spiritual subjects*, Rockville, MD, 1995, National Institute for Health Care Research.

Rabins PV, et al.: The emotional impact of caring for the chronically ill, *Psychosomatics* 31(3):331-6, 1990.

Recommended Readings

Aldridge D: Is there evidence for spiritual healing? *Advances, Journal of Mind-Body Health* 9(4):1993.

Benson H and Stark M: *Timeless healing: the power and biology of belief*, New York, 1996, Scribner.

Coulter AH: Tapping the soul's healing potential: an interview with Carlos Warter, *Alternative and Complementary Therapies* 2(5):283-288, 1996.

Coons D and Mace N: *Quality of life in long-term care*, New York, 1996, Haworth Press.

Cutcliffe JR: How do nurses inspire and instill hope in terminally ill HIV patients? *Journal of Advance Nursing* 22(5):888-895, 1995.

Czerwiec M: When a loved one is dying: families talk about nursing care, *American Journal of Nursing* 96(5):32-36, 1996.

Doherty DS: Keeping body and soul together, *Journal of Christian Nursing* 13(3):36, 1996.

Dunkle RM: Parish nurses help patient: body and soul, *RN* 59(5):55-58, 1996.

Fulford RC: *Dr. Fulford's touch of life: the healing power of natural life force*, New York, 1996, Pocket Books.

Gaynor ML: *Healing essence: a cancer doctor's practical program for hope and recovery*, New York, 1995, Kodansha International.

Kodish E and Post SG: Oncology and hope, *Journal of Clinical Oncology* 13(7):1817-1822, 1995.

Kuhn CC and Driscoll C: Humor yourself II: more lessons on laughter, *Real Living with Multiple Sclerosis* 1(5):12-15, 1994.

Kumasaka L and Miles A: My pain is God's will, *American Journal of Nursing* 96(6):45-47, 1996.

Leifer R: Psychological and spiritual factors in chronic illness, *American Behavioral Scientist* 39(6):752-67, 1996.

Lorig K, et al.: *Living a healthy life with chronic conditions*, Palo Alto, CA, 1994, Bull Publishing Co.

Maffeo R: To live until I die, *Journal of Christian Nursing* 13(3):28, 1996.

Michael SR: Integrating chronic illness into one's life, *Journal of Holistic Nursing* 14(3):251-267, 1996.

Miller JF: *Coping with chronic illness: overcoming powerlessness*, ed 2, Philadelphia, 1992, FA Davis Co.

Partners in Caregiving: *Life after diagnosis*, Winston-Salem, NC, 1995, Wake Forest University.

Sanker A: *Dying at home: a family guide for caregiving*, Baltimore, MD, 1991, Johns Hopkins University Press.

Taylor PB: Fostering farewell: giving children the chance to let go, *Nursing 96* 26(1):54-57, 1996.

Thompson M: Nurturing hope: a vital ingredient in nursing, *Journal of Christian Nursing* 11(4):10-17, 1994.

Walton J: Spiritual relationships: a conceptual analysis, *Journal of Holistic Nursing* 14(3):237-250, 1996.

Index